# Evidence-Based
# Practice
# With Women

# Evidence-Based Practice With Women

Toward Effective Social Work Practice With Low-Income Women

## Martha Markward
*University of Missouri–Columbia*

## Bonnie Yegidis
*University of South Florida–Tampa*

 EVIDENCE-BASED PRACTICE IN SOCIAL WORK

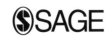

Los Angeles | London | New Delhi
Singapore | Washington DC

*For information:*

SAGE Publications, Inc.
2455 Teller Road
Thousand Oaks, California 91320
E-mail: order@sagepub.com

SAGE Publications Ltd.
1 Oliver's Yard
55 City Road
London EC1Y 1SP
United Kingdom

SAGE Publications India Pvt. Ltd.
B 1/I 1 Mohan Cooperative Industrial Area
Mathura Road, New Delhi 110 044
India

SAGE Publications Asia-Pacific Pte. Ltd.
33 Pekin Street #02-01
Far East Square
Singapore 048763

Printed in the United States of America

*Library of Congress Cataloging-in-Publication Data*

Markward, Martha J.
Evidence-based practice with women : toward effective practice with low-income women / Martha Markward, Bonnie Yegidis.
    p. cm.
Includes bibliographical references and index.
ISBN 978-1-4129-7575-9 (pbk.)
    1. Social work with women. 2. Psychiatric social work. 3. Poor women—Mental health. 4. Poor women—Mental health services. 5. Poor women—Services for. I. Yegidis, Bonnie L. II. Title.

HV1444.M37 2011
362.2'0425082—dc22                          2010026695

This book is printed on acid-free paper.

10   11   12   13   14   10   9   8   7   6   5   4   3   2   1

| | |
|---|---|
| *Acquisitions Editor:* | Kassie Graves |
| *Editorial Assistant:* | Courtney Munz |
| *Production Editor:* | Brittany Bauhaus |
| *Permissions Editor:* | Adele Hutchinson |
| *Copy Editor:* | Alan J. Cook |
| *Typesetter:* | C&M Digitals (P) Ltd. |
| *Proofreader:* | Laura Webb |
| *Indexer:* | Sheila Bodell |
| *Cover Designer:* | Gail Buschman |
| *Marketing Manager:* | Dory Schrader |

# Brief Contents

# Detailed Contents _____

# Foreword

During the past decade there has been growing recognition of and reliance on evidence-based practice in the professions of medicine, psychology, social work, nursing, criminal justice, and public health. Advances in health and mental health care have resulted in a complex system of care in which professionals are confronted on a daily basis with issues of time management. The application of technological advances such as evidence-based knowledge and intervention strategies places an increasing burden on the care provider. This burden is intensified in the provision of services to low-income women. Most providers of care to low-income women labor under stressful conditions of high caseloads, unmanageable paperwork, and poor working conditions. Their commitment to this work is indeed commendable.

In *Evidence-Based Practice With Women: Toward Effective Practice With Low-Income Women*, Markward and Yegidis provide a wealth of information on empirically supported assessments and intervention strategies for the practitioner working with low-income women and their families who are experiencing mental health disorders and substance abuse in their lives. The authors combine the empirical evidence with a discussion of environmental factors to provide a comprehensive and rich contextual framework for understanding and providing a comprehensive and effective approach to treatment.

As the authors note, for too long women, especially poor women, have received substandard care—often being treated for their physical symptoms with little attention to their emotional or mental health needs. This book is consistent with the mission and values of social work: to improve the biopsychosocial well-being of clients and to promote the provision of the best assessment and treatment possible for all persons, especially for those who are vulnerable, oppressed, or living in poverty.

This book will most certainly facilitate the training of practitioners and future practitioners in the provision of services to low-income women. Focusing on the most prevalent mental health issues facing women, the authors provide cross-cultural and cross-generational information on trauma and post-traumatic stress disorder, depression, generalized anxiety disorder, substance use and abuse, and borderline personality disorder. Data on prevalence and etiology, screening and rapid assessment approaches, and empirically based clinical practices are provided for each disorder. Additionally, each chapter contains discussion questions, case vignettes, and illustrative readings. In the final chapter, the authors provide a framework for advancing the agenda for more effective treatments for low-income women.

Markward and Yegidis have successfully compiled a remarkably comprehensive book that captures the required comprehensive nature of practice while simultaneously focusing on the specific knowledge and skill needed to provide high-quality mental health services to poor women. This book skillfully and seamlessly integrates research evidence, practice, and knowledge while simultaneously focusing on the environmental factors affecting the scope and prevalence of these disorders among poor women.

I am excited about this new book and its potential to move the field forward in providing a higher level of services to women and their families who are affected by mental illness and substance abuse. I have no doubt that current practitioners in the field will find this resource to be invaluable in their practice. This book will most certainly prove to be an extremely valuable resource for students, clinicians, supervisors, administrators, and educators. Markward and Yegidis have produced an extraordinary resource for all social workers and clinicians either working in the field or concerned with the plight of disadvantaged women.

*—Karen Sowers*

Dean of the College of Social Work

University of Tennessee, Knoxville

# Preface

Recognizing that we are fortunate in the 21st century to have made significant gains in developing research knowledge that is applicable to women, we developed this book to share this knowledge with social work educators and students alike. The authors have both taught a women's course in social work practice at different universities and have had difficulty locating a single text specifically dedicated to empirically-based practice with poor women. In an attempt to limit the scope of the book, we decided to focus on the mental health problems most prevalent in this population of women across the nation and worldwide, and as such, we chose to address post-traumatic stress disorder (PTSD), depression, generalized anxiety disorder (GAD), substance use disorder (SUD), and borderline personality disorder (BPD). In doing so, we do not presume that other disorders are less important, but we believe that women in low-income families have higher rates of these disorders than do women in the general population. Evidence suggests that women in low-income families increasingly engage in abuse and misuse of substances as well.

There are few full-length monographs in the social work literature specifically devoted to the assessment and treatment of mental health disorders in women, though there are two leading books on social work practice with women, both of which are edited books of readings that have been in print for several years. The first edited book is by Peterson and Lieberman (2001), *Building on Women's Strengths: A Social Work Agenda for the 21st Century*. Both the first and second editions of this book offer a strengths-based perspective on feminist social work practice. The second is *Feminist Practice in the 21st Century* (Van Den Bergh, 1995). It is distinctive in its organization, focusing on methods, fields of practice, and special populations. Neither book, however, provides empirical data on assessing and treating the mental health disorders that are typical among economically disadvantaged women.

Women experience PTSD, depression, and GAD at significantly higher rates than do men. Since poor women experience those disorders at even higher rates than women in the general population and social workers often provide services for this population of women, we chose to emphasize the prevalence, etiology, screening, and treatment of those disorders in women. We also chose to address substance abuse and misuse in light of its increasing prevalence in low-income families and due to its association with child abuse and intimate partner violence. Similarly, we address borderline personality disorder due to its prevalence among poor women.

In Chapter 1 of the book, we highlight the fact that many women in the U.S. live in or near poverty, and how the lack of income is most often the stressor that amplifies or mediates women's predispositions to mental health problems. In Chapters 2 through 6, we focus on evidence-based knowledge about addressing the mental health problems found to be most prevalent among women, and we infuse each chapter with the available cross-cultural and cross-generational information. Each chapter presents a definition of the disorder, data on its prevalence and etiology, screening and rapid assessment approaches that can be used in identifying the disorder, and the clinical practices that have been proven to work. In addition, each chapter is accompanied with discussion questions, case vignettes, and illustrative readings. In Chapter 7, we propose how social workers can move toward more effective practice with low income women.

We agree with the authors of the two competing social work texts that environmental factors play a very large role in shaping the mental health of women and men. However, we posit that people present for mental health treatment as complex individuals and that their biological, psychological, social, and environmental characteristics, as well as their strengths and limitations, must be assessed and treated with the best possible science known. It is in the scientific and empirical literature that these best practices may be found, when they are available. We are fortunate that we could draw on literature from the disciplines of psychology, counseling, psychiatry, and medicine, as well as social work.

For example, there are a number of outstanding edited textbooks that address the treatment of specific mental health disorders in women, such as *The Handbook of Addictions Treatment for Women* (Straussner & Brown, 2002). This text provides a comprehensive approach to treating specific substance abuse disorders in women in a range of practice settings. Similarly, *Mood and Anxiety Disorders in Women* (Castle, Kulkarni, & Abel, 2006) provides a biopsychosocial and developmental approach to mood and anxiety disorders in women and presents empirically-based treatment implications. *Gender and PTSD* (Kimerling, Ouimette, & Wolfe, 2002) and *Understanding Depression in Women: Applying Empirical Research to Practice and Policy* (Mazure & Keita, 2006) are instructive in treating PTSD and depression.

We believe our book is important in the field of social work because social workers are often employed in settings where they assess and provide direct services to women who have few resources. Women often present to their primary care physicians with physical symptoms, such as low energy, insomnia, and headaches, and are treated for these symptoms without a full mental

health assessment. Women are also treated for physical and emotional ill-
nesses in urgent care or walk-in medical facilities, hospital emergency rooms,
substance abuse settings, rape crisis or domestic violence shelters, child protective services units, and agencies that serve the needs of elders, including
nursing homes and extended care facilities.

In these circumstances, social workers regularly have the opportunity to
make a critical and substantial difference in the lives of female consumers,
especially low-income consumers, if they are well versed in the clinical social
work literature about effective interventions. This book is intended to meet
that need. We hope that it will provide social work faculty and students with
evidence-based material about assessing and treating the most common mental health disorders among women, particularly low-income women. We
identify the implications for policy, practice, and research needed to enhance
further evidence-based social work practice with economically disadvantaged
women, as well as make recommendations for service provision. Thus, the
book should be relevant for social work practice courses in both master of
social work and bachelor of social work programs, and could also have utility as a supplemental text in policy, diversity, and human behavior courses.

# Acknowledgments

The authors and SAGE gratefully acknowledge the contributions of the
following reviewers:

Kathryn Betts Adams, *Case Western Reserve University*

Julia Archer, *University of Kansas*

E. Joan Looby, *Mississippi State University*

Jennifer Pepperell, *Minnesota State University, Mankato*

Mark S. Perez-Lopez, *Virginia Tech University*

Lynda R. Ross, *Athabasca University*

Min Zhan, *University of Illinois*

# 1

# Introduction

S ocial workers are challenged to meet the mental health needs of women at a time when women are taking on increased responsibilities in both the home and workplace. In accepting this challenge, social workers must provide women, especially low-income women, with the most effective practice possible. Given that effective practice relies on knowing which psychosocial interventions have been proven to work, social workers require knowledge about which interventions bring about the most positive, measurable changes in the lives of low-income women, regardless of etiology. Those insights have particular policy, practice, and research implications for those concerned about the well-being of all women, particularly when one considers that women are the primary consumers of mental health services.

## Explaining Women's Poverty

One definition of poverty suggests simply that individuals are in poverty when they lack necessities, including food, shelter, medical care, and safety (Bradshaw, 2007). Even though some argue that basic needs are relative to each individual (Sen, 1999), others perceive poverty as simply a matter of inequality (Valentine, 1968). However, the most typical definition of poverty is the statistical measure known as the *poverty line* that Orshansky created in 1963 for the Department of Agriculture. In 2000, the poverty line for a family of four was $17,500 (United States Census Bureau, 2000), though Quigley has noted that this measure of poverty is problematic inasmuch as it fails to account for the various views of family, cash income, work-related expenses, and regional differences in the cost of living (Bradshaw, 2007). Regardless of definition, the theories used to explain poverty are perhaps more important than definition to our text.

The cumulative and cyclical interdependencies theory of poverty provides an explanation of why a disproportionate number of women live in poverty in the United States. The theory builds on the following traditional theories of poverty: Individuals are inherently to blame in some way for living in poverty (Bradshaw, 2007; Gwartney & McCaleb, 1985; Maskovsky, 2001; Weber, 2001); cultural belief systems support subcultures of poverty (Asen, 2002; Chaturvedi, Chiu, & Viswanathan, 2009; Lewis, 1998); economic, political, and social distortions or discriminations result in poverty among certain groups (Abramovitz, 1996; Alinsky, 1945; Blank, 2003; Chubb & Moe, 1996; Jencks, 1996; Quigley, 2003); and geographical disparities, such as rural versus urban circumstances, account for poverty (Goldsmith & Blakely, 1992; Pruitt, 2007; Weber & Jensen, 2004). The cumulative and cyclical interdependencies theory of poverty posits that these various explanations of poverty are interconnected and linked.

This interdependency theory of poverty explains how women become disadvantaged in the midst of poverty, and in turn, become psychologically disabled at the individual level. When women lack opportunities to be self-sufficient, this circumstance results in little, if any, motivation and often in depression in individuals (Bradshaw, 2007). Most important, the theory allows for the possibility that if any of the links between individual, cultural, socio-economic, and geographic aspects of poverty are broken, then the poverty cycle can be broken as well. This can be accomplished by identifying elements of self-sufficiency and addressing them via income and economic assets, education and skills, safe housing, access to health care, social services, close personal ties, or personal resourcefulness and leadership skills (Miller, Mastuera, Chao, & Sadowski, 2004).

## Women in Poverty

Nearly 60% of Americans who live in poverty are women (Cawthorne, 2008). While poverty rates for men and women are the same in childhood, the rates increase for women in the childbearing years and in old age (Weiss, 2009). Interestingly, the gap between the rates of poverty for women (13%) and men (11.1%) is greater in the U.S. than in any other country in the Western world, and this gap is reflected across ethnic groups. A quarter of Black women and nearly a quarter of Latina women are poor, and both groups of women are twice as likely as White women to live in poverty (Cawthorne, 2008; United States Census Bureau, 2008). The following rates reflect poverty among married and unmarried women with and without children: married women with dependent children (54%); single women with dependent children (26%); single women with no children (12%); and married women with no dependent children (Cawthorne, 2008; Weiss, 2009).

The number of single mothers has increased significantly since 2000 (Weiss, 2009). This trend does not take into account the number of unmarried mothers who are close to being in poverty or who have inadequate incomes that fall above the poverty line. Women are paid less than men, are segregated into lower-paying occupations, provide more unpaid caregiving than men, bear the costs of raising children, and are often pushed into a cycle of poverty due to domestic and sexual violence. As a result of these long-term circumstances, one in five women living in poverty are elderly women 60 years of age and older (United States Census Bureau, 2008; Weiss, 2009).

Even though most women on welfare live in poverty, many women with children who are underemployed, as well as many women who are unemployed without children, live in or near poverty. In addition, many unmarried women who are widowed, divorced, separated, or never married are on their own (Weiss, 2009), and these groups of women comprise three fourths of women who live in poverty. The rate of poverty among this group of women is 20.8%, compared to the 6.2% rate of poverty among married women. In sum, based on the poverty line, many women are at or near poverty, and nearly half of those women are unmarried.

Pruitt (2007) noted that poverty in rural areas is a serious problem for female-headed households. In 2003, 36.3% of families headed by females in rural areas were living in poverty, compared to 28.9% of families headed by females in urban areas. In rural areas, single female heads of households with children are more likely than single female heads of households without children to live in poverty. As a result, the children in these households are twice as likely to live in poverty as children who live in suburban areas, and thus the cycle of poverty will likely continue, especially for females.

Several authors have presented the faces of women who live in poverty. Berrick (1997) described the lives of five women on welfare. For example, she described Darlene, a woman on welfare who had become immobilized by deep depression that kept her from wanting to wake up in the morning, primarily because she feared social contacts with social workers, her children's teachers, social workers, and other parents (Berrick, pp. 94–95). Connelly (2000) provided a glimpse of the lives of homeless women with children and how they negotiated daily living without a home. Raphael (2000) told the story of Bernice, a woman from a violent background who became the victim of domestic violence. Ehrenreich (1996) presented the face of many women underemployed in the secondary labor force. She stated:

> When poor single mothers had the option of remaining out of the labor force on welfare, the middle and upper middle class tended to view them with impatience, if not disgust. The welfare poor were excoriated for their laziness, their persistence in reproducing in unfavorable circumstances, their presumed addictions, above all for their "dependency." Here they were, content to live off "government handouts" instead of seeking "self-sufficiency," like everyone else, through a job. They needed to get their act together, learn how to wind an alarm clock, and get to work. (Ehrenreich, 1996, p. 220)

# Poverty and Women's Mental Health

A mental disorder is a state of emotional and psychological well-being in which an individual is unable to use his or her cognitive and emotional capabilities, function in society, and meet the ordinary demands of everyday life (American Heritage Dictionary, 2000). The National Institute of Mental Health (NIMH) National Advisory Mental Health Council's Workgroup on Basic Science placed emphasis on gender differences in the developmental, social, and environmental contributions to mental health (National Institute of Mental Health, 2004). Equally important, however, is the connection between poverty and women's mental health.

Belle (1990) highlighted the association between poverty and women's mental health, particularly the association between poverty and depression. Estimates suggest that between one fourth and one third of women on welfare experience some combination of post-traumatic stress disorder (PTSD), depression, generalized anxiety disorder (GAD), or substance abuse or misuse (see Anderson & Gryzlak, 2002; Coiro, 2001; Danziger, Kalil, & Anderson, 2001; Lens, 2002; Meara, 2006; Montoya, Bell, Atkinson, Nagy, & Whitsell, 2002). More recently, Cook et al. (2009) found that among single mothers on welfare, 61% of mothers reported a lifetime rate of any disorder listed in the fourth edition of the *Diagnostic and Statistical Manual of Mental Disorders (DSM-IV)*; 46.8% of mothers reported at least one disorder in the past 12 months. The lifetime and 12-month rates for specific disorders were substance use disorder (SUD; 29.1%, 9%), mood disorders (28.8%, 20.1%), and anxiety disorders (47.1%, 39.0%).

Similarly, in the National Household Survey of Drug Abuse (NHSDA), 19% of welfare recipients met the criteria for depression and had used illicit drugs in the past year (Jayakody, Danziger, & Pollack, 2000). Barusch, Taylor, Abu-Bader, and Derr (1999) found that nearly 43% of welfare recipients scored positively for clinical depression, 15% scored positively for PTSD, and approximately 7% scored positively for GAD. In another study, welfare program directors surveyed believed that 65% of recipients needed substance abuse treatment (Cordozo & Sussman, 2001).

Wenzel, Tucker, Hambarsoomian, and Elliott (2006) examined violence among 869 women randomly selected from shelter settings and low-income housing in one California metropolitan county. They found that 23% of women in shelters and 9% of women in low-income housing reported experiencing physical violence. For sheltered women, the perpetrators were especially diverse, including sexual partners and family members, as well as strangers; furthermore, the violence was severe. The researchers suggest that impoverished women should be screened specifically for safety. Goodman, Smyth, Borges, and Singer (2009) highlighted that intimate partner violence (IPV) and poverty intersect to shape women's mental health and ways of coping.

In this regard, Goodman et al. (2009) proposed that poverty *does* contribute to IPV, despite the attempt of those involved in the early domestic violence movement to portray IPV as a classless phenomenon. Poverty contributes to IPV primarily in that poor women are more likely than middle- to upper-class women to remain financially dependent on an abusive partner. Reciprocally, IPV contributes to persistent poverty inasmuch as it often leads to mental health-related unemployment and homelessness. Taken together, the mutually reinforcing effect of IPV and poverty results in stress, powerlessness, and social isolation for women, a context in which women must cope very differently than other battered women (Goodman et al., 2009).

The Substance Abuse and Mental Health Services Administration (SAMHSA; 2008) noted that cultural disparities place certain groups of women at even greater risk of poor mental health, particularly due to the lack of economic resources. Women from ethnic minority groups often face racism, discrimination, and violence in their social environments, and those women who have recently come to the United States as immigrants or refugees are at risk of mental disorders due to the additional stresses and traumas that are related to acculturation and assimilation expectations. Also, women from ethnic and cultural minority groups may not seek help for mental health problems because of the stigma attached to mental illness within their cultures.

Several researchers have found that stress among low-income women is associated with mental health problems (Vandergriff-Avery, 2002; Vogel & Marshall, 2001). In the National Survey of American Families (NSAF), parents in stressful family environments were four times more likely than other parents to report symptoms of mental health problems, and low income in families is highly associated with stress (Moore & Vandivere, 2000). The dual role of breadwinner and nurturer undoubtedly places stress on women, particularly those making the transition from welfare to work and who have joined the ranks of the working poor (Cancian, 2001). Sadly, public policy leaders have disenfranchised poor women, especially those in rural areas, from meaningful discussions about the challenge of both working and caring for children (Cancian, Haveman, Meyer, & Wolfe, 2002; Cocca, 2002; Lens, 2002; Pruitt, 2007).

Due to mental health problems, some women on welfare who want to be employed may be unable to understand or conform to the instructions of agencies, or be able to find and keep a job (Cordozo & Sussman, 2001, p. 5). If they do find jobs, the disorders may interfere with interpersonal relationships and functioning in ways that cause them problems in the workplace (Cordozo & Sussman, 2001). This may be especially true for many women whose mental or learning disorders go untreated or undertreated prior to their entering the labor force. The stress of trying to be effective in the workplace may be amplified when women must assume the roles of breadwinner and nurturer.

Ultimately, mental illness and psychological distress can impact the daily functioning and work life of individuals with these conditions. Symptoms such as severely depressed affect, low energy, feelings of hopelessness and worthlessness and suicidal thoughts can make functioning in the work place, even at a basic level, extremely difficult for a person suffering from clinical depression. Other disorders, such as anxiety related conditions, post-traumatic stress disorder and obsessive-compulsive thinking can make regular work environments intimidating, and even overwhelming. A person with a psychiatric illness often feels challenged by even the most fundamental tasks, such as getting out of bed in the morning, tending to personal activities of daily living and parenting. These struggles often preclude seeking work outside the home, and certainly constrain work performances and impair long-term consistency and effectiveness (Cordozo & Sussman, 2001, p. 1).

# Poor Women, Mental Health, and Social Work Practice

Many authors have focused on topics that range from men's abuse of women to poverty among women (Abramovitz, 1996; Amott & Matthaei, 1996; Burden & Gottlieb, 1987; Davis, 1994; Gutierrez & Lewis, 1999; Hanmer & Statham, 1989; Loseke, 1992; Roberts, 1998; Stout & McPhail, 1998; Van Den Bergh, 1995; Van Den Bergh & Cooper, 1986; Van Wormer, 2001; Van Wormer & Bartollas, 2000). However, few authors have focused on the mental health of poor women. As a result, much more information is needed to understand how social workers can practice more effectively with poor women.

First, the literature suggests that the most prevalent disorders among low-income women are PTSD, depression, GAD, and SUD. Given the fact that low income and gender are predictors of borderline personality disorder (BPD) and the lethality of this disorder is so great, this disorder is also important to consider when practicing with poor women. The evidence also indicates that these particular disorders often exist in combination, and as such, it is plausible, for example, that low-income women may use substances to treat symptoms of other mental health disorders. By comparison, eating disorders are not prevalent among low-income women.

Second, individual predispositions to these mental health disorders must be taken into consideration. For example, in the case of PTSD, trauma may actually change the brain in a way that contributes to ongoing symptoms of PTSD, and as such, weight may be given to internal processes rather than external stressors. In the future, it may be that pharmacological intervention will account for more positive outcomes than psychosocial interventions for women who have experienced traumatic events, including childhood sexual abuse, domestic violence, and war experiences. As more research is conducted using technology, such as the use of magnetic resonance imaging, the extent to which biochemical and genetic factors contribute to mental health disorders will determine the extent to which psychosocial versus pharmacological interventions are effective in addressing particular disorders and in what proportions.

Third, much more interest must be paid to the stressors that amplify and exacerbate women's predispositions, especially when one considers the ongoing impact of poverty on mental health. Among drug-addicted women, Kubiak (2005) explored the cumulative effect of women's exposure to stress and found that PTSD increased 40% with each trauma, and that adding chronic stressors increased the likelihood of PTSD. The results of one study indicate that among low-income African American women in an urban Midwestern county, IPV increased women's odds of receiving welfare benefits in a year whereby previous welfare receipt did not (Yoshihama, Hammock, & Horrocks, 2006).

Fourth, routine screening of low-income women who social workers perceive to be at risk of particular disorders seems warranted in order to identify the presence of mental health problems and needs in particular areas. For example, Pruitt (2007) noted the prevalence of depression among low-income women in rural areas. Clark et al. (2008) found that poor women who witnessed community violence in urban neighborhoods were twice as likely as women who did not witness such violence to experience anxiety as well as depressive symptoms. This may mean that social workers develop self-anchored screening measures that reflect the norms in particular areas (Jordan & Franklin, 2003).

Fifth, it is important for social workers to gain insight into the cultural and ethnic factors that affect the mental health of poor women. In this regard, how poor women from ethnic minority groups make sense of mental health problems in terms of causes may reflect the stigma and prejudice that exacerbate these problems. It is imperative to understand more precisely how mental health problems determine whether or not women seek help from formal versus informal caregivers. Perhaps most importantly, women from ethnic minority groups are likely to respond in unique ways to traditional and nontraditional screening measures and interventions (Bhui & Dinos, 2008).

Last, evidence-based interventions that focus on the mental health needs of all women are important in gaining insight into how programs and services can be developed that meet the mental health needs of poor women. While it is especially important to assess accurately the client's situation quantitatively, (Meyer, 1992; Jordan & Franklin, 2003), inferential thinking about and interpretation of data about the client are important skills that allow clinicians to determine the most effective treatment for particular clients (Meyer, 1992). Evidence-based practice (EBP) incorporates what social workers know from their experiences as clinicians and what consumers know from their own life experiences (Gambrill, 1999, 2001; Rosen & Proctor, 2002; Webb, 2001; Witkin & Harrison, 2001).

With this in mind, Gilgun (2005) proposed the following cornerstones of evidence-based practice: (a) what we know from research and theory, (b) what we learn from consumers of our services, (c) what social workers know from their own experience, and (d) what the consumer brings to the situation. In this context, we focus on what we know from the research and theory on treating the mental health disorders prevalent among low-income women. We assume that students who use this text will have a basic understanding of theories that explain mental health problems and of both qualitative and quantitative measures used in screening for mental health disorders, and are willing to use interventions that have been proven to work in addressing the mental health needs of individuals.

## Summary

We noted that the cumulative and cyclical interdependencies theory explains women's poverty by linking the individual, cultural, socioeconomic, and geographic factors that contribute to poverty. We found that in order to reduce poverty, elements of self-sufficiency must be identified and addressed through income and economic assets, education and skills, safe housing, access to health care, social services, close personal ties, and personal resourcefulness and leadership skills. In this context, we noted the considerable numbers of women who live in poverty or near poverty, and how poverty contributes to mental health problems (specifically, PTSD, depression, GAD, SUD, and borderline personality disorder) among many women.

In the remaining chapters of this text, we examine those disorders relying primarily on the Ovid databases, using the Cochrane Central Registry of Clinical Trials, the Cochrane Database of Systematic Reviews, Medline, and Psych INFO. The descriptors used to identify salient literature varied by disorder but included *women, low-income women, poor women, etiology, prevalence, screening, assessment, evidence-based practice*, and *effective practice*. In addition, information was utilized that is available on the webpages of the American Psychological Association, the National Institutes of Health, the National Institutes of Mental Health, and SAMHSA.

# 2

# Women, Trauma, and Post-Traumatic Stress Disorder

Darlene is a young woman in her early twenties of Puerto Rican descent who has never married and has three young children, though the children are currently in foster care. She is employed at McDonald's in a suburban shopping area, rents a small apartment, and takes care of her basic needs. Darlene dropped out of high school during her junior year and has not obtained her GED. She had one sibling, an older brother, who was murdered while in his teens. Darlene reports using alcohol, marijuana, and crack cocaine in the recent past. Darlene states that she was physically, emotionally, and sexually abused as a child and spent most of her life in foster care. She was emancipated at age 16. The murder of her brother was a very traumatic event for her, and she states that she feels powerless and hopeless with regard to getting the children returned to her care. Darlene reports that she has had continual thoughts about suicide. She has few friends or sources of emotional support in the community.

Post-traumatic stress disorder (PTSD) includes the symptoms that occur in the short or long term following exposure to a traumatic event, whether by experiencing or by witnessing the event. Vogel and Marshall (2001) concluded that socioeconomic status contributes more than ethnicity to women's vulnerability to abuse and symptoms of stress, though it is important to note that many women who have a low income or who live in poverty are not abused. Due to an inability to afford housing in less violent neighborhoods, many women are exposed to both community and interpersonal violence. Browne and Bassuk (1997) concluded that, among homeless mothers receiving welfare, PTSD was the main contributor to substance abuse and depression (Browne and Bassuk, 1997).

# Clinical Description

Numerous symptoms are commonly seen when the trauma is an interpersonal stressor, specifically childhood sexual abuse, physical abuse in childhood, or domestic battering (American Psychiatric Association, 2000). Those symptoms include, but are not limited to: self-destructive and impulsive behavior; somatic complaints; and feelings of shame, despair, and hopelessness. In young children, however, PTSD may present in the form of nightmares about monsters and of rescuing others or of threats to self or others. It is noteworthy that PTSD may also be associated with general medical conditions that can be measured in terms of changes in vital signs, such as increased heart rate and glandular activity.

# Prevalence

Findings in community-based studies show that the lifetime rate of PTSD is 8% among adults in the United States (American Psychiatric Association, 2000). By comparison, Breslau and Davis (1992) found in a large community sample that women are at greater risk than men of developing PTSD after exposure to trauma (see also Breslau, Davis, Andreski, Peterson, & Schultz, 1997). Although Breslau and colleagues noted that the risk of PTSD among all individuals is 9%, the risk for women is 13% and for men 6%. Exposure to multiple trauma experiences places both men and women at greater risk of developing PTSD; it is women's exposure to sexual assault that contributes to the gender difference in risk (Breslau et al., 1997).

In the Trauma Recovery Project, a large epidemiological study designed to examine multiple outcomes after major trauma, including PTSD, researchers found that, depending on whether full or partial *DSM* diagnostic criteria were used, women in the general population were 2.4 to 2.8 times more likely than men to experience PTSD (Holbrook, Hoyt, Stein, & Sieber, 2002). Moreover, the researchers found that being female, perceiving threat to one's life, and symptoms of acute stress disorder (ASD) significantly and independently predict risk of PTSD. The prevalence of PTSD among women takes on salience when one considers its well-documented comorbidity with depression, generalized anxiety, and substance use and abuse disorder (SUD).

It is important to note that ASD may precede PTSD and that panic disorder (PD) often co-occurs with PTSD. ASD refers to symptoms that one might experience within the first month following a traumatic event and prior to the PTSD diagnosis (see Bryant, 2006). Dissociation, or the feeling of being disconnected from one's surroundings, may occur, and this may include having no memories for an extended period of time. In addition to experiencing a traumatic event and reacting to it with strong feelings of fear, one must experience three of the following symptoms: numbness or detachment; being dazed or unaware; feelings that people, places, and things are not real;

feelings of separateness; and being unable to recall key aspects of the traumatic experience. Seeking treatment for ASD is critical in preventing PTSD.

PD is more likely than ASD to co-occur with PTSD, as well as with depression and SUD (see Nixon, Resick, & Griffen, 2004). A panic attack is the experience of intense fear or discomfort and must actually be experienced before a diagnosis can be made. For the diagnosis, four of the following symptoms must be reported: pounding heart or increased heart rate; sweating; trembling or shaking; feeling of suffocation; choking; chest pain; abdominal problems; dizziness; detachment; loss of control; fear of death; numbness; and chills or hot flashes.

One must also have experienced an unexpected attack, and at least one attack must be followed by a month or more of either concern about having an additional panic attack, worry about the consequences of a panic attack, or a change in behavior due to the attack. It is possible to have panic attacks without having the disorder. Approximately 13% of women with PTSD develop PD as compared to 7% of men with PTSD, which is likely due to high rates of childhood sexual abuse and physical abuse among women with panic disorder. In addition, women are more likely than men to be raped.

## Etiology

Genetic factors may influence the risk of exposure to some forms of trauma, specifically as a result of differences in personality that contribute to environmental and behavioral choices of individuals (Gilbertson et al., 2002; Stein, Jang, Taylor, Vernon, & Livesley, 2002). If this is so, genes that influence one's vulnerability to assaultive trauma may also influence susceptibility to PTSD. In monkeys, researchers have found that serotonin may modulate the effect of adversity in females but not in males (Barr et al., 2004), which may be helpful in understanding responses of humans in certain stress-related syndromes, including PTSD. In the case of childhood sexual abuse, researchers have found that the trauma may induce abnormal blood flow to the hippocampus, the part of the brain associated with memory, processing emotions, and visual perception (Bremner et al., 1999; Shors et al., 2001). In one study, researchers found that early trauma in women may result in a sensitized stress system that responds in an overly active way to subsequent stresses (Heim et al., 2000).

Using naturalistic, qualitative studies, researchers have explored the possibility that dissociation during and immediately following the trauma predicts PTSD. The research indicates that if one has an out-of-body experience *at the time* the trauma occurs in order to protect herself or himself from being emotionally overwhelmed by the traumatic event, that specific, acute dissociation predicts PTSD (Brewin & Holmes, 2003; Ozer, Best, Lipsey, & Weiss, 2003). In contrast, using multivariate analysis, Briere, Scott, and Weathers (2005) found that *persistent* trauma-related dissociation is the best predictor of PTSD, and thus, they concluded that what happens at the time of trauma is less important than what happens afterward (see also Halligan, Michael, Clark, & Ehlers, 2003; Murray, Ehlers, & Mayou, 2002).

Within the context of cognition, evidence indicates that individuals have normative schemas that allow them to make sense of experiences relative to established norms of behavior and affect. However, traumatic experiences damage and violate expectations and emotions inherent in these basic schemas (see Kronenberger & Meyer, 2001, pp. 260–261), and as a result, individuals who experience PTSD often perceive the world as an unsafe place and themselves to be incompetent (Foa & Jaycox, 1999). If the discrepancy between memories of the experience and normative schemas goes unresolved, individuals find mechanisms for coping with the discrepancy, such as dissociating, that result in mental disorders, specifically PTSD. This cognitive discrepancy could explain both immediate and prolonged onset of PTSD (Holbrook et al., 2002).

For girls and women, the antecedents to abuse-related traumatic events are most often external stressors, including physical or sexual assault in childhood (PA/CSA), adult sexual assault (ASA), and domestic battering. Elliot, Mok, and Briere (2004) found that, among 941 participants, 22% of women reported ASA, as compared to 3.8% of men, and when multivariate analysis was conducted, the risk factors for ASA were: being of younger age, being female, being divorced, having experienced CSA, and having experienced PA in adulthood. It is also noteworthy that PTSD and stressful life events are associated with greater odds of chronic medical conditions among women, particularly among women who were sexually assaulted both as children and adults (see also Dobie et al., 2004; Ouimette et al., 2004; Ulman & Brecklin, 2003). In a sample of 1,225 women who were members of an urban HMO, health care costs doubled among women whose PTSD scores were high (Walker et al., 2003). It is a reasonable conclusion that low-income women suffering from PTSD often have additional health problems or issues that contribute to difficulties in functioning and self-sufficiency.

## Screening and Assessment Measures

Given the emotional and financial costs associated with PTSD among women, assessment in the form of both structured clinical interviews and objective, self-report measures take on special importance in identifying the disorder in child, adolescent, and adult females. Females with whom social workers practice may have been sexually assaulted in childhood and adulthood, so it is especially important that they screen females for PTSD as early as possible. Moreover, the measures we identify in the following sections are ones that social workers can administer with relative ease, speed, and reliability.

## Clinician Structured Interviews

Most experts argue that there is no substitute for a good clinical interview, and we agree. This is especially true with respect to assessing PTSD. The structured interview schedule allows for in-depth exploration of any information that women are willing and able to share about a traumatic event, as well as their emotional responses to it. It is important to note that this assessment approach has potential to reveal multiple traumatic events, including a woman's experience of sexual assault as a child and as an adult. Although we have identified three schedules that social workers might use in identifying the extent to which women have experienced trauma or PTSD, structured interview schedules may be developed and standardized for particular client populations if desired.

---

**Adult Female**

Structured Clinical Interview for *DSM-TR* (SCID-RV)

Post Traumatic Stress Disorder Interview (PTSD-I)

Clinician-Administered PTSD Scale (CAPS-1)

**Young Female**

Clinician Administered PTSD Scale for Children and Adolescents (CAPS-CA)

Clinician Administered PTSD Scale (CAPS-1)

---

### SCID, PTSD-I, and CAPS-1

The SCID (Spitzer & Williams, 1985) requires that a social worker ask specific questions about the client's symptoms. The instrument has a PTSD component that has been shown to be a clinically valuable measurement of the construct. The SCID-RV reflects the latest revisions; information about the instrument can be obtained at http://www.scid4.org/contact.html.

The PTSD-I (Watson, Juba, Manifold, Kucala, & Anderson, 1991) is comprised of 20 DSM-related items. The questions assess whether the respondent has experienced a traumatic event and various symptoms of mental disorders subsequent to the event. With an alpha coefficient of .92 and test-retest reliability coefficient of .95, the instrument has utility in cross-validating other measures of PTSD. In addition to the SCID and PTSD-I, the CAPS-1 (Blake, Weathers, Nagy, Kaloupek, Klauminzer, Charney, & Keane, 1990) also measures current PTSD status. The instrument measures the frequency and intensity of distress associated with PTSD, such as the occurrence of unpleasant dreams about the event.

## CAPS-CA

The CAPS-CA was adapted from the CAPS-1 in order to screen for PTSD among children and adolescents between 8 and 15 years of age (Newman, Weathers, Nader, Kaloupek, Pynoos, et al., 2004). In using this measure, the clinician asks the client to rate the frequency and intensity of 17 symptoms of PTSD that are consistent with a formal diagnosis. The CAPS-CA is also helpful in evaluating the impact of the symptoms on the child's social, occupational, and developmental functioning, as well as the level of subjective distress, global severity, and the validity of the interview. The instrument allows for assessing lifetime PTSD even when there is no diagnosis of current PTSD.

## Objective Measures

Self-report, objective measures also have utility in assessing PTSD. Several measures are described in this section, though this may not include all measures of the construct, primarily because many instruments include some component or components of PTSD. It is important to note that some of the instruments are in the public domain while others must be purchased. From among the numerous instruments that can be used to assess trauma, we have selected for discussion several rapid assessment instruments that have utility in screening for PTSD in females.

**Adult Female**

> PTSD Symptom Checklist (PCL)
> PTSD Symptom Scale (PSS)
> Impact of Events Scale-Revised (IES-R)
> Harvard Trauma Questionnaire (HTQ)
> Beck's Depression Inventory (BDI/BDI-II)

**Young Female**

> Child Post-Traumatic Stress Disorder Reaction Index (CPSD-RI)

## PCL

The PCL is a 17-item brief self-report instrument that can be used to screen for PTSD (Weathers, Litz, Herman, Huska, & Keane, 1993). It was first administered to motor vehicle accident and sexual assault victims using diagnoses and scores from the CAPS as the criteria. As a whole, the PCL is highly correlated with the CAPS (.93), providing a measure of its concurrent validity. The purpose in using the PCL is to screen for PTSD rather than for diagnosis, and its utility is in its use as a rapid assessment instrument.

## PSS

The PSS (Foa, Cashman, Jaycox, & Perry, 1997) contains 17 items that assess the severity of PTSD symptoms. An interview and self-report version of the PSS were administered to a sample of 118 recent victims of sexual and nonsexual assault. The results indicate that both versions of the PSS have satisfactory internal consistency, high test-retest reliability, and good concurrent validity. The interview version yielded high interrater agreement when administered separately by two interviewers and excellent convergent validity with the SCID. When used to diagnose PTSD, the self-report version of the PSS was somewhat more conservative than the interview version (Foa, Riggs, Dancu, & Rothbaum, 2005).

## IES-R

The IES-R (Weiss, 1994) is a self-administered, 22-item questionnaire based on three clusters of symptoms that indicate PTSD. The instrument is not a diagnostic or screening tool for PTSD, but is used to obtain a respondent's report of symptoms in response to a traumatic event within 2 weeks of the event. In this regard, it can be used to measure and evaluate recovery as well. Respondents are asked to rate the degree of distress for each of 22 symptoms on a 5-point Likert-type scale (*0 = not at all; 1 = a little bit; 2 = moderately; 3 = quite a bit; 4 = extremely*). A version of the instrument is also available for use with children and adolescents.

## HTQ

The HTQ has four parts that address traumatic events, description of events, events leading to head injury, and trauma symptoms (Mollica & Caspi-Yavin, 1991). Part IV is used to screen for PTSD and consists of 16 items that focus on key symptoms of PTSD. Those items as a whole have good reliability and internal consistency; in particular, the test-retest reliability on the HTQ ranges between 0.89 and 0.92. The fourth part of the HTQ has special utility in assessing PTSD because it has been used extensively across cultures and in numerous countries.

## BDI/BDI-II

The BDI/BDI–II consists of 21 items to assess the intensity of depression in clinical and normal patients (Beck, 1967). Each item is a list of four statements arranged in increasing severity about a particular symptom of depression. Several items on the original instrument have been replaced on the BDI-II, primarily to address loss of energy, as well as the increases and decreases in sleep and appetite. Respondents are now asked to respond regarding symptoms experienced during the preceding two weeks, as opposed to one week on the original BDI. These new items bring the BDI–II into alignment with *DSM–IV* criteria. With the new items added, the coefficient alpha for the BDI-II is .92 versus .86 for the original version.

### CPTSD-RI

The CPTSD-RI was developed for use with individuals 5 years of age and older (Pynoos et al., 1987). The instrument asks children and youth to report the extent to which they have experienced 20 symptoms of PTSD during the week prior to completing the measure. This instrument has good internal consistency, with alpha coefficients that range from 0.74 to 0.84 and interrater reliability of 0.88. The CPTSD-RI was developed to screen for fear and anxiety and for disturbances in sleep and concentration.

In sum, the measures identified herein are ones that social workers can administer quickly and with relative ease in a variety of settings. When one considers the prevalence of childhood and adult sexual assault among women, it is critical that much more attention be given to screening for PTSD. This is especially true regarding screening for PTSD among young girls, so that they can be referred to appropriate programs and services as soon as possible.

## Effective Treatment

In general, Bradley, Greene, Russ, Dutra, and Westen (2005) found that the majority of patients treated with psychotherapy for PTSD in randomized trials recover or improve, though they noted several caveats when treatment is applied to consumers in the community. First, most consumers have numerous symptoms that may indicate disorders apart from PTSD, so it may be difficult to generalize positive results of studies to the population of PTSD consumers. Second, there are few studies that follow consumers for an extended period of time, and consumers may have residual symptoms. With these caveats in mind, more research is needed that follows consumers for at least two years (Bradley, et. al. 2005).

In the field of social work, it is important that practitioners are able to assess PTSD in women and refer them to appropriate clinicians, or, when feasible, intervene themselves to address PTSD. The results of nonsystematic and systematic reviews indicate that the most effective interventions in treating PTSD are trauma-focused cognitive behavior therapy (TF-CBT; Bisson & Andrew, 2007; Bisson, Ehlers, & Matthews, 2007; Bradley, Greene, Russ, Dutra, & Westen, 2005; Kornør et al., 2008; Seidler & Wagner, 2006) and eye movement desensitization and reprocessing (EMDR) (Bisson & Andrew, 2007;

Bisson et al., 2007; Bradley et al., 2005; Davidson & Parker, 2001). Even though the results of nonsystematic reviews indicate that prolonged exposure (PE) and stress inoculation training (SIT) are effective in treating PTSD when compared to therapies such as psychoanalysis and unmodified psychodynamic therapy (Nemeroff et al., 2006), the results of the most current systematic reviews show that TF-CBT and EMDR are the most effective evidence-based interventions to use with women in cases of childhood sexual abuse, battering, and rape.

---

Trauma-Focused Cognitive Behavioral Therapy (TF-CBT)

Cognitive Trauma Therapy-Battered Women (CTT-BW)

Prolonged Exposure (PE)

Eye Movement Desensitization and Reprocessing (EMDR)

Stress Management or Stress Innoculation Therapy (SIT)

---

## TF-CBT

TF-CBT is a Substance Abuse and Mental Health Services Administration (SAMHSA) model program and psychotherapeutic intervention designed to help children and adults address the negative effects of traumatic life events, including sexual or physical abuse, loss of a loved one, various types of violence, disasters, and terror attacks. This intervention blends cognitive and behavioral interventions with a focus on empowerment and trust. TF-CBT targets the depression and behavioral problems that often co-occur with PTSD. TF-CBT alleviates poor self-esteem, mood instability, and self-injurious behavior by encouraging children and adults to talk directly about their traumatic experience in a supportive environment where they feel safe. Guidelines for implementing the intervention are as follows:

- Intervention can be divided into 12 to 16 sessions, on average, including several sessions for parents of children.
- Each session lasts 60 minutes to 90 minutes and a session is provided weekly.
- Even though the process may be completed in 16 sessions, the process may take longer, depending on the circumstances.

The results of initial studies of TF-CBT validate its effectiveness, particularly with traumatized children (Cohen, Deblinger, & Mannarino, 2004; Deblinger, Lippman, & Steer, 1996). While TF-CBT is recommended for use with young children, particularly young females who have been sexually abused, this intervention can be used with adult females as well (Kornør et al., 2008). In sum, social workers should use this intervention for addressing childhood sexual abuse among young females or adult women who were sexually abused as children. If social workers are not in a position to implement the intervention, they can and should make a referral to a clinician who uses TF-CBT.

## CTT-BW

Cognitive trauma therapy for battered women (CTT-BW), a variation on TF-CBT, has been proven to be effective in the treatment of PTSD among battered women (Kubany, Hill, & Owens, 2003; Kubany et al., 2004). CTT-BW involves the use of several cognitive approaches, including trauma history exploration, education, stress management, exposure, self-monitoring of negative self-talk, and cognitive therapy for guilt. Kubany et al. (2004) randomly assigned 125 ethnically diverse women to immediate or delayed CTT-BW. They found that PTSD remitted in 87% of women who completed CTT-BW, and the gains were maintained at 3- and 6-month follow-ups. The gains included decreases in depression and guilt, as well as a substantial increase in self-esteem. There were no differences in benefits between clients who were White and those from ethnic minority groups, or between those treated by therapists with different levels of education and training.

## EMDR

EMDR is a comprehensive, integrative psychotherapy approach that includes aspects of several therapies, including psychodynamic, cognitive-behavioral, interpersonal, experiential, and body-centered therapies (Shapiro, 2002). Despite the debate about the effectiveness of EMDR, it is an information processing therapy that allows individuals to accurately process information associated with a traumatic or negative event wherein strong negative feelings or dissociation may interfere with processing information. The technique involves the patient moving her eyes back and forth while she concentrates on the event.

Usually, the clinician waves a stick or light in front of the patient and expects her to move her eyes to follow the stick or light. EMDR involves an eight-phase approach to processing past experiences that trigger negative feelings, beliefs, and emotions related to a traumatic event. With successful treatment, individuals identify the positive experiences that are needed to enhance future adaptive behaviors and mental health, and the proposed explanation is that rapid eye movements somehow unblock the information-processing system in such a way that patients can process information more effectively. The eight phases of the treatment are as follows:

- **Phase 1:** Take a history and develop a treatment plan targeting distressing events, current situations that elicit emotional disturbance, and development of skills and behaviors needed to cope.

- **Phase 2**: Stabilize the individual sufficiently to be able to handle emotional distress.
- **Phase 3**: Focus the individual on a negative belief about the traumatic event; simultaneously, focus individual on a preferred positive belief. After the intensity of both are rated, the individual is instructed to focus on the image of the event, as well as on negative thoughts and sensations associated with the event, while simultaneously moving eyes back and forth following the therapist's fingers as they move across his or her field of vision. The time needed for this may vary depending on the circumstance, and the process is repeated numerous times in a session until the individual experiences no distress in thinking about the image that is the focus of the session.
- **Phase 4**: Focus on different negative belief.
- **Phase 5**: Focus on a second different negative belief.
- **Phase 6**: Focus on third different negative belief.
- **Phase 7**: Closure: the therapist asks the client to keep a journal during the week to document any related material that may arise and reminds the client of the self-calming activities that were mastered in Phase 2.
- **Phase 8**: Re-evaluate previous work, as well as progress since the previous session. EMDR treatment ensures processing of all related historical events, current incidents that elicit distress, and future scenarios that will require different responses (anticipation).

Rothbaum, Astin, and Marsteller (2005) compared the efficacy of EMDR and exposure therapy in work with female rape victims. While these researchers found that both interventions were equally effective, primarily because they are both exposure interventions, they believed that the "blanking" component of EMDR allowed women a break from the exposure. Similarly, Edmond and colleagues have used EMDR with adult female survivors of childhood sexual abuse (Edmond, Rubin, & Wambach, 1999; Edmond, Sloan, & McCarty, 2004). Researchers have also found EMDR to be effective in treating Iranian girls who were sexually abused (Jaberghaderi, Greenwald, Rubin, Dolatabadim, & Zand, 2004).

## SIT and PE

Despite findings in the most recent systematic reviews and meta-analyses, Foa, Rothbaum, Riggs, and Murdock (1991) examined the extent to which stress inoculation training (SIT) and prolonged exposure (PE) positively impacted PTSD among 45 rape victims. Within the context that SIT includes a combination of strategies, including relaxation, restructuring thinking, and role-playing, PE involves activating and fully experiencing the fear associated with a traumatic event albeit in a safe setting. The researchers found that directly after intervention, 50% of women who received SIT improved, 26% of women who received PE improved, and 20% of women in a waiting list control group (supportive counseling) improved. At a 3-month follow-up, PE reduced symptoms in 60% of women compared to symptom reduction in 49% of women who received SIT, while supportive counseling reduced symptoms in 36% of women. Foa et al. (1999) conducted additional research with 96 female assault victims and found that PE was significantly more effective than SIT, a combination of both treatments, and no treatment among women in a wait list group. Even so, the relative gains in all groups of women were maintained at a 12-month follow-up.

Exposure therapies include step-by-step desensitization and flooding, and thus, require that women face their fears via images and memories just enough to avoid being overwhelmed. In general, cognitive therapy per se utilizes strategies that address the discrepancies between the damaged and violated expectations that result from a traumatic event, such as sexual abuse or assault, and the normative schemas that allow young girls and women to make sense of the experiences. In conjunction, managing the anxiety associated with a traumatic event involves using relaxation techniques, as well as distraction, primarily to manage anxiety associated with fears. It is noteworthy that interpersonal therapy, or the focus on relationship interactions, may also be used as well in treating women who have experienced traumatic experiences (Bleiberg, & Markowitz, 2005; Resick, Neshith, Weaver, Astin, & Fuer, 2002).

## Summary

Several conclusions can be drawn from the review of literature on evidence-based practice with females who experience trauma and subsequently PTSD. First, it is important for social workers to understand that trauma may actually change brain functioning as a response to stress, and thus affect long-term functioning in terms of PTSD (as well as depression and other disorders). Second, the extent to which social workers can determine how PTSD has developed over time may be important in determining which intervention is most efficacious. Third, social workers can and should screen for PTSD among the women with whom they work, especially low-income women who may be exposed more often to trauma in their families and communities than other women. Finally, some social workers may have the education and training to be able to effectively address PTSD, but those who are unable to provide intervention should make every effort to refer women to appropriately trained service providers.

### Discussion Topics

1. Explain why the rate of PTSD among women is greater than the rate among men in the general population.

2. Delineate between ASD and PTSD, and discuss why it is important to screen women for ASD shortly after the experience of a traumatic event.

3. Discuss the importance of researchers understanding at what point in time the onset of PTSD occurs. Consider why women with PTSD who live in low-income neighborhoods have more health problems than other women.

4. Clearly explain the differences in using the following treatments to address PTSD: CBT, PE, SIT, CTT-BW, and TF-CBT. Use additional research to learn more about each type of intervention.

## CASE STUDY 2.1

Emily is 16 years of age and was brought to the clinic by her adoptive mother. Her biological parents were drug users and neglected to adequately meet Emily's needs, and as a result, their parental rights were terminated. While between the ages of 8 and 12, Emily was sexually abused by her father and an adoptive brother, and she was sexually assaulted at age 13 by an adult male who broke in through her bedroom window. In addition, Emily was hospitalized at age 13 for a methamphetamine overdose. At about 14 years of age, Emily began having flashbacks related to her sexual assault, occasional auditory hallucinations, and episodes of depersonalization. She expresses intense anger with men. Her adoptive mother reports that Emily has poor personal boundaries with males, is defiant toward authority figures, has been self-injurious, and has also attempted to overdose on her prescription medication. During the interview at the clinic, Emily expressed shame and hopelessness, and she complained of having headaches and stomachaches.

### Discussion Questions: Emily

How would you go about selecting an assessment instrument for Emily given her multiple experiences of sexual assault; her physical illness and complaints; and her feelings of anger, shame, and hopelessness?

Given the instruments you administer and the resulting assessment(s) you make, how would you prioritize her treatment needs? What would be the advantages and disadvantages of using cognitive behavioral therapy? Are both forms of treatment equally appropriate for her?

Is her self-injurious behavior independent of her other symptoms? If not, how might they be related with respect to etiology and possible treatment?

What unmet needs does Emily's case suggest, and how would you go about assessing and prioritizing these?

## Illustrative Reading

# Resource Loss and Naturalistic Reduction of PTSD Among Inner-City Women

Kristen H. Walter

*Kent State University*

Stevan E. Hobfoll

*Kent State University Summa Health System*

**Authors' Note:** This research was supported by Grant 5 R01 MH045669–12 National Institute of Health, NIMH Office of AIDS Research. We express our special thanks to Dr. Dawn Johnson who provided helpful suggestions and feedback on the manuscript prior to submission. Correspondence concerning this article should be addressed to Kristen H. Walter, Kent Hall 136, Kent State University, Kent, OH 44242; e-mail: Kwalter2@kent.edu.

Halting the process of psychosocial and material resource loss has been theorized as being associated with the reduction of post-traumatic stress disorder (PTSD). This study examines how the limiting of resource loss is related to alleviation of PTSD symptoms among 102 inner-city women, who originally met diagnostic criteria for PTSD after experiencing interpersonal traumatic events such as child abuse, rape, and sexual assault. Participants whose PTSD symptoms improve and become nondiagnostic for PTSD are compared with those who remain diagnostic. The two groups are not significantly different at pretest. However, at the 6-month time point, those who become nondiagnostic for PTSD report less resources loss in three of four domains. This pattern suggests that as PTSD symptoms decrease, women's material and psychosocial resource loss diminishes, which in turn, may aid their recovery process.

**Keywords:** PTSD; resources; symptom reduction

Considerable research has examined the etiology and treatment of post-traumatic stress disorder (PTSD). Epidemiological studies have estimated that the lifetime prevalence of PTSD ranges from 8% to 12% (Kessler, Sonnega, Bromet, Hughes, & Nelson, 1995; Resnick, Kilpatrick, Dansky, Saunders, & Best, 1993). Although there is a well-established relationship between traumatic events and the risk for developing PTSD, not everyone exposed to traumatic events will develop PTSD or continue to have resulting symptoms (Kulka et al., 1990; Wolfe, Keane, Kaloupek, Mora, & Wine, 1993). Studies of PTSD have identified risk factors for onset and chronicity of the disorder (Koenen, Stellman, Stellman, & Sommer, 2003), but little is known about how circumstances in people's lives might influence the waxing or waning of their symptoms. This is especially important to study among inner-city women and women of color because both are more likely to be exposed to childhood and adult trauma (Breslau, Chilcoat, Kessler, Peterson, & Lucia, 1999; Switzer et al., 1999) and are less likely to obtain mental health treatment if they develop PTSD (Cooper-Patrick et al., 1999; Kessler et al., 1999).

Although risk factor studies provide essential information relating to who does and does not develop PTSD, they have seldom examined the course of PTSD once present. This is particularly important because PTSD is a persistent disorder, especially in the context of multiple traumas (Kessler, 2000). The typical person with PTSD experiences active symptoms of the disorder for approximately two decades in duration (Kessler, 2000). Yet only about 38% of individuals with PTSD seek treatment (Kessler et al., 1999). This relatively low rate of treatment seeking may be related to avoidance, but it is possible that natural symptom remission processes, even if temporary, occur and also decrease motivation and in some cases the need for treatment. Consequently, it is imperative to determine the course of symptoms of PTSD and the factors that influence the alleviation of symptoms once a person develops the disorder.

A few recent studies examined the course of PTSD symptoms (Koenen et al., 2003; Orcutt, Erickson, & Wolfe, 2004). Most individuals with PTSD do not experience consistent, stable PTSD symptoms continually for a long duration but rather experience a fluctuation of symptoms over the course of their disorder (Orcutt et al., 2004). Various symptom trajectories are possible for individuals with PTSD. Studies have shown a tendency toward decreasing the rate of symptoms over time (Blanchard et al., 1996; Ehlers, Mayou, & Bryant, 1998). However, other studies have indicated that symptoms may actually increase over time (Southwick et al., 1995) and/or display a variable time course (Mayou, Tyndel, & Bryant, 1997). Clearly, further understanding of the factors that influence the course of PTSD symptom trajectories is an important endeavor.

Research, albeit scant, has demonstrated evidence for factors related to the longitudinal fluctuation of PTSD symptoms. Orcutt et al. (2004) found two growth curves that described the course of PTSD among Gulf War veterans.

The first symptom course was characterized by low levels of PTSD symptoms that barely increased over time. The second symptom course revealed a pattern where veterans had higher levels of initial PTSD symptoms that subsequently increased further. Veterans in the lesser symptomatic course group had higher levels of education, less combat exposure, and were more likely to be White and male. Given that education and being from the ethnic majority group are associated with having greater access to material resources (D. R. Williams & Jackson, 2005), the influence of material resource factors may be relevant.

Another study examined the longitudinal process of psychological disorders among Dutch Cambodia veterans. Veterans who had greater self-efficacy and perceived control over situations were found to have a reduction in psychological disorder symptoms, including PTSD, than those who were lower in self-efficacy and perceived control (de Vries, Soetekouw, Van Der Meer, & Bleihenberg, 2001). This suggests that personal resources, such as self-efficacy and a sense of personal control, contribute to improvement of psychological symptoms, even though these same resources are vulnerable to loss owing to PTSD and the nature of the original trauma experience.

One way to conceptualize the onset and maintenance of PTSD, as evidenced by these studies, is that the disorder is accompanied by a rapid loss of material and psychosocial resources (Hobfoll, 1991). The loss of these resources may contribute to further stress, decreasing the probability for easing symptoms. In turn, the halting of these resource loss

*(Continued)*

(Continued)

cycles may be a key to alleviating symptoms. Just as psychological treatment frequently focuses on increasing patients' resources such as social support, employment, and self-esteem, the natural course of PTSD may be related to similar factors.

This process, whereby resources are theoretically connected to PTSD, is illustrated by the conservation of resources (COR) theory (Hobfoll, 1989; Hobfoll & Lilly, 1993). Resources are defined in the COR theory as things that people value or that assist in obtaining what is valued (Hobfoll, 1989; Hobfoll & Lilly, 1993). The COR theory posits that stress can be conceptualized in terms of resource loss and asserts that there is a basic human motivation to obtain, retain, and protect resources. Because humans desire to obtain, retain, and protect these resources, they act to minimize loss and maximize resource gain. Stress results, in particular, from a loss of resources, and this process may lead to a downward spiral as the resources needed to cope with the trauma are also depleted (Baumeister, Bratslavsky, Muraven, & Tice, 1998). Hence, trauma causes both a rapid decline of resources, and the resultant state of resource loss, in turn, undermines recovery processes (Hobfoll, 1991).

A key principle of the COR theory is that people must invest in resources to retain resources, protect against resource loss, recover from losses, and gain further resources. Hence, those who lack resources are at additional risk because they have fewer resources to invest in recovery (Ennis, Hobfoll, & Schröder, 2000; Hobfoll, Johnson, Ennis, & Jackson, 2003). They may experience loss spirals, as initial coping efforts cycle into further resource loss (Benight et al., 1999; Hobfoll et al., 2003; Norris & Kaniasty, 1996). Thus, those with PTSD will have depleted resource reservoirs; however, to the extent that they can halt the resource loss process, they can enhance their chances of reducing symptoms of PTSD (Schumm, Hobfoll, & Keogh, 2004).

The importance of halting or reversing resource loss cycles has been noted. Holahan, Moos, Holahan, and Cronkite (1999) found that over the course of 10 years, those with initial depression who continued to experience resource loss also continued to report continued depression. In comparison, those who reversed resource loss cycles no longer reported depressive symptoms. Similarly, women who were able to halt resource loss cycles had diminished likelihood of PTSD stemming from childhood and adult trauma history (Schumm et al., 2004). This process is also cited in the social support deterioration deterrence model (Kaniasty & Norris, 1997; Norris & Kaniasty, 1996), which asserts that after traumatic circumstances, social relationships are crucial to coping with the subsequent stressors but are themselves often lost in the process.

Halting of resource loss cycles has also been shown to be related to PTSD in U.S. veteran samples and following disaster. In a longitudinal examination of 348 Gulf War returnees, PTSD symptoms increased over time, whereas resources decreased (Benotsch et al., 2000). In the same study, even after controlling for Time-1 resources, PTSD symptoms predicted later coping and relationship efforts, alluding to a reciprocal effect of halting resource loss and PTSD symptoms (Benotsch et al., 2000). In another study of 775 Persian Gulf War troops, PTSD diagnosis was related to resource loss areas, including less commitment, less family cohesion, and lower satisfaction with social support (Sutker, Davis, Uddo, & Ditta, 1995). Similarly, Arata, Picou, Johnson, and McNally (2000) found that among Alaskan fisherman affected by the *Exxon Valdez* oil spill, 6 years postdisaster, resource loss still predicted PTSD and depression. These studies indicate the critical role of halting resource loss for reducing PTSD.

We examined naturalistic PTSD symptom remission among a sample of 102 women receiving gynecological medical care at two inner-city clinics to achieve a reasonably representative sample because such a high percentage of women receive gynecological care. It was hypothesized that those women whose PTSD symptoms decreased over time and became nondiagnostic would experience a halting of resource loss compared with those whose symptoms did not show improvement and remained diagnostic for PTSD. Although these women might again increase in PTSD symptoms, we know that symptom remission is accompanied by less emotional suffering and might opportune women to improved quality of life and even further symptom relief.

## Method

### Participants

A total of 102 women who met diagnostic criteria for probable PTSD were selected from a larger sample of 940 women involved in a study of stress and health. The use of the sample for this study was approved by the institutional review boards of Kent State University and Summa Health System. The original sample of 940 women was selected because single, inner-city women are known to be at risk for violence and trauma (Horowitz, McKay, & Marshall, 2005; Urquiza, Wyatt, & Root, 1994). The selected subsample included participants who met *Diagnostic and Statistical Manual of Mental Disorders* (*DSM*) diagnostic criteria for probable PTSD at the pretest assessment (diagnosis based on the Posttraumatic Stress Scale–Interview [PSS-I]). Participants experienced interpersonal trauma such as childhood physical abuse, childhood sexual abuse, physical assault, and sexual assault/rape.

Participants were, on average, 22.37 (*SD* = 4.22) years of age, 66% were unemployed, and 69% had annual household incomes under US$10,000. Forty-four percent of the sample had some high school education, with an additional 32% earning a high school diploma. The large majority of the sample had never been married, comprising 88% of the respondents. African Americans constituted 62% of the sample, and 27% of the sample were European American. The remaining 11% of respondents were Hispanic, Asian, or of other ethnic backgrounds. Only 2 participants did not provide assessment data at the 6-month follow-up. The initial sample consisted of 104 participants, but the 2 participants who did not attend the 6-month follow-up assessment point were removed from the analyzed sample.

### Measures

*Demographic questionnaire.* A self-report demographic questionnaire was used to collect information relating to age, racial group, education, employment status, marital status, income, religion, and pregnancy status.

*PSS–I version.* The PSS-I (Foa, Riggs, Dancu, & Rothbaum, 1993) is a 17-item scale that contains items which correspond to PTSD symptom criteria found in the *Diagnostic*

*(Continued)*

(Continued)

*and Statistical Manual of Mental Disorders,* fourth edition, text revision (*DSM-IV-TR;* American Psychiatric Association, 2000). The PSS-I is the interview version of the Posttraumatic Stress Scale–Self-Report version (PSS-SR; Foa et al., 1993). Each symptom criterion is rated in terms of frequency or severity on a 0 (*not at all*) to 3 (*very much*) scale. The Cronbach's alpha for the PSS-I ranges from .65 to .86 (Foa & Tonlin, 2000). Cronbach's alpha for this study was .81, and probable PTSD was scored as having a minimum of one re-experiencing symptom, three avoidance symptoms, and two hyperarousal symptoms. A symptom was recorded if the respondent reported a 1 (*a little*), 2 (*moderately*), or 3 (*very much*) in terms of severity. In addition, women were provided with a list of A1 criterion events to ensure that the reported interpersonal event met this criterion before administering the PSS-I.

*Conservation of Resources–Evaluation* (*COR-E;* Hobfoll & Lilly, 1993). We selected 45 resources relevant for inner-city women's lives from the full 74-item measure. Resource categories were gleaned from broader categories of resources. Resource item categories included material resources (i.e., money for transportation), energy resources (i.e., financial assets), nonfamilial interpersonal resources (i.e., loyalty of friends), family resources (i.e., intimacy with spouse/partner), and work resources (i.e., necessary tools for work). The loss variables were rated on a scale from 1 (*no loss* or *threat of loss*) to 3 (*a great deal of loss*). Cronbach's alpha was found to be .86 in this study.

## Study Procedures

Women were recruited at two community obstetrics/gynecological clinics in a medium-sized midwestern city serving low-income populations. Obstetrics/gynecological clinics were selected because women coming for such care reflected the general population of all but the most severely disenfranchised, as medical care is covered by welfare benefits at these clinics. Previous studies showed this method to produce samples that were broadly representative of inner-city women (Hobfoll, Jackson, Lavin, Johnson, & Schröder, 2002).

When women showed interest, a female interviewer explained the content of the study and offered US$25 for participating in interviews. They were assured that their participation was voluntary and would not affect their medical care. Study inclusion criteria comprised being single and not cohabitating with a partner, currently not being in the third trimester of pregnancy (out of respect for women's time and commitment), participating in risky sexual behavior, and being in the 16 to 29 years age range, to identify women at risk for violence and ongoing sexual disease risk. Risky sexual behavior included situations such as suspecting that a partner was unfaithful, having unprotected sex, or having multiple partners in the past 6 months. Minors could participate with their assent and their parent or guardian's informed consent. Interviewers were trained in multicultural sensitivity by two clinical supervisors who were women of color and experts on multicultural interviewing. Supervision of the interviewers occurred weekly throughout the project.

Female interviewers followed a written protocol of an interview questionnaire. Questionnaires were administered at pretest and 6-month follow-up. Interviewers were trained to ask questions and to clarify responses when misunderstandings or inconsistencies arose. Care was taken not to prompt a certain response, and women were assured that their honest response was appreciated.

After women were initially interviewed, they were randomly assigned to one of two health promotions or a standard care control condition (for a further detailed description see Hobfoll et al., 2002). The health promotion groups focused primarily on AIDS prevention, which included an emphasis on safer sex behaviors and interpersonal negotiation skills designed to reduce the risk of HIV/AIDS. The control group condition received individual sessions with a master's-level clinical psychology graduate student that focused on safer sexual and general health behaviors. The health promotion groups consisted of 5 to 8 women, which were again led by master's-level clinical psychology graduate students. Women in the health promotion groups received both health education and psychoeducation combined with negotiation skill training targeted to reduce the physical and psychological impact of unsafe sexual behaviors. Women engaged themselves in role-plays to practice specific skills and to increase empowerment in areas related to positive health behaviors and the prevention of sexually transmitted diseases. These groups might have indirectly affected recovery from PTSD; however, there were no significant health intervention group differences on probable PTSD diagnosis.[1] Although there were no significant health group differences, health group was used as a control group to focus entirely on its impact. The information obtained at pretest and 6-month follow-up provided the data for analysis.

**Table 1** Intercorrelations Between Resource Variables at Pretest Assessment ($n = 102$)

| Resource Loss Variable | 1. | 2. | 3. | 4. |
|---|---|---|---|---|
| 1. Energy | 1 | .63* | .62* | .74* |
| 2. Family | | 1 | .72* | .63* |
| 3. Nonfamilial interpersonal | | | 1 | .60* |
| 4. Material | | | | 1 |

*$p$ <.01 level.

**Table 2** Intercorrelations Between Resource Variables at 6-Month Follow-Up Assessment ($n = 102$)

| Resource Loss Variable | 1. | 2. | 3. | 4. |
|---|---|---|---|---|
| 1. Energy | 1 | .67* | .63* | .77* |
| 2. Family | | 1 | .65* | .69* |
| 3. Nonfamilial interpersonal | | | 1 | .59* |
| 4. Material | | | | 1 |

*$p$ <.01 level.

(Continued)

(Continued)

## Analysis Plan

The multivariate analysis of covariance (MANCOVA) procedure was selected for the analysis as multiple dependent variables can be examined in the context of the independent variable while also controlling for covariates. The four resource variables, that is, energy, material, nonfamilial interpersonal, and family interpersonal resources, constituted the dependent variables in the analyses. Work resources were not included in the analyses as the majority of the sample were unemployed. The dependent variables were all normally distributed at both time points in the study. Although all variables were significantly correlated at the $p < .01$ level, the variables were not correlated highly enough to be multicollinear (i.e., $r \geq .80$; see Tables 1 and 2 for correlations). Tolerance and variance inflation factor (VIF) values were reviewed to further examine multicollinearity. Tolerance values were greater than .2 and VIF values were less than 4, indicating that multicollinearity is not evident (Hutcheson & Sofroniou, 1999). Mahalanobis distance values were used to identify any multivariate outliers in the sample; however, no multivariate outliers were present in this analysis.

*PTSD symptom groups.* Probable PTSD diagnosis (improved vs. nonimproved) served as the independent variable. The improvement/alleviation course of PTSD symptoms was defined as a reduction in symptoms from PTSD at the 6-month follow-up. Thus, the improved group met criteria for PTSD at pretest but did not meet criteria at 6-month follow-up. The non-improved group consisted of individuals who met diagnostic criteria for PTSD at both pretest and 6-month assessments. To eliminate those individuals who improved only slightly, half of the standard deviation (*SD* =9.30, cutoff =5) was used as a cutoff to include individuals. Therefore, those individuals who improved by 5 points or less on the PSS-I were not included in the analyses, even if they no longer met criteria for PTSD, so as to make the sample more reflective of those whose symptoms were likely to represent true alleviation. Fifty-nine women comprised the improved symptom group and 43 women were included in the nonimproved symptom group in the analyses.

## Results

### Pretest MANCOVA Analysis

Independent samples *t* tests were used to compare women who experienced a decrease in symptoms from probable PTSD and those who did not experience symptom alleviation on continuous-scaled demographic variables, at pretest when both groups experienced probable PTSD. The groups significantly differed in terms of age, $t(105) = 54.59$, $p < .001$. As a result, age was entered as a covariate in the analyses. In addition to independent *t* tests, chi-square tests were conducted to assess the differences on categorical demographic variables between individuals whose PTSD symptoms alleviated and those whose symptoms did not. No significant differences were found on racial group, employment status, or education level between the two groups. Demographic variables were comparable between groups on factors other than age in this sample.

A MANCOVA analysis was conducted to determine the differences in pretest resources between those participants who experienced symptom alleviation from PTSD and those who did not, although controlling for age. Intercorrelations between variables for the analysis can be found in Tables 1 and 2. Analyses examined the level of resource loss including material, energy, interpersonal, and family interpersonal resources. The MANCOVA analyses failed to yield significant results on any of these resources, indicating the two groups did not differ on the level of resources, $F(4, 96) = 0.50$, NS ($p > .70$), at the initial pretest assessment (see Figure 1).

**Figure 1**   Pretest Resource Loss Means

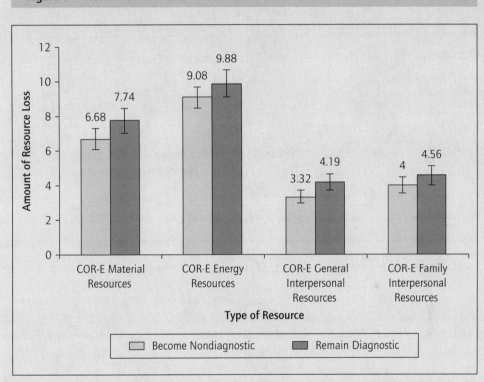

*Note:* COR-E = Conservation of Resources Evaluation.

## Six-Month Follow-Up MANCOVA Analysis

A MANCOVA was conducted to determine mean differences between individuals whose symptoms improved from probable PTSD and individuals whose symptoms did not at 6-month follow-up. Specifically, material, energy, family, and nonfamilial interpersonal losses were entered as dependent variables. Time-1 resource loss, age, and intervention group were entered as covariates, and symptom improvement was entered as the predictor variable. Controlling for Time-1 levels of resource loss, the overall analysis was significant, indicating differences among the level of resource loss between those whose symptoms improved and those whose symptoms did not improve from probable PTSD, $F(4, 91) = 4.59$, $p < .01$ (see Figure 2).

*(Continued)*

(Continued)

**Figure 2**   Six-Month Follow-Up Resource Loss Means

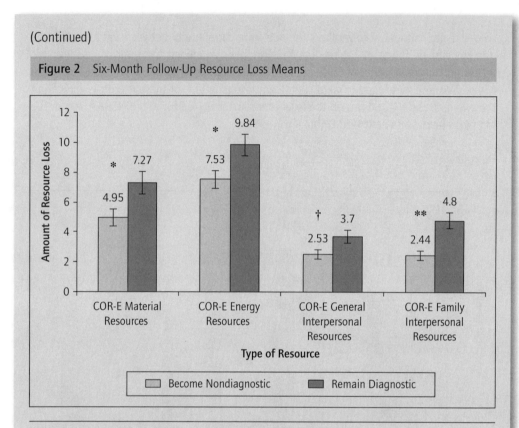

*Note:* COR-E =Conservation of Resources Evaluation. *$p$ <.05. **$p$ <.001. †Trend.

Follow-up examination of resource loss categories indicated that those who no longer met the criteria for PTSD did not experience as many resource losses on three of the four resource variables as compared with those who continued to meet the criteria for PTSD. This was significant for material resources, $F (1, 94) = 6.08$, $p <.05$; partial eta squared ($\eta^2_p$) $=.03$; family interpersonal losses, $F (1, 94) = 16.87$, $p <.001$; $\eta^2_p = .11$; and energy resources, $F (1, 94) = 4.58$, $p <.05$; $\eta^2_p = .03$. Although nonfamilial resource losses were not significant in the follow-up analysis, they did reveal a trend in the data, $F (1, 94) = 2.70$, $p <.10$, such that those who became nondiagnostic reported less resource loss in this domain as compared with women who remained diagnostic.

## Discussion

The hypothesis that women whose PTSD symptoms lessened would have less resource loss over the course of 6 months than those whose symptoms did not improve was supported. Specifically, women whose PTSD symptoms improved had significantly less resource loss at 6-month follow-up controlled for earlier loss levels than women whose symptoms did not improve. Hence, halting resource loss cycles separated the groups with regard to their symptom course at 6-month follow-up. Material, energy, and familial interpersonal resources were significantly different between the groups, with nonfamilial interpersonal resources indicating a trend in the same predicted direction.

This pattern of halting resource loss cycles in women who showed improvement in symptoms of PTSD attests to the contribution of resources to psychological functioning. The maintenance of family relationships, personal energy resources, and material resources appear to foster psychological well-being. These findings among inner-city women support recent work examining the relationship between halting of resource loss cycles and psychological well-being among Dutch Cambodian veterans (de Vries et al., 2001), PTSD among Alaskan fisherman affected by the *Exxon Valdez* oil spill (Arata et al., 2000), Gulf War returnees (Benotsch et al., 2000), Persian Gulf War troops (Sutker et al., 1995), and individuals with depression (Holahan et al., 1999). This suggests the importance of an array of psychosocial resources in not just promoting resistance to psychological distress but perhaps by fostering symptom improvement in those who have experienced significant psychological distress. As noted by King, King, Foy, Keane, and Fairbank (1999) and Holahan et al. (1999), although stress depletes resources, those who preserve resources are more likely to experience a decrease in PTSD symptoms.

Not only is it important to improve our knowledge about the impact of resources on preventing psychological distress, but the course of PTSD also needs further exploration. Given that the majority of individuals with PTSD do not seek treatment for the disorder (Kessler et al., 1999), the findings of the study illuminate possible naturalistic processes that help individuals reduce their symptoms without professional psychological treatment. Prior research has examined resiliency factors that clarify who does and who does not develop PTSD; however, very few studies have focused on the variables that assist people in recovery once they develop the disorder. This examination thus increases this body of literature by going beyond risk/resiliency factors of developing PTSD. The mechanisms that contribute to and, most importantly, sustain halting resource loss cycles and symptom reduction now need to be explored as there are most certainly complex processes involved (Norris, Perilla, Riad, Kaniasty, & Lavizzo, 1999).

This study has several strengths. First, the study employs a longitudinal design. This longitudinal approach allowed for demonstration of the variable nature of resource loss and how it is not necessarily a static phenomenon but one that changes as those with PTSD attempt to cope with their psychological distress. This is critical as most resource models depict resiliency resources as static, rather than varying under stress as has been noted by Norris et al. (1999) and Monnier, Cameron, Hobfoll, and Gribble (2002).

A second strength of the study is the ethnic composition of the sample, with African Americans constituting 62% of the sample. Furthermore, the majority of these women live below the poverty line, thus allowing for an analysis of a demographic group potentially affected by resource loss and gain to a great extent. As these women are at high risk for PTSD (Horowitz et al., 2005; Urquiza et al., 1994), such information is especially important. It should be recognized, however, that African Americans were oversampled with respect to the population of the United States and thus can affect the generalizability of the sample. Nevertheless, this population is largely understudied and often lacks access to resources, making the focus of the study especially pertinent.

Another strength of the study is that the majority of studies examining the relationship between resources and PTSD have used samples of male veterans (Benotsch et al., 2000;

*(Continued)*

(Continued)

de Vries et al., 2001; Sutker et al., 1995), and this study explores the link between the variables in inner-city women. Although it may be inappropriate to compare samples with vastly different demographic and traumatic event characteristics, our findings support previous research findings using veteran samples (Benotsch et al., 2000; de Vries et al., 2001; Sutker et al., 1995). Thus, it is possible that although there are differences between the samples, these findings allude to the important relationship between resources and PTSD symptoms.

Limitations of this research should also be noted. First, although the study employs a longitudinal design, the results cannot be used to imply causality between the variables. The two groups experienced similar levels of resource loss at pretest; however, exactly when these levels changed is unclear. It may be as likely that naturalistic recovery from PTSD preceded halting of resource loss cycles, as it is that halting of resource loss cycles that resulted in naturalistic recovery from PTSD. For example, when people experience an alleviation of PTSD symptoms, they may be more likely to engage in their environment and to obtain additional resources. The improvement in symptoms may lead to the acquisition of resources such as renewed interpersonal relationships or improved work performance. These resources may then create an "upward spiral" resulting in further resource gain. The alternative hypothesis also presents a possibility; individuals attain initial resources that aid in reducing the symptoms of PTSD. The initial resource gains may help ease stressors in peoples' lives contributing to the reduction of PTSD symptoms. Resource gains could explain why naturalistic recovery occurs—people are able to halt their loss cycles and, as a result, decrease their PTSD symptoms. In a therapeutic setting, perhaps resources obtained in psychotherapy, such as increased self-esteem, hope, and support, provide a pathway to the reduced PTSD symptoms that clients experience. Importantly, these findings nevertheless support the notion, argued by Holahan et al. (1999), that resources are not necessarily stable factors in individuals' lives and that fluctuations are common. Results should only be interpreted as an association between halting resource loss and naturalistic recovery outcome. Additional assessment points would help solve this problem in future research and shed light on the directionality of the role of resources in the alleviation of PTSD symptoms.

Another limitation is that PTSD diagnosis and naturalistic recovery were assessed and determined based on the PSS-I scale. The PSS-I contains one question for each of the 17 criteria items found in the *DSM* and as such may not be sufficient for placing individuals in a diagnostic category. The PSS-SR correctly classified 86% of individuals when the Structured Clinical Interview for the *DSM-IV-TR* (SCID; J. B. Williams et al., 1992) was used as criterion reference. However, this scale still does not correctly classify individuals as well as the SCID.

This research has important implications. Clearly, resources play a part in the healing efforts following a traumatic event. In psychotherapy, treatment often focuses on emotions and cognitions, which are integral to alleviating psychological distress. However, considering other psychological resources, as well as social and material resources, can provide additional tools for both assessment and treatment of PTSD. By facilitating psychological resource acquisition and reversing resource loss cycles of material and tangible resource possessions, this could have an impact on affected individuals and provide them an enhanced ability to decrease PTSD symptoms.

Further understanding of the course of PTSD is an important endeavor. Recognizing the natural mechanisms that ameliorate symptoms of PTSD should be further examined. The course of PTSD symptoms and its relation to resources may help clarify people's adaptive strengths, capacity for resilience, and personal growth in the face of difficulty and challenge (Bonanno, 2004; Holahan & Moos, 1991). These mechanisms further our knowledge of the spirit of human recovery and the ability to find strength after the devastating effects of trauma.

## Note

1. Only specific psychological treatments have acquired empirical support in alleviating post-traumatic stress disorder symptoms including exposure therapy, stress inoculation training, cognitive-behavioral therapy, and eye movement desensitization/reprocessing (Chemtob, Tolin, van der Kolk, & Pitman, 2000; Foa et al., 1999; Rothbaum, Meadows, Resick, & Foy, 2000).

## References

American Psychiatric Association. (2000). *Diagnostic and statistical manual of mental disorders* (4th ed., Text Revision). Washington DC: Author.

Arata, C. M., Picou, J. S., Johnson, G. D., & McNally, J. S. (2000). Coping with technological disaster: An application of the conservation of resources model to the *Exxon Valdez* oil spill. *Journal of Traumatic Stress, 13*, 23–39.

Baumeister, R. F., Bratslavsky, E., Muraven, M., & Tice, D. M. (1998). Ego-depletion: Is the active self a limited resource? *Journal of Personality and Social Psychology, 74*, 1252–1265.

Benight, C. C., Ironson, G., Klebe, K., Carver, C. S., Wynings, C., Burnett, K., et al. (1999). Conservation of resources and coping self-efficacy predicting distress following a natural disaster: A causal model analysis where the environment meets the mind. *Anxiety, Stress and Coping, 12*, 107–126.

Benotsch, E. G., Brailey, K., Vasterling, J. J., Uddo, M., Constans, J. I., & Sutker, P. B. (2000). War zone stress, personal and environmental resources, and PTSD symptoms in Gulf War veterans: A longitudinal perspective. *Journal of Abnormal Psychology, 109*, 205–213.

Blanchard, E. B., Hickling, E. J., Barton, K. A., Taylor, A. E., Loos, W. R., & Jones-Alexander, J. (1996). One-year prospective follow-up of motor vehicle accident victims. *Behaviour Research and Therapy, 34*, 775–786.

Bonanno, G. A. (2004). Loss, trauma, and human resilience: Have we underestimated the human capacity to thrive after extremely aversive events? *American Psychologist, 59*, 20–28.

Breslau, N., Chilcoat, H. D., Kessler, R. C., Peterson, E. L., & Lucia, V. C. (1999). Vulnerability to assaultive violence: Further specification of the sex difference in posttraumatic stress disorder. *Psychological Medicine, 29*, 813–821.

Chemtob, C. M., Tolin, D. F., van der Kolk, B. A., & Pitman, R. K. (2000). Eye movement desensitization and reprocessing. In E. Foa, T. Keane, & M. Friedman (Eds.), *Effective treatments for PTSD* (pp. 60–83). New York: Guilford.

Cooper-Patrick, L., Gallo, J. J., Powe, N. K., Steinwachs, D. M., Easton, W. W., & Ford, D. E. (1999). Mental health service utilization by African American and Whites: The Baltimore epidemiologic catchment area follow-up. *Medical Care, 37*, 1034–1045.

*(Continued)*

(Continued)

de Vries, M., Soetekouw, P. M. M. B., Van Der Meer, J. W. M., & Bleihenberg, G. (2001). Natural course of symptoms in Cambodia veterans: A follow-up study. *Psychological Medicine, 31,* 331–338.

Ehlers, A., Mayou, R. A., & Bryant, B. (1998). Psychological predictors of chronic posttraumatic stress disorder after motor vehicular accidents. *Journal of Abnormal Psychology, 107,* 508–519.

Ennis, N., Hobfoll, S. E., & Schröder, K. E. E. (2000). Money doesn't talk it swears: How economic stress and resistance resources impact inner-city women's depressive mood. *American Journal of Community Psychology, 28,* 149–173.

Foa, E. B., Dancu, C. V., Hembree, E., Jaycox, L. H., Meadows, E. A., & Street, G. P. (1999). The efficacy of exposure therapy, stress inoculation training, and their combination for reducing posttraumatic stress disorder in female assault victims. *Journal of Consulting and Clinical Psychology, 67,* 194–200.

Foa, E. B., Riggs, D. S., Dancu, C. V., & Rothbaum, B. O. (1993). Reliability and validity of a brief instrument for assessing posttraumatic stress disorder. *Journal of Traumatic Stress, 6,* 459–473.

Foa, E. B., & Tonlin, D. F. (2000). Comparison of the PTSD symptom scale-interview version and the Clinician-Administered PTSD Scale. *Journal of Traumatic Stress, 13,* 181–191.

Hobfoll, S. E. (1989). Conservation of resources: A new attempt at conceptualizing stress. *American Psychologist, 44,* 513–524.

Hobfoll, S. E. (1991). Traumatic stress: A theory based on rapid loss of resources. *Anxiety Research, 4,* 187–197.

Hobfoll, S. E., Jackson, A. P., Lavin, J., Johnson, R. J., & Schröder, K. E. E. (2002). Effects and generalizability of communally oriented HIV-AIDS prevention versus general health promotion groups for single, inner-city women in urban clinics. *Journal of Consulting and Clinical Psychology, 70,* 950–960.

Hobfoll, S. E., Johnson, R. J., Ennis, N. E., & Jackson, A. P. (2003). Resource loss, resource gain, and emotional outcomes among inner-city women. *Journal of Personality and Social Psychology, 84,* 632–643.

Hobfoll, S. E., & Lilly, R. S. (1993). Resource conservation as a strategy for community psychology. *Journal of Community Psychology, 21,* 128–148.

Holahan, C. J., & Moos, R. H. (1991). Life stressors, personal and social resources, and depression: A 4-year structural model. *Journal of Abnormal Psychology, 100,* 31–38.

Holahan, C. J., Moos, R. H., Holahan, C. K., & Cronkite, R. C. (1999). Resource loss, resource gain, and depressive symptoms: A 10-year model. *Journal of Personality and Social Psychology, 77,* 620–629.

Horowitz, K., McKay, M., & Marshall, R. (2005). Community violence and urban families: Experiences, effects, and directions for intervention. *American Journal of Orthopsychiatry, 75,* 356–368.

Hutcheson, G. D., & Sofroniou, N. (1999). *The multivariate social scientist: Introductory statistics using generalized linear models.* Thousand Oaks, CA: Sage.

Kaniasty, K., & Norris, F. (1997). Social support dynamics in adjustment to disasters. In S. Duck (Ed.), *Handbook of personal relationships* (2nd ed., pp. 595–619). London: Wiley.

Kessler, R. C. (2000). Posttraumatic stress disorder: The burden to the individual and society. *Journal of Clinical Psychiatry, 61,* 4–12.

Kessler, R. C., Sonnega, A., Bromet, E., Hughes, M., & Nelson, C. B. (1995). Posttraumatic stress disorder in the National Comorbidity Survey. *Archives of General Psychiatry, 52,* 1048–1060.

Kessler, R. C., Zhao, S., Katz, S. J., Kouzis, A. C., Frank, R. G., Edlund, M., et al. (1999). Past year use of outpatient services for psychiatric problems in the national comorbidity survey. *American Journal of Psychiatry, 156,* 115–123.

King, D. W., King, L. A., Foy, D. W., Keane, T. M., & Fairbank, J. A. (1999). Posttraumatic stress disorder in a national sample of female and male Vietnam veterans: Risk factors, war-zone stressors, and resilience-recovery variables. *Journal of Abnormal Psychology, 108,* 164–170.

Koenen, K. C., Stellman, J. M., Stellman, S. D., & Sommer, J. F. (2003). Risk factors for course of posttraumatic stress disorder among Vietnam veterans: A 14-year follow-up of American legionnaires. *Journal of Counseling and Clinical Psychology, 71,* 980–986.

Kulka, R. A., Schlenger, W. E., Fairbank, J. A., Hough, R. L., Jordan, B. K., Marmar, C. R., et al. (1990). *Trauma and the Vietnam War generation.* New York: Brunner/Mazel.

Mayou, R., Tyndel, S., & Bryant, B. (1997). Long-term outcome of motor vehicle accident injury. *Psychosomatic Medicine, 59,* 578–584.

Monnier, J., Cameron, R. P., Hobfoll, S. E., & Gribble, J. R. (2002). The impact of resource loss and critical incidents on psychological functioning in fire-emergency workers: A pilot study. *International Journal of Stress Management, 9,* 11–29.

Norris, F., & Kaniasty, K. (1996). Received and perceived social support in times of stress: A test of the social support deterioration deterrence model. *Journal of Personality and Social Psychology, 71,* 498–511.

Norris, F. H., Perilla, J. L., Riad, J. K., Kaniasty, K., & Lavizzo, E. A. (1999). Stability and change in stress, resources, and psychological distress following natural disaster: Findings from Hurricane Andrew. *Anxiety, Stress, and Coping, 12,* 363–396.

Orcutt, H. K., Erickson, D. J., & Wolfe, J. (2004). The course of PTSD symptoms among gulf war veterans: A growth mixture modeling approach. *Journal of Traumatic Stress, 17,* 195–202.

Resnick, H. S., Kilpatrick, D. G., Dansky, B. S., Saunders, B. E., & Best, C. L. (1993). Prevalence of civilian trauma and posttraumatic stress disorder in a representative national sample of women. *Journal of Consulting and Clinical Psychology, 61,* 984–991.

Rothbaum, B. O., Meadows, E. A., Resick, P., & Foy, D. W. (2000). *Effective treatments for PTSD.* New York: Guilford.

Schumm, J. A., Hobfoll, S. E., & Keogh, N. J. (2004). Revictimization and interpersonal resource loss predicts PTSD among women in substance use treatment. *Journal of Traumatic Stress, 17,* 173–181.

Southwick, S. M., Morgan, C. A., Darnell, A., Bremner, D., Nicolauou, A. L., Nagy, L. M., et al. (1995). Trauma-related symptoms in veterans of operation desert storm: A 2-year follow-up. *American Journal of Psychiatry, 156,* 1150–1155.

Sutker, P. B., Davis, J. M., Uddo, M., & Ditta, S. R. (1995). War zone stress, personal resources, and PTSD in Persian Gulf War returnees. *Journal of Abnormal Psychology, 104,* 444–452.

Switzer, G. E., Dew, M. A., Thompson, K., Goycoolea, J. M., Derricott, T., & Mullins, S. D. (1999). Posttraumatic stress disorder and service utilization among urban mental health center clients. *Journal of Traumatic Stress, 12,* 25–39.

Urquiza, A. J., Wyatt, G. E., & Root, M. P. P. (1994). Introduction. *Violence and Victims, 9,* 203–206.

Williams, J. B., Gibbon, M., First, M. B., Spitzer, R. L., Davies, M., Borus, J., et al. (1992). The structured clinical interview for *DSM-III-R* (SCID): II. Multi-site test-retest reliability. *Archives of General Psychiatry, 49,* 630–636.

Williams, D. R., & Jackson, P. B. (2005). Social sources of racial disparities in health. *Health Affairs, 24,* 325–334. Wolfe, J., Keane, T. M., Kaloupek, D. G., Mora, C. A., & Wine, P. (1993). Patterns of positive stress adjustment in Vietnam combat veterans. *Journal of Traumatic Stress, 6,* 179–193.

Wolfe, J., Keane, T., Kaloupek, D., Mora, C., & Wine, P. (1993). Patterns of positive readjustment in Vietnam combat veterans. *Journal of Traumatic Stress, 6*(2), 179-183. DOI: 10.1002/jts.2490060203.

## About the Authors

**Kristen H. Walter**, MA, is currently a 3rd-year clinical psychology graduate student at Kent State University in Kent, OH. She is also the project director for an NIH-funded grant

*(Continued)*

(Continued)

examining the effects of women's health intervention on the physical and mental health of inner-city women. In addition, she is a research assistant on an NIMH-funded randomized clinical trial studying mental health outcomes of female domestic abuse survivors at the Summa-Kent State Center for the Treatment and Study of Traumatic Stress. Walter has presented research on the topic of post-traumatic stress disorder (PTSD) at national and international conferences. Her research interests focus on the influence of trauma and PTSD on specific populations, such as victims of interpersonal violence. Specifically, her current research examines the relationship of resource loss and PTSD symptoms in survivors of interpersonal violence.

**Stevan E. Hobfoll** has authored and edited 11 books, including *Traumatic Stress, The Ecology of Stress,* and *Stress, Social Support and Women.* In addition, he has authored over 160 journal articles, book chapters, and technical reports. He is currently Distinguished Professor of Psychology at Kent State University and Director of their Applied Psychology Center and the Summa-KSU Center for the Treatment and Study of Traumatic Stress.

# 3

# Women and Depression

Latika is a black female who is 30 years of age with two children who are 6 and 8 years of age. Recently, she was admitted to a mental health unit due to alcohol intoxication. She reported that she became depressed after the birth of her first child 8 years ago and was treated successfully with antidepressant medicine. Latika reported that she has been experiencing insomnia and a decrease in appetite, and has lost approximately twenty pounds. She believes she "feels down" due mostly to the fact that her children were removed from the home and placed in foster care. Latika was charged with child endangerment because she drove one time while intoxicated with the children in the car. Although she is currently married, she and her husband are separated after only a year of marriage. Her husband is currently incarcerated for physical assault with a deadly weapon and will be eligible for parole in six months. Latika indicated that her drinking has increased because she is depressed over the loss of her children. She would like to get help so she can regain custody of her children.

Experts generally agree that depression affects many women in the United States. However, lack of income is perhaps the major stressor in the lives of women, and across racial and ethnic groups, poverty is a major risk factor for major depression. The rate of major depressive disorder among persons living in poverty is approximately 1.5 times that among the general population, and this rate is significantly associated with the prevalence of major depressive disorder in White persons (Riolo, Nguyen, Greden, & King, 2005). Belle and Doucet (2003) posited that poverty is a consistent predictor of depression in women, and specifically, that poverty is a major contributor to depressive symptoms in women who reside in rural areas of the United States (Simmons, Braun, Charnigo, Havens, & Wright, 2008).

Given the link between poverty and depression, it is easy to see that poor women are at particular risk of dysthymic disorder or major depression. Corcoran, Danziger, and Tolman (2003) examined the mental and physical health of welfare recipients across four waves of testing (from 1997–2002). Women included in the study were selected for participation in the Women's Employment Survey in 1997 and were representative of African American and White single mothers in the state of Michigan. At each wave of interviews, between 16% and 25% of recipients met the diagnostic screening criteria for major depressive disorder (MDD), which was approximately twice the rate of recipients in the general population. Hyman (2006) noted that depression also disproportionately affects women globally and is considered a leading disability for women.

# Definitions

Depression is a medical illness that affects the mind as well as the body, and stressful life experiences often trigger depression. The illness may be characterized in a variety of ways that include: (a) persistent sad mood, (b) constant feelings of sadness, (c) excessive crying, (d) low energy, (e) feelings of worthlessness, (f) difficulty concentrating or making decisions, (g) loss of interest in pleasurable activities, (h) sleep disturbances, (i) appetite and weight changes, (j) thoughts of death or suicide, and (k) physical symptoms that do not respond to treatment (Alexander, LaRosa, & Bader, 2001, pp. 50–76). It should be noted that depression may also be a side effect of another illness, medication, or a consequence of substance abuse.

Although major depression is linked to anxiety disorders in both males and females, the rates of anxiety disorders associated with major depression are higher for women than for men (Breslau, Chilcoat, Peterson, & Schultz, 2000). More important, major depression is linked with pre-existing anxiety disorders, particularly post-traumatic stress disorder (PTSD). In addition, depression is related to several other disorders that women typically experience, though depression may be secondary to those disorders (Breslau et al., 2000; Conway, Compton, Stinson & Grant, 2006; Kessler, Barker, et al., 2003).

## Dysthymia

Kornstein et al. (2002) noted that depression can be chronic in the form of MDD, dysthymic disorder (chronic mild depression for at least 2 years), double depression (MDD superimposed on an episode of dysthymia), or recurrent MDD without complete recovery (cited in Cyranowski & Frank, 2006, p. 90; see also Kornstein, 2002). Chronic forms of depression are associated with suicide attempts and hospitalization, as well as with impairments in the public and private spheres of functioning (Cyranowski & Frank, 2006). Chronically depressed women fare less well than chronically depressed men in terms of symptoms and social adjustment (Kornstein et al., 2002).

## Atypical Depression

Atypical depression occurs when one is unable to respond to a positive event and the condition is accompanied by two of the following symptoms: overeating, excessive sleep, a feeling of sluggishness in the limbs, or vulnerability to rejection. This type of depression tends to be prevalent in the adolescent years, and it is likely to occur with social phobia, a disorder that is often comorbid with generalized anxiety disorder. Although called "atypical" depression, this disorder is actually more typical than other types of depression, because situations in the adolescent years often exacerbate stressors in the lives of females. In a sample of 1500 patients, Nosvick et al. (2006) found that over 18% of the sample met criteria for atypical features, and this group was more likely to be female and have an earlier age at onset.

## Bipolar Disorder

Bipolar disorders are cyclical disturbances in mood, thought, and behavior (see Jacobson & Jacobson, 2001). A diagnosis of bipolar I disorder must consist of at least one episode of mania or mixed episodes (both depression and mania) during the same period of time. For a diagnosis of bipolar II disorder, both hypomania (mild mania) and major depressive episodes must occur. In comparison, cyclothymia refers to chronic changing between hypomania and subclinical depression. Given that it is the manic episode that delineates bipolar disorder from MDD, an episode of mania must have lasted at least a week and an episode of hypomania must have lasted at least four days.

McDermott, Quanbeck, and Frye (2007) found that women with bipolar disorder are at special and significant risk for arrest as compared to women without bipolar disorder, and it seems that women with both bipolar disorder and substance use disorder are at an even greater risk of arrest. The odds of having a comorbid substance use diagnosis for arrested female patients was more than 38 times that for community female patients. Women were more likely to have been arrested for violence and substance use charges, whereas men were more likely to have been arrested for theft and miscellaneous charges.

## Premenstrual Dysphoric Disorder

Premenstrual dysphoric disorder (PMDD) is the depressive syndrome that some women experience the week before menstruation. Women who experience PMDD typically are depressed, anxious, irritable, and moody during the week before menstruation to the point that these symptoms interfere with daily activities. While the etiology of PMDD is unclear, it may be related to the response of particular women to environmental or hormonal changes or may also be related to a history of mood disorders or biochemical changes (Dreher et al., 2007).

## Prevalence and Age of Onset

The results of national surveys show that nearly 22% of women compared to 13% of men have a lifetime prevalence of MDD (Kessler, Barker et al., 2003; Kessler, Berglund et al., 2003; Kessler, McGonagle et al., 1993; see also Conway et al., 2006). Miranda (2006) noted that the rates of MDD are similar for White women (17%) and African American women (15%), though when classified by race, ethnicity, education, and gender, White and Black females with 8 or fewer years of education had higher rates of dysthymic disorder than Mexican females with the same amount of education (Riolo et al., 2005). Although more education, at least to the middle school level, was associated with a lower rate of dysthymic disorder among White females, education had a lesser effect on dysthymic disorder among Black and Mexican females.

With respect to populations of women who have immigrated to the U.S, the rate of major depression appears to increase for Mexican immigrant women after they have been here for at least 13 years, and the rate for Mexican women born in the United States is similar to that for White women (Vega et al., 1998; Vega, Kolody, Aguilar-Gaxiola, & Catalano, 1999). By comparison, Chinese American immigrant women have a 7% lifetime rate of major depression, which is about half that of White women (Takeuchi et al., 1998). While Korean women also appear to be more vulnerable to depression than white women, Chinese and Vietnamese women seem to be more resilient and less likely to experience depression due to life stress (Jiang, 2004).

It is noteworthy that there are no obvious gender differences in depression until early adolescence (Keita, 2007; Kovacs, Obrosky, & Sherrill, 2003; University of Michigan Depression Center, 2007). However, the rate of depression for females increases to twice the rate for males between the ages of 10 and 16 (Keita, 2007; Twenge & Nolen-Hoeksema, 2002). It is also interesting to note that the rate of depression is due to first-onset depressive episodes rather than to duration or recurrence (Kovacs et al., 2003). When one considers prevalence, it is important to recognize that women experience premenstrual, perinatal (prenatal, antenatal, and postpartum), and menopausal depression whereas men do not.

The results of a meta-analysis that included 21 studies show that nearly 11% of pregnant women experience depression across the antenatal period (Dennis, Ross, & Grigoriadis, 2009). While 7.4% of women experience depression in the first trimester, nearly 13% experience depression in the second trimester (Dennis et al., 2009). These researchers suggest that low income, lack of social support, stressful life events, and poor interpersonal relationships place women at risk of antenatal depression. Researchers have found that 13% of women experience postpartum depression (PPD; Wisner, Parry, & Piontek, 2002).

Although both major depression and depressive symptoms diminish with age, in general, the rate of depression in females remains twice that of their male counterparts (Pennix, 2006). Hormonal changes increase during the transition between premenopause to menopause, and as a result some women are at risk of depression. While some women may experience no mood problems as they move into menopause, others are at increased risk for depression. This seems to occur even among women without a history of depression (Cohen et al., 2006; Freeman, Sammel, Lin, & Nelson, 2006). It is important to note, however, that older women are less likely than men to recover from depression, even though they are more likely to receive treatment for depression (Barry, Allore, Guo, Bruce, & Gill, 2008). The gender difference in depression and depressive symptoms takes on special salience in view of the fact that women tend to outlive men (Pennix, 2006). Depression among women results in great economic burden to society, especially with respect to productivity in the home and workplace (Greenberg, Kessler, et al., 2003).

## Etiology

There are five key explanations for the rate of depression in women. First, biochemical and genetic processes may explain a proportion of women's depression. Second, women experience numerous stressful life events associated with rearing children and family caregiving responsibilities. Third, many women experience interpersonal violence in their lives from a very early age. Fourth, many women live in poverty, and low income is a key predictor of depression. Fifth, the extent to which women are depressed seems contingent on the interaction between their life experiences and their ability to deal with those experiences.

The relative significance of external stressors versus predispositions in part determines the intervention that is needed to enhance an individual's mental health. For example, greater weight may be given to genetic influences or biological processes. On the other hand, greater weight may be given to an environmental circumstance, such as low income or poverty, and this may indicate the use of either pharmacology or psychosocial interventions to address mental health problems.

### Genetic and Other Biological Contributions

Kendler and Prescott (1999) found in twin studies that major depression is equally heritable in men and women and that most genetic risk factors influence MDD similarly in the two sexes (see also Kendler, Thornton, & Prescott, 2001). However, the researchers concluded that genes may exist that act uniquely to create risk for MDD in different ways for men and women. Additional genetics research indicates that the risk for developing depression likely involves the combination of multiple genes with environmental or other factors (Tsuang, Bar, Stone, & Faraone, 2004).

In animal studies, several researchers have found that levels of estrogen may also influence women's response to stress, a finding that seems to explain depressive symptoms in women at various points in their lives. Shors and Leuner (2003) found that high levels of estrogen impair females' performance in response to stress compared to males' performance. Shansky et al. (2004) found that estrogen amplifies the stress response in the prefrontal cortex, which in turn, may make women more susceptible to stress-related disorders, including depression (see also Cohen et al., 2006; Dreher et al., 2007; Freeman et al., 2006). Some evidence also suggests that hormones may play a role in premenstrual depression (Schmidt, Nieman, et al., 1998).

In general, the evidence from twin studies regarding the direct genetic influence on women's depression is inconclusive (Kendler, Gardner, Neale, & Prescott, 2001; Kendler & Prescott, 1999; Silberg et al., 1999). However, Zubenko and colleagues contend that a specific gene might predispose women to deficits in cognition, neural plasticity (early brain development), and long-term memory (Zubenko et al., 2002; Zubenko, Hughes, Stiffler, Zubenko, & Kaplan, 2002). In turn, these deficits may trigger certain endocrine responses to stress that may ultimately result in women's depression.

Along these lines, Nolen-Hoeksema (2006) suggested that women's endocrine system may become overreactive and dysregulated in response to stress via the hypothalamic-pituitary-adrenal (HPA) feedback system. When humans experience stress, the HPA axis becomes overactive, but when they no longer experience stress, the HPA axis should return to homeostasis. Given that individuals with depression often show chronic hyperactivity in the HPA axis, it may be that women's exposure to numerous stressors may result in dysregulation of the HPA system, and in turn, in depression.

## Stressful Life Events

While men experience stress related to job loss, legal problems, robbery, and work problems, women experience stress related to housing, loss of a confidant, relationship problems, and illness in their social network (Kendler, Thornton, & Prescott (2001). Women are more likely than men to become depressed after stressful life events (Maciejewski, Prigerson, & Mazure, 2001). Work may also be a stressful event for women, particularly for women in the secondary labor market, where they often experience both sex and racial discrimination (Belle & Doucet, 2003) as well as sexual harassment (Gutek & Done, 2001). In this regard, all types of discrimination in the workplace may be associated with depressive symptoms and risk of major depression for women (Dansky & Kilpatrick, 1997).

## Interpersonal Violence

Women are more likely than men to experience interpersonal violence in their lives. The lifetime rate of depression for victims of completed rape in childhood (52%) is twice that for nonvictimized women (Saunders, Kilpatrick, Hanson, Resnick, & Walker, 1999), though childhood physical abuse has been found to be a key risk factor for depression in women from all backgrounds (Springer, Sheridan, Kuo, & Carnes, 2007). Nearly half of battered women experience depression (Golding, 1999); of particular interest is the finding that between 40% and 50% of battered women experience marital rape, and between 10% and 14% of all married women have experienced marital rape (Martin, Taft, & Resick, 2006).

Interpersonal violence is especially prevalent in the lives of particular populations of women. For example, Evans-Campbell, Lindhorst, Huang, and Walters (2006) surveyed American Indian and Alaska Native (AIAN) women in New York City and found that 65% of participants had experienced some form of interpersonal violence; 28% reported childhood physical abuse, 48% reported rape, 40% reported domestic violence, and 40% reported multiple victimizations. As one might expect, this history of interpersonal violence is associated with depression, as well as other physical and mental health problems (see Smith, A., 2005).

## Cognitive-Personality Factors

Cognitive-personality factors may also contribute to the prevalence of depression in women as compared to men (Nolen-Hoeksema, 2006). The findings suggest that women experience negativity, hopelessness, and lack of futuristic thinking more often than men (Abramson et al., 2002). This may be especially important for both adolescent and adult females with same-sex, bisexual, and transgender issues relative to their identity acquisition (Eubanks-Carter, Burckell, & Goldfried, 2005). In addition, the evidence indicates that women's preoccupation with what others think of them may be related to depressive symptoms (Mazure, Bruce, Maciejewski, & Jacobs, 2000; Nolen-Hoeksema & Jackson, 2001). Girls and women tend to ruminate about themselves or think about their inadequacies more than boys and men do (Nolen-Hoeksema, 2004), and this tendency may begin at an early age (Schmidt, Nieman, Danaceau, Adams, & Rubinow, 1998).

## Screening And Assessment Measures

Social workers can play a key role in screening adolescent and adult females for depression, primarily because social workers are often the first persons who interact with depressed women in various environments, including the home, school, mental health center, or hospital. Zucherbrot et al. (2007) reviewed adolescent screening instruments and found that none are "perfect" (p. e1303). However, it is important that social workers be aware of the screening and assessment instruments that address the etiological factors related to depression in women, particularly hopelessness.

## Adolescence/Young Adulthood

Zucherbrot et al. (2007) noted that the most commonly used instruments to screen for depression in adolescents and young adults include the Beck's Depression Inventory (BDI-II) and the Reynolds Adolescent Depression Screen (RADS; Reynolds & Graves, 1989). We also include the newer Kutcher Adolescent Depression Scale (KADS; Brooks, Krulewicz, & Kutcher, 2003) that has been used with a school population, which makes it especially useful for screening purposes. In light of cognitive-personality factors that contribute to depression in adolescent females, additional screening measures are useful, particularly in early adolescence. For example, females are more likely than males to score high on measures of hopelessness in early adolescence. We also recommend using the Children's Depression Inventory (Kovacs, 2003) and the Beck's Hopelessness Scale (Beck, Weissman, Lester, & Trexler, 1974), though it is noteworthy that there are many more instruments that have specific use in screening for depression in girls and young women.

---

Beck Depression Inventory-II (BDI-II)

Reynolds Adolescent Depression Scale (RADS-2)

Kutcher Adolescent Depression Scale (KADS)

Children's Depression Inventory (CDI)

Beck Hopelessness Scale (BHS)

---

### BDI-II

The BDI-II is a 21-item multiple-choice self-report inventory that is widely used to measure the severity of depression (Beck, Steer, & Brown, 1996). It was designed for individuals aged 13 and over and is composed of items relating to cognitive, physiological, and somatic symptoms of depression. The BDI-II was administered to 105 male and 105 female outpatients between 12 and 18 years old who were seeking psychiatric treatment; the mean score for girls was significantly higher than that of boys (5 points), suggesting that females were more depressed than males. The internal consistency of the BDI-II is quite good, with an 0.92 alpha coefficient.

## RADS-2

The RADS-2 is a 10-item short form designed to screen for depression in adolescents (Reynolds, 2005; Reynolds & Graves, 1989). The RADS-II asks adolescents to rate how often they experience a particular symptom on a 4-point Likert-type scale. The instrument was standardized with 3,300 adolescents who were well matched with the United States demographics relative to age, gender, and race/ethnicity. Moreover, reliability and validity studies were conducted in a school-based sample. The internal consistency alpha coefficients range from .91 to .96, and the test-retest reliability is approximately .80. The RADS-II short form can be administered in 2–3 minutes with individuals or groups and provides information about affective status and depressive symptomatology.

## KADS

The KADS is a 6-item self-report measure used to screen for depression in adolescents 12 to 17 years of age (Brooks et al., 2003). There are also 16-item and 11-item versions of the KADS available, though the 6-item version can be used very quickly as a screen. Adolescents are asked to rate the frequency of symptoms using a 4-point Likert-type scale (*hardly ever, much of the time, most of the time, all of the time*), and the ratings are summed to obtain a score. The Cronbach's alpha for this version of the KADS is .80, and there is a moderate correlation between the three versions of KADS and clinician-rated depression range between 0.37 and 0.42. The cutoff score of 6 on the 6-item version has a sensitivity of 92% and specificity of 71%.

## CDI

The CDI is a 10-item self-rating measure that can be used as a quick screen for depression in children 7 through 17 years of age (Kovacs, 2003). The CDI identifies negative mood, interpersonal problems, ineffectiveness, anhedonia (lack of interest in pleasure), and low self-esteem. For each item, the child or adolescent has three possible answers regarding the presence of depressive symptoms (absent, mild, definite), and the ratings are summed to obtain a possible summed score of 30 for the short version of the CDI. The normative sample consisted of 1,266 public school students from Florida in grades 2 through 8, which included 592 boys between 7 and 15 years of age and 674 girls between 7 and 16 years of age. Even though the Cronbach's alpha for the CDI total score was .88 for one sample, the reliability seems to increase with age. Because its major value is as a screen for depression, the CDI should be used with other assessment instruments for diagnosis.

### BHS

The BHS is a 20-item self-report instrument developed to measure the negative expectations of adolescents regarding the future based on their thoughts in the week prior to completing the questionnaire (Beck et al., 1974). This instrument has been used with high school students and other nonclinical populations, as well as with inpatient and outpatient adolescent psychiatric patients. Adolescents are asked to use a true/false format to identify expectations, and the summed scores range from 0 to 20, with higher scores indicating a greater degree of hopelessness.

## Pregnant Teens and Adults

Screening for postpartum depression has become a controversial issue. The Melanie Blocker Stokes Postpartum Depression Research and Care Act (Mothers Act) passed the House of Representatives and was being considered in the Senate as of this writing. The intent of the law, if passed, is to mandate funding for research, education, and public service announcements about postpartum depression. However, opponents of the bill are concerned that screening for depression in pregnancy will result in medication use that primarily benefits the pharmaceutical companies. In addition, one opponent, Michael O'Hara, University of Iowa professor, contends, "Women who have been healthy all their lives, who haven't suffered lots of anxiety and depressive symptoms, are unlikely to have problems in the postpartum period" (cited in Elton, 2009, p. 55). On the other hand, psychiatrist Katherine Wisner at the University of Pittsburgh Medical Center notes that we screen all infants for phenylketonuria, which is extremely rare, and that this raises the question "why would we not screen for PPD" (cited in Elton, p. 56).

From the perspective of social workers who frequently work with women who have little access to primary care and whose children may be at risk of harm due to mothers' depressive symptoms or major depression, screening for depression during and after pregnancy may be in the best interest of both mothers and their children. From the perspective of optimum child development, perinatal depression can interfere with the quality of child-rearing and positive parent-child interactions. The responsiveness of mother to infants' vocalizations and gestures is essential. Given that early detection can improve outcomes for both mothers and children, we offer several psychometrically sound measures that have utility in screening for depression in women during pregnancy and postbirth. However, we also recommend that social workers rely on clinical judgment and social histories prior to screening.

---

Patient Health Questionnaire-9 (PHQ-9) Patient Health Questionnaire-2 (PHQ-2)

Edinburgh Postnatal Depression Scale (EPDS)

Beck Depression Inventory (see description in previous section)

The PHQ-9 is the 9-item depression scale of the Patient Health Questionnaire (Spitzer, Kroenke, & Williams, 1999) and is recommended as a screening tool for depression that has 88% sensitivity and specificity in identifying symptoms of and impairment due to depression in primary care settings. Staff can administer the PHQ-9; it is in the public domain at the website of the McArthur Initative (an initiative to enhance the ability of primary care providers to identify and manage depression). Likewise, a social worker can administer and score it. It is noteworthy that the 2-item version has greater sensitivity (96%) but less specificity (56%) than the 9-item version of the PHQ-9 (Thibault & Steiner, 2004). The two questions asked of respondents regarding feelings in the past month are:

(a)  Have you often been bothered by feeling down, depressed, or hopeless?

(b)  Have you often been bothered by little interest or pleasure in doing things?

If the answer to either is *yes*, the screen is positive. Both the 9- and 2-item PHQ versions can be downloaded in English directly from the Utah Department of Health website at http://health.utah.gov.

The EPDS (Cox, Holden, & Sagovsky, 1987; Eberhard-Gran, Eskild, Tambs, Opjordsmoen, & Samuelsen, 2001) is a quick 10-item screening tool for maternal depression. Respondents are asked to use various 4-point Likert-type scales to rate their experiences in the past 7 days. For example, they are asked to rate the extent to which they have been able to laugh and see the funny side of things, to look forward to things, and to feel scared or panicky. The maximum score is 30, and mothers who score above 13 are likely to be suffering from a depressive illness of varying severity. The ranges for sensitivity (65–100%) and specificity (49–100%) on the EPDS are wide, and as a result, the use of this score for any diagnosis should not take the place of clinical judgment if the clinician believes a woman should be referred for diagnosis.

## Middle and Elder Adult Years

It is especially important to assess and treat depression in women's middle years, when they are having and raising children and in some cases also working. As we have established, depression in women is highly correlated with external stressors, particularly income and intimate partner violence (IPV), which is most prevalent between 25 and 45 years of age. Koss, Bailey, Yuan, Herrera, and Lichter (2003) argued that depressive symptoms may better reflect the range of responses of abuse victims than do symptoms and criteria for PTSD, particularly for women who suffer repeated abuse in such forms as incest and IPV. Until postmenopause, many women also experience premenstrual depression, and given that depression is associated with many physical health problems in women

(Birnbaum, Leong, & Greenberg, 2003), it is extremely important for social workers to consider screening the women with whom they practice for depression. We recommend three measures that are quick to use, moderately reliable, and valid for use with this population.

> Brief Screen for Depression (BSD)
>
> Center for Epidemiologic Studies Depression Scale (CES-D)
>
> Geriatric Depression Scale (GDS)

The BSD is a 4-item measure that has use in screening for depression. Respondents are asked to use a 5-point Likert-type scale to rate the frequency with which they have been preoccupied by thoughts of hopelessness, helplessness, pessimism, intense worry, or unhappiness. They are asked to use a 9-point Likert-type scale to rate (a) how relaxed they have been compared to how relaxed they normally are, (b) the extent to which they have difficulty starting and following through on ordinary jobs and tasks, and (c) how satisfied they are with their ability to perform usual domestic duties. This screening measure has only fair reliability but correlates well with the BDI-II.

The CES-D (Radloff, 1977) is a 20-item self-report instrument developed for use in initially identifying depressive symptoms in the general population. Adults over 18 years of age are asked to use a 4-point Likert-type scale to rate the frequency or duration of time (in the past week) that they have experienced certain feelings or situations (some or a little of the time, some of the time, good part of the time, most or all of the time). Examples of items include *I did not feel like eating, I thought my life had been a failure,* and *I have nightmares.* The CES-D has been used with large and varied populations and has good reliability and validity (Fischer & Corcoran, 1994). Because the CES-D does not assess the full range of depressive symptoms (for example, it does not assess suicidal behavior) and because it assesses the occurrence of symptoms only during the past week, users are cautioned against relying on the CES-D exclusively. No training is required to administer the CES-D. It should be noted that the CES-D can also be used with adolescents.

Holroyd and Clayton (2002) compared the Hamilton Rating Scale for Depression (HAM-D; Hamilton, 1960), the Zung Self-Rating Depression Scale (SDS; Zung, 1965), the Montgomery-Asberg Depression Rating Scale (MADRS; Montgomery & Asberg, 1979), and the Geriatric Depression Scale (GDS; Yesavage et al., 1983) to determine which one is best to use in screening elderly women for depression. The researchers found that the GDS is the best measure for social workers to use in screening for depressive symptoms in elders who are not cognitively impaired. However, one should be *very* cautious in using any depression rating scale with the elderly for any reason apart from screening, given the various presentations of depression in the elderly, such as withdrawal, agitation, and anxiety.

The GDS is a 15-item measure developed as a minimal screen for geriatric affective disorder (Yesavage et al., 1983). This version has tolerability in out-patient family practice settings, and it is highly correlated to the longer GDS version, so it has special use as a rapid screening device. Using a cutoff of 5 to 6, the short form GDS shows a sensitivity of 85% and specificity of 74% (Herrman et al., 1996). The long form of the GDS has been used extensively in a variety of settings, and researchers have found that the short form is an adequate substitute for the long form (Lesher & Berryhill, 1994).

## Evidence-Based Interventions

Prior to discussing evidence-based approaches to treating depression in women, it is important to identify qualifiers. First, as Hollon (2000) has pointed out, there are few studies that specifically examine gender differences in treatment, primarily because the majority of individuals who participate in studies of depression are women (Sinha & Rush, 2006). Second, many of the efficacy studies (or those that are randomized, controlled trials) have been conducted in primary care settings rather than in community health facilities (Miranda et al., 2005), thus limiting generalizability of the findings. Third, in the absence of specialized clinicians to implement efficacious interventions within the community, it is difficult to know how well those interventions work, especially with women from ethnic and racial minority groups. Last, while medication may be warranted to address depression, we address only psychosocial interventions here.

With these qualifiers in mind, Sinha and Rush (2006) noted that, on average, cognitive-behavioral therapy (CBT; see Butler, Chapman, Forman, & Beck, 2006; Klein, Jacobs, & Reinbeck, 2007) and interpersonal psychotherapy (IPT; Butler et al., 2006; see also Parker, Parker, Brotchie, & Stuart, 2006) are the most efficacious psychosocial interventions for treating depression in women of all ages. Although few researchers have examined the effects of CBT or IPT on depression in members of racial and ethnic minority groups, Miranda et al. (2005) examined evidence in studies of depression and depressive symptoms in members of those groups. The researchers concluded that depressive symptoms are reduced when CBT and IPT modalities are culturally adapted to a particular ethnic minority group. This takes on salience when one considers that a large percentage of women from ethnic minority populations are impoverished. Psychosocial interventions used to treat depression in women can and should be tailored to gender, culture, and age.

With an emphasis on problem-solving, CBT is a short-term therapy based on the notion that change in the way an individual thinks about an event or situation will affect how he or she feels emotionally. By comparison, IPT is a short-term therapy that focuses on an individual's relationships, under the assumption that peers and family members must be involved in therapy in order for the consumer to decrease depressive symptoms. The use of IPT usually involves 20 sessions (1 hour per week) with the first several sessions addressing assessment and identification and subsequent sessions addressing change in relationships. The evidence indicates that CBT and IPT are especially helpful in preventing relapse and for maintenance purposes. The American Psychological Association supports behavioral therapy and behavioral activation (Coffman, Martell, Dimidjian, Gallop, & Hollon, 2007; Cuijpers, van Straten, & Warmerdam, 2007). From this perspective, depression is regarded as a result of the lack of positive reinforcement for prosocial behavior. In turn, individuals withdraw and avoid others. With this in mind, these therapies focus on increasing sense of mastery, social skills, and decreasing aversive experiences. In addition, the American Psychological Association approves the use of the Cognitive Behavioral Analysis System of Psychotherapy for Depression (CBASP; McCollough, 2000, 2006). This is integrative therapy used with chronically depressed persons that combines cognitive, behavioral, interpersonal, and psychodynamic theories, and as such, focuses on situational analysis and behavioral skill training.

Problem-solving therapy (PST) is an excellent intervention that can help women to more effectively identify solutions for problems (Cuijpers et al., 2007; Gellis & Kenaley, 2008). This therapy utilizes the following steps: identify the problem, identify possible solutions, choose the best solution, make a plan for implementing the solution, implement the solution, and evaluate the extent to which the solution works. Problem-solving may emphasize social problems, problem-solving in agency and primary care settings (paraprofessionals); and self-problem-solving. PST is short-term therapy (8–16 sessions, on average) that can be provided individually or in groups. It might require fewer or greater number of sessions, depending on the circumstances.

## Adolescence

Vitiello (2009) examined the evidence on the treatment of adolescent depression. Results of clinical trials suggest that pharmacological interventions are most effective, but CBT seems to help when used in combination with appropriate medication. Since the effect size in treatments is small, it may be that a "more personalized approach to the treatment of adolescent depression" (Vitello, 394) is warranted—one that accounts for the correspondence between individual characteristics and stressors. For example, results in one study show that group jogging may improve depressive symptoms, hormonal response to stress, and physiological fitness in adolescent females (Nabkasorn et al., 2006).

With adolescent females, prevention of depression should be a major goal, primarily because the first episode of depression tends to result in a chronic course (Le, Munoz, Ippen, & Stoddard, 2003). Preventing the first episode of depression is even more important when one considers that depression also places females at risk of smoking, misusing substances, and becoming mothers at an early age (Le et al., 2003). Moreover, Le and colleagues suggest that prevention programs should be available to those at risk of experiencing depressive symptoms who have little access to mental health services, such as low-income women, as well as women who are members of ethnic minority groups.

The literature on evidence-based interventions with youth who are members of ethnic minority groups suggests that culturally adapted interventions tend to be as effective as traditional interventions with majority youth (Miranda et al., 2005). In addition, clinicians should also become aware of their attitudes toward adolescent females who are struggling with sexual orientation at a time when they may experience depressive symptoms as a function of predispositions and other stressors (Eubanks-Carter et al., 2005). School-based interventions that target all youths (rather than particular youths) seem to lower depressive symptoms and suicidal ideation among all youth (Miranda et al., 2005); therefore, prevention programs will likely be effective in addressing depression among young females. As a specific example of this, the Resolve Project in Alberta, Canada offer data on gender-specific violence prevention programs for females that social workers can implement in schools with relative ease (online at www.ucalgary.ca/resolve/violenceprevention).

On average, violence and substance abuse prevention programs require 12 to 16 group or classroom sessions of intervention that focus on cognitive and behavioral factors, such as problem-solving and coping skills. Social workers who serve adolescent females either within the school or from outside the school (community-based agencies) can play a key role in implementing prevention programs, assuming school personnel are willing to sanction the implementation of these types of programs. Therefore, we encourage social workers to access information on gender-specific programs that have been proven to be more effective with females than males, as well as to implement prevention programs to identify gender differences in particular locations and geographic settings

## Young and Middle Adulthood

Approximately 13% of all new mothers experience postpartum depression (O'Hara & Swain, 1996). In the results from 9 trials involving 956 women, Hodnett (2007) found that both psychosocial interventions such as peer support and nondirective counseling and psychological interventions such as CBT and IPT are effective in reducing symptoms of postpartum depression. In terms of prevention, Dennis (2005) found in 15 trials involving 7,697 women that (1) intensive postpartum support from a health professional had a preventative effect, (2) interventions with only a postpartum component were more effective than those that included an antenatal component, and (3) interventions for individuals are more effective than those for groups. However, it is also noteworthy that Bledsoe and

Grote (2006) found that both medication only and medication in combination with CBT were more effective than other interventions in treating depression during pregnancy and postpartum. Both CBT and ITP have been found to be effective in preventing depression in low-income pregnant women and pregnant women from racial and ethnic minority groups (Le et al., 2003; Munoz et al., 2007; Spinelli & Endicott, 2003; Zlotnik, Miller, Pearlstein, Howard, & Sweeney, 2006).

As with adolescent females, CBT and IPT are effective in treating depression in women who are members of ethnic minority groups (Lara, Navarro, & Rubi, 2003). However, many studies have been conducted in primary care centers, and as a result, physicians have acknowledged the importance of maintenance and monitoring in treating depression. In this regard, the collaborative and stepped care models are effective and cost-saving means of achieving positive results in treating depression (Gilbody, Bower, Fletcher, Richards, & Sutton, 2006; Patel et al., 2007).

Collaborative care is structured care that involves roles for nonmedical professionals to augment primary care; the configuration of professionals involved varies from program to program. In analyzing the results of 37 studies including 12,355 patients with depression in primary care settings, Gilbody et al. (2006) found that collaborative care is more important than standard care in improving both short- and long-term depression outcomes, and that case or care manager supervision is a key determinant in achieving positive outcomes. For example, pharmacists and nurses may be involved as members of the collaborative team if the primary intervention is medication, and with respect to treating depression in women using psychosocial interventions, care management holds promise for social work involvement in the process.

In using a review of findings in narrative literature, Bower and Gilbody (2005) concluded that stepped care, which includes briefer, more minimal services, shows promise in treating depression. Seekles, van Straten, Beekman, van Marwijk, and Cuijpers (2009) implemented stepped care in a randomized, controlled trial in the Netherlands. Although the study was conducted in a primary care setting, this is an intervention wherein social workers could play a key role in many of the steps. The steps include:

(a) *watchful waiting*: a period of 4 weeks that has utility to see if individuals recover spontaneously over time (see Spijker et al., 2002);

(b) *guided self-help:* This begins with six 30-minute weekly sessions with a care manager in which the care manager excludes a diagnosis of severe depression, gives psychoeducation, and explains self-help interventions. In this process, arrangements are made for how feedback will be given every 3 days (i.e., by e-mail, telephone, or texting);

(c) *problem-solving treatment*: a sequence of 45-minute sessions once a week for 5 weeks (see Mynors-Wallis, 2005); and

(d) *pharmacological or more specialized mental health care*: the final step, in which the care manager sets up an appointment with a mental health specialist.

## Elderly Women

Treating depression in elderly women may be challenging due to the variable etiology of the disorder in elderly individuals (Cyranowski & Frank, 2006) or to the possibility that structural changes in the brain may result in vascular depression (Gatz & Fiske, 2003). Moreover, elderly women may not report depressive symptoms, per se, but they may report somatic symptoms instead. Scogin, Welsh, Hanson, Stump, and Coates (2005) reviewed evidence-based psychological treatments for geriatric depression and found that in addition to CBT and IPT for maintenance (Reynolds et al., 1999), behavioral therapy, bibliotherapy, problem-solving, and reminiscence therapy are effective.

Reynolds and colleagues suggest that clinicians use a variety of interventions to address depression in elderly women. However, they must understand how to change behavior using strategies such as the use of a token economy to reward appropriate behavior and extinguish less appropriate behavior. Likewise, bibliotherapy involves the use of topical and relevant books to identify and address aspects of women's lives that result in depressive symptoms. While clinicians are familiar with problem-solving and finding solutions to problems as a function of CBT, reminiscence therapy may require that clinicians have specialized training in order to utilize information about which women reminisce in a way that reduces depressive symptoms.

# Alternative Therapies

Within the context that many individuals fail to respond to pharmacological or psychosocial interventions, alternative therapies hold some promise for the treatment of depression in women (Manber, Allen, & Morris, 2002). Those therapies include: exercise, particularly in older adults (Blumenthal et al, 1999) and adolescents (Nabkasorn et al., 2006); yoga, mindfulness, and meditation for chronic, recurring depression (Segal, Williams, & Teasdale, 2002); acupuncture (Gallagher, Allen, Hitt, Schnyer, & Manber, 2001); and herbal remedies (Hypericum Depression Trial Study Group, 2002). Although bright light exposure seems to be effective in treating seasonal affective disorder in women, it is significantly less effective in treating MDD.

The evidence suggests that CBT and IPT are interventions proven to be effective in addressing depression in all women, particularly if they are adapted culturally to specific groups of women. Prevention programs may be beneficial forms of intervention for adolescent females and pregnant women, and in this regard, social workers could implement prevention programs in schools with relative ease. Perhaps most important, collaborative care and stepped care models hold potential for addressing depression in women of all ages, and in turn, the potential for social workers to participate as members of an interdisciplinary team in various steps of the process.

## Summary

In this chapter, the focus has been on the prevalence, etiology, screening, assessment, and evidence-based treatment of depression in women. First, it seems that depression and depressive symptoms are prevalent enough among women that social workers might anticipate that some number of women with whom they practice are depressed. Second, it seems necessary that social workers become familiar with the explanations of women's depression in an attempt to understand how biochemical and genetic factors interact with external stressors. This is particularly important as low income and interpersonal violence intersect to contribute to women's depression. Third, social workers may suspect from data they collect via interviews and narratives that women consumers with whom they work are experiencing depressive symptoms; therefore, they should consider using brief psychometrically acceptable measures to screen for depression as a means of providing appropriate intervention themselves or making referrals to clinicians or physicians they believe to be well-trained in the evidence-based treatment modalities. Last, the evidence suggests that CBT and IPT are psychosocial interventions proven to work in treating depression in women, and if these interventions are culturally adapted, they seem to work with women from racial and ethnic minority groups as well. Given the prevalence of depression in women, collaborative and stepped types of care seem to be viable options in identifying, monitoring, and maintaining mental health in women, especially among low-income women.

### Discussion Topics

1. Discuss at what age in the lifespan atypical depression is most typical, and speculate why this is so.

2. Discuss why women with bipolar disorder are at greater risk of arrest than women without bipolar disorder, and also why bipolar disorder is highly comorbid with substance abuse.

3. Debate the extent to which the etiology of depression is due to internal processes (biochemical and genetic factors) versus external stressors, and suggest the proportion that one might speculate each contributes to depression among women.

4. Discuss how and why the hypothalamic-pituitary-adrenal (HPA) feedback system may be especially important in explaining depression in low-income women.

5. Explain why depression is difficult to identify in elderly women and why CBT may not be the most effective intervention for elderly women with depression.

---

## CASE STUDY 3.1

Lorraine is a Caucasian female 78 years of age who was referred for evaluation by the county DHSS worker. The DHSS worker was concerned about Lorraine's depressed mood, as well as the stress she is under while providing care for her husband, who has mild dementia and a host of chronic health problems. The couple is on social security and Medicaid and receives mobile meals daily, as well as in-home assistance with cleaning and laundry. Lorraine complains about feeling very sad and tired. She has been interviewed by several social service workers, each of whom has reported some concerns for her, including noting her slow speech, very low volume, and poor inflection. Lorraine's movements are also very slow and deliberate, and she shows little emotion and facial expression. When questioned about the duration of her feelings, Lorraine indicated that she has struggled with feelings of intense sadness for as long as she can remember. She complained that she feels a general sense of hopelessness, inability to make decisions or concentrate, lack of energy, constipation, and irritability. In addition to this, Lorraine is relatively isolated, indicating she has no energy to go to church or visit with friends. While she has two adult children, they are both married and living out of state. These are her only living family members.

### Case Questions

What is your preliminary assessment of the etiology of Lorraine's depression?

Would Lorraine be a good candidate for a short, self-report assessment measure of her depression and if so, which measure might you recommend?

What are the relative advantages and disadvantages of administering the GDS to Lorraine, and would it make any difference if you administer the shorter or longer form in assessing her depression?

How would you go about treating her symptoms, including the stress and depression she experiences because she is her husband's caregiver?

What forms of intervention and treatment might be most effective for treating Lorraine?

## Illustrative Reading

# In-Home Cognitive Behavior Therapy for a Depressed Mother in a Home Visitation Program

Robert T. Ammerman

Amy L. Bodley

Frank W. Putnam

Wendi L. Lopez

Lauren J. Holleb

*Cincinnati Children's Hospital Medical Center, University of Cincinnati College of Medicine, Cincinnati, Ohio*

Jack Stevens

*Columbus Children's Hospital, The Ohio State University College of Medicine and Public Health, Columbus, Ohio*

Judith B. Van Ginkel

*Cincinnati Children's Hospital Medical Center, University of Cincinnati College of Medicine, Cincinnati, Ohio*

**Authors' Note:** Supported by a grant from The Health Foundation of Greater Cincinnati and support from the Kentucky HANDS Program. Wendi Lopez is now at the University of Oklahoma Health Sciences Center. Lauren Holleb is now at the University of Maine. Address correspondence to Robert T. Ammerman, PhD, Cincinnati Children's Hospital Medical Center, 3333 Burnet Avenue, Cincinnati, OH 45229; e-mail: robert.ammerman@cchmc.org.

Depression is frequently observed among young mothers who are low income who participate in home visitation programs that are focused on optimizing child development. Maternal depression can undermine such prevention programs, and mothers are faced with significant barriers to obtaining concurrent effective mental health treatment. This case study describes In-Home Cognitive Behavior Therapy (IH-CBT), an adapted treatment for depressed mothers in home visitation. IH-CBT provides an empirically-based treatment in the home setting that is tightly integrated with ongoing home visitation. The treated mother presented with major depressive disorder in the postpartum period and poor attachment with her baby. After 15 sessions of IH-CBT, provided in conjunction with home visitation, significant improvement occurred in mood, self-sufficiency, and her relationship with her baby.

**Keywords:** maternal depression; cognitive behavior therapy; home visitation

## Theoretical and Research Basis

### Maternal Depression

Major depressive disorder (MDD) is a potentially devastating condition that affects a significant proportion of pregnant women and new mothers. Lifetime prevalence of MDD in women is about 14% (Kessler et al., 2003). Prevalence of depression during pregnancy and postpartum is equally high. For example, Evans, Heron, Francomb, Oke, and Golding (2001) found that 13.5% in a sample of 9,028 women who were pregnant reported clinically elevated levels of depression. In a meta-analysis of prevalence studies, O'Hara and Swain (1996) reported that 13% of women experience MDD postpartum. Women who are at risk have higher rates, as demonstrated by the 27.6% prevalence during pregnancy and 23.4% postpartum in inner-city women who are low income (Hobfoll, Ritter, Lavin, Hulsizer, & Cameron, 1995).

Major depressive disorder results in considerable functional impairment. In the National Comorbidity Survey Replication, Kessler et al. (2003) reported that 87.4% of persons who were depressed experienced impairments in home, work, relationships, and social roles. The greatest impairments were in home (90.8%) and social (87.9%), which increased with greater clinical severity. In the general population, although 57.3% of adults who are depressed receive some type of treatment, only 21.6% receive minimally acceptable treatment. The proportion of women who are pregnant, postpartum, and depressed who receive treatment is dramatically lower (20% to 30%). This is because of, in part, difficulties identifying the disorder during a time in which normative features of pregnancy and the postpartum period (e.g., fatigue, sleep problems) overlap with symptoms of depression. Among women who are low income, there are numerous barriers to obtaining mental health services (e.g., transportation needs), which further decrease their accessibility to effective treatment.

A sizable body of evidence has accrued linking maternal depression to negative development outcomes in children (Goodman & Gotlib, 2002). Maternal depression undermines nurturing and effective parenting (Lovejoy, Graczyk, O'Hare, & Newman, 2000), which in turn disrupts developmental processes in affective, social, and cognitive systems. Poor short- and long-term child outcomes include insecure attachment formation, emotional dysregulation, impaired early socialization, cognitive delays, and behavior problems (Martins & Gaffan, 2000). The deleterious effects of maternal depression on children are more severe and more durable if the depression occurs early in life, if there are multiple episodes, and if the episodes are severe (Hay, Pawlby, Angold, Harold, & Sharp, 2003; O'Hara, 1997). Clearly, early detection and treatment is essential to ameliorate maternal depression and mitigate the negative effects of exposure to children's development.

### Depression in the Context of Home Visitation

Home visitation has emerged as a promising prevention strategy for young children and their families (Guterman, 2001). In home visitation, a home visitor (who, depending on the program model, is a nurse, social worker, or paraprofessional) provides psychoeducational training and case management services to mothers and children. Designed primarily to prevent

*(Continued)*

(Continued)

child abuse and neglect, home visitation seeks to promote optimal child development and prevent negative outcomes, including academic underachievement, psychological maladjustment, and antisocial behavior. Home visits, which can begin during the prenatal period and last until the child reaches age 2 to 5 years, target diverse areas such as parenting skills, mother-child relationship, home safety, maternal health, and infant nutrition.

It is widely recognized that mental illness, and particularly maternal depression, interferes with the effective delivery of home visitation (Margie & Phillips, 1999; Stevens, Ammerman, Putnam, & Van Ginkel, 2002). The symptoms of depression (poor concentration, poor memory, fatigue) interfere with learning, challenge home visitors who have limited training with women who are depressed, and divert home visitors' attention from the primary goal of delivering child-focused prevention curricula (LeCroy & Whitaker, 2005). The prevalence of depression in mothers participating in home visitation has not been extensively researched, although preliminary data indicate that it is a significant problem. For example, Ammerman, Putnam, Altaye, et al. (2005) reported that almost one half (45%) of first-time mothers in home visitation obtained elevated scores on the Beck Depression Inventory-II (BDI-II; A. T. Beck, Steer, & Brown, 1996) in the first year of service. Despite the growing recognition of maternal depression as a significant challenge in home visitation, no systematic approach to identification and intervention has been developed.

### In-Home Cognitive Behavior Therapy: An Innovative Treatment for Mothers Who are Depressed and in Home Visitation

In-Home Cognitive Behavior Therapy (IH-CBT) was developed to provide treatment of depression in first-time mothers enrolled in home visitation programs (Putnam, Ammerman, Stevens, Novak, & Holeb, 2005). In-Home Cognitive Behavior Therapy is provided in the home, thereby reaching mothers who otherwise would not receive consistent and effective mental health treatment. In-Home Cognitive Behavior Therapy is an adapted treatment in that it relies on an empirically proven approach to depression (cognitive behavior therapy [CBT]; see Gloaguen, Gottraux, Cucherat, & Blackburn, 1998) but contains specialized features that are designed to meet the needs of new mothers (Whitton & Appleby, 1996) and to integrate seamlessly with ongoing home visitation services. In-Home Cognitive Behavior Therapy utilizes the practices and procedures of CBT as developed by Beck and colleagues (A. T. Beck, Rush, Shaw, & Emery, 1979; J. S. Beck, 1995). These include identification of maladaptive thought patterns through daily monitoring, elucidation of irrational thought processes (e.g., overgeneralization), and their replacement with more rational beliefs. Behavioral activation, a key feature of effective CBT, is used to increase involvement in productive activities (Jacobson, Martell, & Dimidjian, 2001).

In-Home Cognitive Behavior Therapy consists of 15 weekly sessions provided in the home and lasting 60 minutes. A booster session is administered 1 month following treatment. Sessions are standardized to include assessment of mood, homework review, examination of data collected during the week, and cognitive restructuring or behavioral activation. Several clinical tools were developed to maximize treatment impact for young mothers who are low income. For example, The Ladder of Success is a diagram of a ladder that documents the mother's progress during treatment and visually shows the relationship between changes in cognitions and symptom relief and functional improvement. It helps mothers understand the connections between cognitive changes and recovery. In addition, the Therapy Summary and Planning for the Future, which is prepared for mothers at the end of treatment, summarizes what was learned during IH-CBT and how to prevent relapse through continued practice.

In-Home Cognitive Behavior Therapy is adapted for home visitation through a series of procedures that link the two approaches. They are meant to work together and in tandem, rather than the more typical lack of coordination between home visitation and mental health treatment provided by outside professionals. By integrating IH-CBT and home visitation, both interventions benefit, and likelihood of success is optimized. The following procedures are used to integrate IH-CBT and home visitation: (a) home visitors attend the 1st and 15th sessions with the therapist and mother; (b) the Therapy Summary and Planning for the Future is shared with the home visitor; and (c) there is frequent written communication between the therapist and home visitor through a Web-based clinical documentation system (see Ammerman et al., in press), and as-needed telephone contacts. Taken together, these procedures build and maintain a strong, collaborative, and supportive relationship between the therapist and home visitor. In addition, frequent contact allows the therapist and home visitor to coordinate their approaches and avoid unnecessary duplicating of efforts.

Preliminary evaluation of IH-CBT has yielded encouraging results. Ammerman, Putnam, Stevens, et al. (2005) examined pretreatment and posttreatment depression and psychosocial functioning in 26 first-time mothers (mean age =22.5 years) in home visitation. Mothers were initially screened based on BDI-II scores ≥20, and offered treatment if they subsequently met criteria for MDD based on a semistructured diagnostic interview. This was a clinically severe sample as evidenced by the facts that 54.5% had a previous depressive episode, 81.8% had a history of significant trauma, 51.5% made a suicide attempt at some point in their lives, and 36.4% had a psychiatric hospitalization. Comorbidity was also high with 61.5% having a comorbid disorder, most often an anxiety disorder or dysthymic disorder. Results indicated that 25 of 26 mothers reported a drop in BDI-II scores, with a mean drop of 16.5 points (pretreatment mean = 30.4, $SD$ = 8.2, posttreatment mean = 13.7, $SD$ = 9.4). At posttreatment, 84.6% of participants no longer met criteria for MDD (full recovery 69.2%, partial 15.4%). This compares favorably to clinical trials of CBT that typically find response rates between 55% and 60% (e.g., Hollon et al., 2005) and is especially impressive given the psychiatric comorbidity, psychosocial adversity, and overall clinical severity of the sample. Mothers also reported an increase in positive attitudes about motherhood and the child, better overall health and functioning, and decreased stress related to child rearing, stress at work or school, financial problems or worries, and social isolation. Mothers and home visitors reported a high degree of satisfaction with the program, and with the strong collaborative relationships between home visitors and the therapist.

### Maternal Depression Treatment Program and Every Child Succeeds

In-Home Cognitive Behavior Therapy is provided as part of the Maternal Depression Treatment Program (MDTP) at Every Child Succeeds (ECS). Every Child Succeeds is a large-scale, community-based home visitation program for first-time mothers and their

*(Continued)*

(Continued)

children. Every Child Succeeds utilizes two national programs of home visitation (Nurse Family Partnership [Olds, 2002] and Healthy Families America [Daro & Harding, 1999]). Eligible mothers are at risk for adverse parenting outcomes based on having at least one of four characteristics: unmarried, low income, age 18 years or younger, and late or no prenatal care. Mothers assigned to the Healthy Families America program also pass through a second level of eligibility determination through completion of a 90-minute assessment interview, which is then used to score the Kempe Family Stress Inventory (KFSI; Orkow, 1985), a measure of risk for negative parenting outcomes (scores of 25 are indicative of elevated risk and subsequent eligibility for home visitation). Mothers are enrolled prenatally through the child reaching age 3 months, and regular home visits are provided by trained nurses, social workers, or related professionals and paraprofessionals. Home visits are provided over a 2½- to 3-year period, starting with weekly visits and tapering to lower frequencies as the program progresses. All mothers are screened for depression at regular intervals throughout the program.

## Case Presentation

Debbie is a 24-year-old, single, White female referred to the Maternal Depression Treatment Program. She resided in public housing with her 11-month-old daughter, Angela. The father of the baby (Alex) was intermittently involved with Debbie and his child, living in the home for several weeks at a time followed by more extended absences. Debbie was referred to ECS by a prenatal clinic during the 7th month of pregnancy, as she met two of the four eligibility criteria (unmarried, low income). She was assigned to the Healthy Families of America program and received an eligibility score of 45 on the KFSI. During the interval between enrollment and the first IH-CBT treatment visit, Debbie received 15 visits with her home visitor. A regularly scheduled screen for depression using the BDI-II (A. T. Beck et al., 1996) revealed a clinically elevated score of 35.

Debbie reported a number of stressors that strained her social and psychological resources, and these had become the primary focus of home visitation. She was enrolled in a job-training program but was not attending regularly because the baby (Angela) was often sick, and she was unable to arrange for child care. She was especially concerned with her financial situation, which included inadequate support from public assistance (this was reduced because of her absences from vocational training), and little support from Alex. Debbie's father was ill and hospitalized at the time of MDTP assessment. The home visitor focused on helping Debbie obtain tangible resources, such as diapers, as she was continuously running out of them. Although she had daily contact with her parents, they were unable to provide substantial support although they occasionally helped her with transportation because she did not own a car. She had few friends, and existing relationships had been strained since the beginning of her relationship with Alex. To increase social support, the home visitor urged Debbie to attend occasional group meetings with other mothers in ECS; however, Debbie was too "overwhelmed" to attend.

The home visitor recommended that Debbie be treated for depression, and on discussing options for obtaining it Debbie expressed interest in talking to someone about her problems rather than receiving medication. She believed that taking medicine would be a sign that she was "crazy," and she also acknowledged that she typically had difficulty remembering to regularly take medications as prescribed. Obtaining treatment at an office-based clinic was problematic given her transportation limitations. On referral to the MDTP, an appointment was made to conduct the assessment to determine if Debbie qualified for IH-CBT. Results (see Assessment) were reviewed, and treatment commenced following determination that Debbie met criteria for MDD.

## Presenting Complaints

Debbie presented with feelings of sadness and hopelessness. Her affect was noticeably dysphoric, and she cried frequently during the assessment and first treatment session. Primary concerns consisted of a loss of interest in being with others, crying easily, irritability, and difficulty sleeping. She reported having thoughts that she would be better off dead, yet she denied having a plan or intent to hurt herself. Debbie had become isolative and often did not get dressed until later in the day. These symptoms, which first emerged during pregnancy and had not improved since that time, were evident every day and worsened later in the day. Disaggregating these symptoms from those that are typical of child rearing in the first year (e.g., sleep problems) indicated that they were minimally related to the demands of caring for her baby, and instead part of the depressive disorder.

Debbie reported having significant relationship problems with Alex. She had a very intense connection to him, characterized by a strong fear that he would leave and "abandon" her. At least weekly, they had heated arguments that typically began with Alex criticizing Debbie and calling her stupid, followed by Debbie reacting angrily. He would then threaten to leave, at which point she would attempt to physically restrain him. The confrontation elevated to mutual choking and throwing objects, ending when Alex left the situation and went to another room in the home. Debbie's fear that Alex would leave prompted her to frequently stay at home on the belief that if she was accessible to him, he would be less likely to leave. Debbie viewed the domestic violence as her fault, a belief that was shared by Alex.

Although Debbie fought with Alex, she stated that she loved him and wanted to be with him. Debbie wanted to work on being able to control her anger better. She expressed desire to get out of the house more and socialize with friends. Debbie also hoped to get a job and return to school. Debbie ultimately wanted to independently take care of her baby and herself. Debbie's goals for therapy were to get a job, do more for herself, and improve her coping during times of depression and anxiety.

## History

Debbie grew up with her mother, father, and younger sister (2 years younger). Her parents worked intermittently, and there were significant financial worries. Debbie describes a household with frequent arguments and physical fighting between her parents. Debbie's father would leave the family after some of these arguments, and this was a source of considerable distress for her. She reported feeling responsible for his leaving. The relationship

*(Continued)*

(Continued)

between Debbie and her father was strained following the revelation of her pregnancy, in part because the father of the baby was African American. After the birth of the baby, the relationship improved, and at the start of treatment Debbie was seeing her parents regularly. She reported having a good relationship with her mother and sister while growing up.

Debbie was enrolled in special education classes through high school. She graduated from high school and enrolled in community college. Debbie met Alex, who was 21 years older, at church. An intimate relationship rapidly ensued, and Debbie quickly dropped out of college and had fewer contacts with friends. Debbie and the father of the baby were together for a year, prior to her pregnancy, which was unplanned. At about 4 months into the pregnancy, the father of the baby left her for another woman. He had since returned and resided with Debbie at the time of assessment. Alex had one adolescent child from a prior marriage. He had a history of domestic violence in previous relationships and had participated in mandatory anger management classes at some point. Religion was important to Debbie and Alex. Debbie reported that he attended church 4 times a week, and she attended a different church twice a week. Debbie stated that her depression emerged during her pregnancy. She denied having any prior psychiatric history or treatment.

## Assessment

The assessment was conducted in Debbie's home. In addition to a brief clinical interview, Debbie was administered the BDI-II, Primary Care Evaluation of Mental Disorders (PRIME MD; Spitzer et al., 1994), the Brief Patient Health Questionnaire (Kroenke, Spitzer, & Williams, 2001), and the Maternal Attitudes Questionnaire (MAQ; Warner, Appleby, Whitton, & Faragher, 1997). Table 1 presents the pretreatment and posttreatment results for Debbie. As noted, Debbie obtained a score of 35 on the BDI-II at referral. Symptoms endorsed at a severe level (3) included past failure, self-dislike, loss of interest (in people or things), irritability, and loss of interest in sex. Items endorsed at the moderate level (2) included feeling guilty, being critical of herself, thoughts of death, propensity of crying, and fatigue. She endorsed several items at the minimal level (1) including feelings of sadness, pessimism, loss of pleasure to agitation, indecisiveness, worthlessness, loss of energy, changes in sleep and appetite, and difficulty concentrating.

On the PRIME MD, Debbie endorsed seven persistent symptoms of major depression (sleeping a lot, having little energy, overeating, feeling down, feeling bad about herself, difficulty concentrating, and wondering if she were better off dead), thereby meeting criteria for MDD. Debbie also reported symptoms of generalized anxiety, indicating that she felt such symptoms most of her life. She indicated experiencing restlessness, fatigue, difficulty sleeping, difficulty concentrating, and becoming easily annoyed. As these symptoms covaried with and emerged after her depression, they were viewed as reflective of MDD, and she was not given a comorbid diagnosis of generalized anxiety disorder. Debbie described experiencing a panic attack, for the first time, while watching television in her home about 3 weeks prior to the assessment. The symptoms were so disconcerting that she went to the hospital emergency room. She did not meet diagnostic criteria for somatization disorder, substance abuse or dependence, or eating disorders. Separate probing for post-traumatic stress disorder (PTSD) indicated that she did not have this diagnosis.

**Table 1**   Pre- and Posttreatment Results for Debbie on Measures of Depression and Associated Functional Domains for Debbie

|  | *Pretreatment* | *Posttreatment* |
|---|---|---|
| BDI-II | 35 | 12 |
| PHQ-9 | 13 (moderate) | 7 (mild) |
| MAQ | 28 | 17 |
| Psychiatric diagnoses | MDD | none |
| Problems at work, home, with others[a] | very difficult | somewhat difficult |
| In last 4 weeks . . .[b] |  |  |
| Worried about health | a lot | a little |
| Worried about weight or appearance | a lot | a lot |
| Difficulties with partner | a lot | none |
| Stress related to care of children | a lot | a little |
| Stress at work and/or school | NA | a little |
| Financial worries | a lot | a little |
| No one to turn to | none | none |

*Note:* BDI-II = Beck Depression Inventory-II; PHQ-9 = Patient Health Questionnaire; MAQ = Maternal Attitudes Questionnaire; MDD = major depressive disorder.

[a]Item 3 from Brief Patient Health Questionnaire.

[b]Item 4 (subitems a,d-h) from Brief Patient Health Questionnaire.

On the Brief Patient Health Questionnaire, Debbie endorsed feeling down, difficulty sleeping, and overeating "nearly every day." She also indicated feeling bad about herself "more than half the days." Debbie acknowledged "several days" of fatigue and thoughts of death. Her score of 13 on the Patient Health Questionnaire (PHQ-9; Spitzer, Kroenke, & Williams, 1999) depression screen was in the moderate range of depression. Overall, Debbie felt her worries and depressive symptoms made her life "very difficult" to manage. Debbie also endorsed other things that "bothered her," including her appearance and/or weight, the father of the baby, parenting, finances, and her health. Debbie confirmed that domestic violence occurred while she was pregnant. Her most stressful thing in her life was described as worrying about taking care of her baby.

Debbie obtained a score of 28 on the MAQ, indicating an emotionally distant relationship with her baby and substantial dissatisfaction with motherhood. For example, Debbie strongly disagreed that "having a baby has made me as happy as I expected" and strongly agreed that "If I love my baby I should want to be with her all the time"; "I have resented not having enough time to myself since having my baby"; and "If I find being a mother difficult, I feel like a failure." She also agreed that her baby was demanding and that her life was restricted since having her baby. Debbie thought she should be able to cope well all the time to be a good mother and that if her baby was unhappy or unwell that it was her fault. She regretted

*(Continued)*

(Continued)

having her child and was disappointed with her maternal role. Debbie was observed to be emotionally distant from Angela, physically intrusive (grabbing her arm suddenly), and interacted with her only when necessary to provide immediate care.

## Case Conceptualization

The conceptualization of Debbie's clinical presentation was guided by CBT frameworks for understanding the development and maintenance of depressive symptomatology. Several cognitive distortions predominated in the way Debbie viewed herself, her relationships with others, and the world. A central feature was Debbie's strong fear of abandonment, particularly by Alex. Debbie engaged in labeling, in which she viewed herself as *incompetent, unworthy,* and *unlovable.* Debbie viewed herself as an ineffective mother, which became self-fulfilling secondary to the effects of depression on parenting (fatigue, loss of interest, failure to read child's cues accurately). Through mental filtering, Debbie focused on negative events and critical comments from others to the exclusion of neutral or positive events and comments. These, in turn, were distorted through magnification and overgeneralization. These cognitive distortions operated against a backdrop of frequent criticism from Alex, a constricted social network of peers that might have otherwise provided support and validation, and unresolved guilt and self-blame regarding Debbie's self-perceived role in her father's abandonment of the family during childhood.

Debbie focused her energy on (a) maintaining her relationship with Alex and (b) managing her depressive affect and anxiety. She was convinced that limiting her contact with others would permit her to concentrate her energies on maintaining her relationship with Alex, and that these efforts would increase the likelihood that he would stay. She used sleep and isolation as ways of coping with general emotional upset. The needs and demands of Angela were potent stressors that were difficult to fulfill. Through the filter of depressive misattributions, Debbie saw Angela as unrewarding, and a reminder of her incompetence as a mother. The focus of treatment was behavioral activation to decrease social isolation, cognitive restructuring to target irrational beliefs that fueled depressive affect and disengagement from natural supports, and increasing Debbie's independence and diminishing her emotional reliance on Alex.

## Course of Treatment and Assessment of Progress

In the first meeting with Debbie, her primary concerns were discussed and core issues were revealed. Shortly after a brief introduction, Debbie broke down in tears, expressing her fear of being overwhelmed. She described her "fear of being alone," and the physical altercations with Alex that emerged from and exacerbated this fear. Overgeneralization was evident in her belief that, if Alex did not "want her," then nobody ever would. She described her sadness resulting from Alex's psychological abuse, and her loneliness emanating in large part from her social isolation and distance from friends.

Goals were developed focusing on Debbie getting out of the house and doing more for herself, getting a job, and improving her coping abilities. Her first homework assignment consisted of contacting a friend that she had not seen for awhile. She expressed fears about being rejected. Through cognitive restructuring, these fears were evaluated and reframed into a more realistic and positive perspective. In the next session, Debbie reported that she had called her friend, who had received her well, and they had plans to go out in the next week.

At this time, Alex continued to intermittently stay with Debbie. Their relationship was more distant, which intensified Debbie's fears of abandonment but provided opportunities in treatment to increase her independence, enhance her management of negative emotions, and work on longer terms goals of resuming her education. To this end, Debbie enrolled in an educational program to obtain certification as a hairdresser, which also included a part-time job in the school's cafeteria. These gains boosted her self-esteem and provided an outlet for additional social interactions.

Debbie maintained a thought record in which depressogenic cognitions were recorded. This exercise revealed a core belief that she was "unlovable" and that she would be alone if Alex left completely. These, in turn, were followed by other negative cognitions, such as "I feel ugly about myself, it's God's fault, and I don't want to be here." This chain of cognitions led to intense dysphoria and anxiety. In examining these thoughts in treatment, Debbie was able to admit that she was not alone in the world. She identified her daughter, her parents, and her sister as important people in her life. Through reaching out to an old friend, she realized that she had a friend who cared about her as well. Debbie also acknowledged that she had good relationships prior to meeting Alex, and that others had loved her in the past. A "coping card" was developed containing replacement thoughts for her irrational cognitions, and Debbie kept the card in a prominent location and referred to it often. This strategy appealed to Debbie and was subsequently used with other cognitive distortions and to help Debbie actively cope with difficult situations and emotions at home and at school and work. Also helpful was the creation of a list of pleasurable activities, from which she attempted to do at least one activity each day. This combination of behavioral activation and thought restructuring was effective in altering negative thinking patterns and engaging her in pleasurable activities that improved her mood.

As Debbie progressed, the therapist communicated improvements to the home visitor through phone calls and notes written in a common case note section of the Web-based system shared with the home visitor. The home visitor, in turn, kept the therapist apprised of issues addressed in home visitation. The home visitor focused on teaching Debbie about Angela's development and worked with her to increase interactions between mother and child. These were reinforced by the therapist, who often used the session to model positive interactions with Angela (e.g., briefly playing with her, setting her up next to Debbie with some toys so that Angela could play quietly while the session progressed).

At the 8th session, the BDI-II was administered, and a score of 16 was obtained. Angela reported improvement in a variety of symptoms, including decreases in crying, sense of failure, and guilt, and corresponding increases in motivation, interest in activities and people, and hopefulness. Furthermore, it was noted that Debbie played more with Angela, was more attentive to cues, paid more attention to her appearance and the cleanliness

*(Continued)*

(Continued)

of her home, and was generally more social and interactive with others. A number of depressive symptoms remained, although they had significantly decreased in severity since the beginning of treatment.

The remainder of treatment focused on reinforcing the use of coping cards, increasing application of alternative cognitions, and helping Debbie continue her momentum of increased social interactions. Debbie's most difficult times were when she was alone, during which she would think about Alex and the possibilities of abandonment (even though she was seeing Alex less). Her inherent worth and the fact that she had reliable supports in her life were reinforced during therapy, and a coping card was made of the people in her life that loved her that she could read and refer to daily. Also around this time, Debbie's home visitor resigned and was replaced by a new home visitor. Debbie had become attached to the home visitor, and the familiar feelings of abandonment emerged. Although it was unfortunate that the home visitor left, it was fortuitous from the perspective of treatment in that Debbie's abandonment concerns could be actively addressed.

Although she continued to argue with Alex, which elicited fears and feelings of being unlovable, Debbie was quick to rebound. Her self-esteem improved, and she became more assertive. She was able to express her anger at Alex's disparaging comments and stopped reacting physically to his threats to leave. As therapy progressed, the Ladder of Success was completed, showing the advances that Debbie had made. Debbie liked this exercise and was surprised and proud of her recent accomplishments. She referred to this worksheet frequently, which further increased her self-esteem. In conjunction with the Ladder of Success, other positives in her life were listed on coping cards. It was suggested she read this twice a day, once in the morning and once in the evening for reinforcement of all she achieved.

The 13th session was notable in that Debbie expressed concerns about having to do an oral presentation in a class, in which she believed that would fail because she believed that she was "stupid." Examination of irrational thoughts, generation of replacement cognitions that were more realistic and supportive, and creation of a coping card were used to address this issue successfully. This experience greatly added to Debbie's confidence, offsetting long-standing beliefs that she was incompetent. At the 15th session, the home visitor joined the session. Progress was reviewed, and successful coping strategies were identified. A plan for continued practice, with the support of the home visitor, was constructed to prevent relapse. During the joint session, the home visitor underscored the improvements that she had observed during treatment. The end of treatment provided another opportunity to address Debbie's concerns about abandonment. Just as the impact of the departure of the first home visitor was lessened by the continuity of treatment provided by the therapist, so was the end of IH-CBT more easily handled by Debbie because of the continuation of home visitation.

At the posttreatment assessment (see Table 1), the pretreatment measures were readministered. Debbie no longer met criteria for MDD. She obtained a BDI-II score of 12, which is under the clinically elevated cut-off of 14. She obtained a PHQ-9 score of 7, indicating mild depressive symptoms. In general, Debbie continued to display some symptoms of depression, although these had decreased in severity and were no longer as persistent.

On the MAQ, she obtained a posttreatment score of 17, reflecting greater emotional closeness with Angela and increased satisfaction with her maternal role. She reported decreased worrying and concerns about health, child care, and finances. She also was a more nurturant mother and clearly derived pleasure from interacting with her daughter. Through separate surveys, Debbie and the home visitor stated that they were pleased with the collaborative relationship between the therapist and home visitor and expressed overall satisfaction with the program.

## Complicating Factors

Comorbid psychiatric disorders are very common in depression. Research suggests that 72.1% have comorbid conditions, most often anxiety disorders (Kessler et al., 2003). Ammerman, Putnam, Stevens, et al. (2005) found a high rate of comorbidity in their sample of mothers participating in IH-CBT and home visitation (61.5%). In addition to MDD, Debbie suffered from generalized anxiety. During the assessment phase, we strived to identify comorbid conditions, determine the relative severity of MDD in comparison to comorbid disorders to ascertain the primary diagnosis, and establish the temporal onset and covariation of MDD with comorbidities to disaggregate their relationships. Through this process, we sometimes determine that another diagnosis other than MDD is primary (and requires a different treatment approach), that other disorders covary with MDD such that successful treatment of MDD may lead to corresponding improvement in comorbidities, or that MDD and comorbidities are largely independent of each other. Comorbidities are monitored throughout IH-CBT treatment. A worsening clinical presentation may require additional concurrent treatment, or referral for different treatments. We maintain our focus on depression throughout IH-CBT. Sometimes, as noted, comorbidities may improve as depression improves. At other times, comorbidities may be directly addressed in treatment if they fit into the CBT model and if the treatment approach also targets depressive symptomatology. In some cases, depression will improve; however, comorbid conditions will remain and will require referral for additional treatment.

Trauma history and domestic violence are frequently found in home visitation populations. There is a strong relationship between interpersonal trauma (sexual abuse, physical abuse, witness of violence) and the development of MDD (Arboleda-Florez, & Wade, 2001). Trauma may play an etiologic role in MDD through its contribution to long-term problems in emotional regulation and in the early development of coping strategies to traumatic experiences that are maladaptive in later stages of development. Ammerman, Putnam, Altaye, et al. (2005) found that 74.5% of mothers in IH-CBT had experienced an interpersonal trauma. Physical and psychological abuse was evident in the case study. Alex frequently criticized Debbie with put downs and insults and manipulated her through threats to leave. As is often the case, Alex saw Debbie as the source of their relationship problems and the sole cause of the physical altercations. He refused to consider treatment for himself, noting that he had already participated in anger management classes, and that was sufficient. As their relationship was already becoming

*(Continued)*

(Continued)

estranged at the time of treatment, we focused on helping Debbie overcome the negative effects of psychological abuse, and to increase her independence in anticipation of the eventual end of their relationship.

Trauma further complicates depression treatment through the manifestation of PTSD, a comorbid condition that may require additional treatment. However, it is noteworthy that, despite the high rate of trauma in their sample, Ammerman, Putnam, Stevens, et al. (2005) found that IH-CBT was effective in reducing depressive symptomatology. Indeed, recent evidence suggests that CBT is more effective than antidepressant medication in depressed women who have been traumatized. Nemeroff et al. (2003) reported that, in the treatment of depression in 681 adults who were chronically depressed, a version of CBT (Cognitive Behavioral Analysis System of Psychotherapy [CBASP]) was superior to nefazodone in those who had been traumatized in childhood (51% remission vs. 34%); the combination of treatments did not significantly enhance response.

Domestic violence is a major contributor to MDD in women and has been found to substantially undermine the benefits of home visitation (Eckenrode et al., 2000). The prevalence of domestic violence in home visitation samples is largely unknown, although anecdotally it is believed to be a sizable problem. Clinically, it poses a significant challenge to therapists. Abusive and controlling partners typically react negatively to the kinds of changes and initiative that are encouraged in therapy and are often the focus of treatment (i.e., getting out of the house, expanding social networks, looking for a job). The threat of violence engenders fear in the mother and a reluctance to make changes, which works against the goals of therapy. Although there are clinical guidelines for addressing domestic violence (e.g., Saunders, 1999), consistently efficacious interventions have not been developed. We assist mothers in developing a safety plan and consult with local shelters about resources and options for mothers who are ready to leave violent relationships. On several occasions, mothers have found refuge in women's shelters and have experienced significant improvements in psychological functioning. In these instances, home visitors have been integral to developing plans, identifying options, and supporting mothers in their transitions. At this point, management of domestic violence consists of attending to the safety of mother and child, maintaining a focus on treatment that promotes recovery from MDD, and supporting mothers in their efforts to leave violent relationships. Each of these was addressed in the current case study.

Several logistical and practical impediments are encountered when providing treatment in the home setting. It is sometimes difficult to find a space in the home that is comfortable, private, and conducive to therapy (see concerns about privacy in Recommendations to Clinicians). Designating a part of the home that is private and workable may require creativity and negotiation with other family members. It is necessary for the therapist to work with the mother to identify times of day in which other family members may be out of the home. Sometimes, it is preferable to find alternative sites (e.g., a relative's home) for conducting therapy. The home setting is also a place with potential distractions. These include interruptions from other family members or friends, telephones, pets, televisions, radios, and inquisitive or crying young children. We work with mothers early in treatment to minimize or eliminate these distractions, and to plan ahead to avoid them. Approaches include turning off all televisions and radios, alerting others in advance that the mother and therapist should not be interrupted, and choosing a time to meet when the child may be napping. There is no single solution for every situation, and the therapist must work closely with the mother to ensure a setting that is acceptable for therapy. For Debbie, there were several challenges to providing therapy sessions free of distractions and interruptions. Alex was unsupportive of Debbie receiving treatment. Sometimes during sessions he would be in the apartment, watching the baby in another room. On occasion, he would interrupt the session, or stop watching the baby thereby requiring that Debbie take over child care needs. In response to these problems, Debbie worked hard at scheduling the session when the father was not present. At other times, child care was unavailable and Debbie would have to tend to her in the session. This was used as an opportunity for the therapist to model nurturing interactions with the baby, which in turn had beneficial effects on Debbie's acquisition of effective parenting skills and an increase in her sense of parenting competence.

## Managed Care Considerations

The MDTP has been funded by a time-limited grant from a local foundation and support from a state public health agency. Efforts to secure long-term funding have been extremely challenging and highlight the lack of a third-party payment infrastructure for this type of in-home, psychological intervention. Third-party payers typically have restrictions in the types of treatment settings that are eligible for reimbursement, and they often discourage the home environment as a place to conduct psychological therapies. There is a growing body of research on the early detection and effective treatment of MDD (e.g., Gilbody, Whitty, Grimshaw, & Thomas, 2003). Yet these initiatives have almost exclusively focused on patients who are middle class, with antidepressant medication as the treatment, and primary care physician offices as the setting. Although MDD affects all class levels, women of lower socioeconomic status are at greatest risk, and they are the most likely participants in home visitation services. As noted, there are numerous barriers facing women who are low income in accessing high-quality and consistent medical care, and in adhering to medication regimens. As a result, these early detection and treatment programs are largely inapplicable to the populations served by home visitation. Because of their low-income status, most women in home visitation rely on Medicaid as their sole insurance coverage. Many mental health practitioners are not Medicaid providers, thereby limiting the pool of available therapists. Reimbursement rates are also problematic in that they are typically too low to support a therapeutic, home-based program that covers a wide geographical area and requires additional time spent traveling.

The extant third-party payment infrastructure is inadequate to meet the mental health needs of women who are low income and depressed, particularly those who are seen in the home in conjunction with ongoing home visitation. Unfortunately, home visitation programs are rarely able to cover the costs of an adjunctive mental health treatment program. Although it is almost universally acknowledged that MDD is a devastating disorder for mothers and children, and is among the most treatable of mental

*(Continued)*

(Continued)

health problems, there is simply no consistent funding support available at this time. Future financial support, which is essential to the viability and sustainability of programs such as the MDTP, will likely have to involve the combined resources of third-party payers, local community mental health boards, and other local and state public agencies that are the primary funders of home visitation and other preventive services.

## Follow-Up

Debbie's booster session was held about a month after treatment ended. Debbie's living situation remained the same, with Alex living in the home although they no longer had a close relationship. School had ended for the semester, and she no longer worked pending resumption of classes. The additional free time was problematic for Debbie, and she spent a considerable amount of time referring to her coping cards and warding off a return of "old" thought patterns. In the booster session, Debbie's accomplishments were reviewed, and proactive coping strategies were reinforced. Behavioral activation was emphasized, stressing the positive impact that pleasurable activities had on her mood. The home visitor arrived at the end of the session, which provided an opportunity to strengthen the connection between therapeutic strategies and home visitation.

## Treatment Implications of the Case

Kessler et al. (2003) found that a slim majority of persons who are depressed receive depression treatment, and only a subportion receives more than minimally accepted treatment. Access to treatment is especially limited for new mothers who are low income. In-Home Cognitive Behavior Therapy reflects an innovative approach to reaching women who are depressed and who otherwise would not receive treatment. First, IH-CBT is offered through and in the context of an early prevention program. Unlike center-based treatments, which rely on clients to take the initiative to contact them, IH-CBT targets new mothers who are already engaged in a prevention program and reaches out to engage them in treatment. By focusing on pregnancy and the postpartum period, effective treatment can be provided in early adulthood and early in the child's life, thereby maximizing benefits for mother and child in subsequent years. And second, bringing treatment into the home circumvents a major barrier to treatment in women who are low income and depressed—transportation.

Coordination between therapists and other service providers is an ideal that is rarely satisfactorily achieved. Numerous forces interfere with coordination, including difficulty reaching and maintaining contact with providers, failure to understand and appreciate different training and professional perspectives, and limited time availability. In-Home Cognitive Behavior Therapy overcomes these challenges by explicitly and systematically building connections between therapists and home visitors. Multiple channels of communication (telephone and written communications), and planned face-to-face contacts between home visitors and mothers, provide the infrastructure for therapists and home visitors to coordinate their efforts and support each other in optimizing the impact of depression treatment and home visitation.

The case study of Debbie reveals an important limitation of IH-CBT and of psychotherapy with this population in general. Although Debbie made significant gains in terms of depressive symptoms and overall functioning, numerous issues and challenges remained (poverty, an uncertain future). The population of new mothers who are young and low income who typically participate in home visitation programs have many needs and concerns that are not readily addressed or resolved by any single intervention. Histories of deprivation and trauma lead to long-term adjustment problems that are not fully amenable to a single, focused treatment. Moreover, poverty, social isolation, underemployment, and undereducation are formidable impediments to sustained psychological health and well-being. In-Home Cognitive Behavior Therapy can help in this process by remediating acute depressive episodes, minimizing recurrence, and helping mothers take the first steps toward improving their lives. In conjunction with home visitation, the chances of continued improvement are further enhanced.

## Recommendations to Clinicians

Although there are several empirically supported treatments for depression, most mothers who are low income have more limited options for treatment than their counterparts who are more affluent. Absent or unreliable transportation and inadequate social resources interfere with obtaining clinic-based treatment. Regular attendance at such settings is often unrealistic for this population. In the current case study, Debbie had not considered obtaining treatment outside of the home; however, with her limited resources and feelings of being overwhelmed, it seems unlikely that she would have sought clinic-based treatment. Yet, in the home setting, Debbie regularly kept weekly appointments. From the first day of treatment, she expressed a commitment to feeling better and working toward positive changes. Debbie utilized her cellular phone to text message the therapist if she needed to cancel, and she made efforts to reschedule these sessions in the same week.

Antidepressant medication is a widely used and effective treatment for MDD in the general population and is often used in conjunction with empirically-based psychotherapies. However, there are numerous barriers for its use with new mothers who are low income. The limited studies available in women who are pregnant and postpartum indicate that they frequently receive suboptimal doses and shorter courses of antidepressant treatment than other women (Altshuler et al., 2001). Evidence has emerged for neurobehavioral disruptions in infants born to mothers using selective serotonin reuptake inhibitors (SSRIs) during pregnancy (Zeskind & Stephens, 2004), although longer lasting effects have yet been identified. This concern appears to limit the dosages that many physicians will prescribe. All of the antidepressant medications are also excreted in breast milk in varying concentrations that are not well-related to type of antidepressant medication, dosage, or maternal blood levels. As with Debbie, some people find medication stigmatizing. Finally, the combined influences of stressors related to new motherhood and poverty, limited social resources, inadequate education, and poor understanding of medication regimens lead to poor adherence. In the MDTP, we have observed mothers

*(Continued)*

(Continued)

who have not taken prescribed medications, failed to take medications at prescribed times and intervals, taken partial doses, and discontinued prematurely. Taken together, it is clear that in-home psychological treatment may be one of the few feasible and effective approaches for this population.

Maintaining client confidentiality is an essential feature of psychological treatment. Conducting treatment in the home, and explicitly integrating treatment into an ongoing prevention program, poses unique challenges to ensuring confidentiality. As noted, finding a private space in the home to conduct treatment may be difficult if others are present. Family members may want to listen to treatment sessions, either through active participation or by surreptitiously monitoring the session from another room. We address these issues in the first session, instructing clients and involved family members in the importance of privacy and confidentiality, and establishing procedures for how sessions will be conducted so that that they are private. This needs to be handled in a clinically sensitive manner, given that other family members in the home may resent efforts by outsiders to restrict their access. Other family members may be concerned that they will be the topic of therapy sessions and are understandably uncomfortable with this prospect. Partners who are abusive are often especially threatened by the loss of control that occurs when mothers enter into a confidential therapeutic relationship. There is no single approach to addressing the above concerns, and the ultimate solution to implementing treatment in a private and confidential setting will be different for each mother. Creativity is important, and we have sometimes alternated the location of therapy in response to repeated pressures that undermine privacy. These include holding the sessions in another family member's home, finding a time when other family members are not in the home, or occasionally meeting out of the home, such as in a room at the home visitation agency or at mother's workplace. In our experience, however, in the vast majority of cases there is a satisfactory solution that permits consistent implementation of IH-CBT in the home. In the case of Debbie, phone contact prior to the session was utilized to determine if there was privacy in the home that day. Rescheduling within that week would occur if needed. Also, sessions were conducted outside on the patio to maintain privacy.

Explicit integration of IH-CBT and home visitation requires regular communication between the therapist and home visitor to ensure coordinated services. Accordingly, we review with mothers the procedures for how and what type of information will be shared between the therapist and home visitor (a written description is contained in the Institutional Review Board (IRB)–approved consent form, a signed copy of which is given to mothers). This is done during the assessment phase, and reviewed again during the first therapy visit. The purpose of sharing information is to improve the therapy and home visitation intervention, so only information that serves this aim is exchanged. Mothers are told that they may ask the therapist not to share certain information with the home visitor, and this request will be honored. In our experience, mothers infrequently ask that information not be shared with home visitors. There are instances where we determine that sharing the information will benefit the relationship between the mother and the home visitor, or the home visitation service. In these cases, we encourage the mother to share the information but avoid pressuring her; ultimately we adhere to the mother's decision. Prior to sharing information with home visitors, the therapist informs the mother of what and how the information will be shared. We regularly review information sharing during clinical supervision to avoid deviating from the above procedures. Debbie was open in regards to this therapist sharing information with the home visitor. A discussion would occur between therapist and Debbie as to what would be discussed with the home visitor prior to doing so. Debbie saw the benefit to the communication between her two workers, specifically when she was provided with additional resources.

## References

Altshuler, L. L., Cohen, L. S., Moline, M. L., Kahn, D. A., Carpenter, D., Docherty, J. P., et al. (2001). Treatment of depression in women: A summary of the expert consensus guidelines. *Journal of Psychiatric Practice, 7,* 185–208.

Ammerman, R. T., Putnam, F. W., Altaye, M., Chen, L., Holleb, L. J., Stevens, J., et al. (2005). *Course of depression in first-time mothers in home visitation.* Unpublished manuscript, Cincinnati Children's Hospital Medical Center, Cincinnati, OH.

Ammerman, R. T., Putnam, F. W., Kopke, J. E., Gannon, T. A., Short, J. A., Van Ginkel, J. B., et al. (2007). Development and implementation of a quality assurance infrastructure in a multisite home visitation program in Ohio and Kentucky. *Journal of Prevention and Intervention in the Community, 34,* (1–2), (89–107).

Ammerman, R. T., Putnam, F. W., Stevens, J., Holleb, L. J., Novak, A. L., & Van Ginkel, J. B. (2005). In-Home Cognitive Behavior Therapy for depression: An adapted treatment for first-time mothers in home visitation. *Best Practices in Mental Health, 1,* 1–14.

Arboleda-Florez, J., & Wade, T. J. (2001). Childhood and adult victimization as risk factor for major depression. *International Journal of Law and Psychiatry, 24,* 357–370.

Beck, A. T., Rush, A. J., Shaw, B. F., & Emery, G. (1979). *Cognitive therapy of depression.* New York: Guilford.

Beck, A. T., Steer, R. A., & Brown, G. K. (1996). *BDI-II manual.* San Antonio, TX: Psychological Corporation.

Beck, J. S. (1995). *Cognitive therapy: Basics and beyond.* New York: Guilford.

Daro, D. A., & Harding, K. A. (1999). Healthy Families America: Using research to enhance practice. *Future of Children, 9,* 152–176.

Eckenrode, J., Ganzel, B., Henderson, C. R., Jr., Smith, E., Olds, D. L., Powers, J., et al. (2000). Preventing child abuse and neglect with a program of nurse home visitation: The limiting effects of domestic violence. *Journal of the American Medical Association, 284,* 1385–1391.

Evans, J., Heron, J., Francomb, H., Oke, S., & Golding, J. (2001). Cohort study of depressed mood during pregnancy and after childbirth. *British Medical Journal, 323,* 257–260.

Gilbody, S., Whitty, P., Grimshaw, J., & Thomas, R. (2003). Educational and organizational interventions to improve the management of depression in primary care: A systematic review. *Journal of the American Medical Association, 289,* 3145–3151.

Gloaguen, V., Gottraux, J., Cucherat, M., & Blackburn, I.-M. (1998). A meta-analysis of the effects of cognitive therapy in depressed patients. *Journal of Affective Disorders, 49,* 59–72.

Goodman, S. H., & Gotlib, I. H. (Eds.). (2002). *Children of depressed parents: Mechanisms of risk and implications for treatment.* Washington, DC: American Psychological Association.

*(Continued)*

(Continued)

Guterman, N. B. (2001). *Stopping child maltreatment before it starts: Emerging horizons in early home visitation services.* Thousand Oaks, CA: Sage.

Hay, D. F., Pawlby, S., Angold, A., Harold, G. T., & Sharp, D. (2003). Pathways to violence in the children of mothers who were depressed postpartum. *Developmental Psychology, 39,* 1083–1094.

Hobfoll, S. E., Ritter, C., Lavin, J., Hulsizer, M. R., & Cameron, R. P. (1995). Depression prevalence and incidence among inner-city pregnant and postpartum women. *Journal of Consulting and Clinical Psychology, 63,* 445–453.

Hollon, S. D., DeRubeis, R. J., Shelton, R. C., Amsterdam, J. D., Salomon, R. M., O'Reardon, J. P., et al. (2005). Prevention of relapse following cognitive therapy vs. medications in moderate to severe depression. *Archives of General Psychiatry, 62,* 417–422.

Jacobson, N. S., Martell, C. R., & Dimidjian, S. (2001). Behavioral activation treatment for depression: Returning to contextual roots. *Clinical Psychology: Science and Practice, 8,* 255–270.

Kessler, R. C., Berglund, P., Demler, O., Jin, R., Koretz, D., Merikangas, K. R., et al. (2003). The epidemiology of major depressive disorder: Results from the National Comorbidity Survey Replication (NCS-R). *Journal of the American Medical Association, 289,* 3095–3105.

Kroenke, K., Spitzer, R. L., & Williams, J. B. W. (2001). The PHQ-9: Validity of a brief depression severity measure. *Journal of General Internal Medicine, 16,* 606–613.

LeCroy, C. W., & Whitaker, K. (2005). Improving the quality of home visitation: An exploratory study of difficult situations. *Child Abuse and Neglect, 29,* 1003–1013.

Lovejoy, M. C., Graczyk, P. A., O'Hare, E., & Newman, G. (2000). Maternal depression and parenting behavior: A meta-analytic review. *Child Psychology Review, 20,* 561–592.

Margie, N. G., & Phillips, D. A. (Eds.). (1999). *Revisiting home visiting: Summary of a workshop.* Washington, DC: National Academy Press.

Martins, C., & Gaffan, E. A. (2000). Effects of early maternal depression on patterns of infant-mother attachment: A meta-analytic investigation. *Journal of Child Psychology and Psychiatry, 41,* 737–746.

Nemeroff, C. B., Heim, C. M., Thase, M. E., Klein, D. N., Rush, A. J., Schatzberg, A. F., et al. (2003). Differential responses to psychotherapy versus pharmacotherapy in patients with chronic forms of major depression and childhood trauma. *Proceedings of the National Academy of Sciences, 100,* 14293–14296.

O'Hara, M. W. (1997). The nature of postpartum depressive disorders. In L. Murray & P. J. Cooper (Eds.), *Postpartum depression and child development* (pp. 3–31). New York: Guilford.

O'Hara, M. W., & Swain, A. M. (1996). Rates and risk of postpartum depression: A meta-analysis. *International Review of Psychiatry, 8,* 37–55.

Olds, D. L. (2002). Prenatal and infancy home visiting by nurses: From randomized trials to community replication. *Prevention Science, 3,* 153–172. Orkow, B. (1985). Implementation of a family stress checklist. *Child Abuse & Neglect, 9,* 405–410.

Orkow, B. (1985). Implementation of a family stress checklist. *Child Abuse & Neglect, 9*(3), 405–10.

Putnam, F. W., Ammerman, R. T., Stevens, J., Novak, A. L., & Holeb, L. J. (2005). *In-Home Cognitive Behavior Therapy (IH-CBT): Treatment manual, v.2.1.* Unpublished manual, Every Child Succeeds, Cincinnati Children's Hospital Medical Center, Cincinnati, OH.

Saunders, D. G. (1999). Woman battering. In R. T. Ammerman & M. Hersen (Eds.), *Assessment of family violence: A clinical and legal sourcebook* (2nd ed., pp. 243–270). New York: John Wiley.

Spitzer, R. L., Kroenke, R., & Williams, J. B. W. (1999). Validity and utility of a self-report version of PRIME-MD: The PHQ Primary Care Study. *Journal of the American Medical Association, 282,* 1737–1744.

Spitzer, R. L., Williams, J. B. W., Kroenke, K., Linzer, M., deGruy, F. V., III, Hahn, S. R., et al. (1994). Utility of a new procedure for diagnosing mental disorders in primary care. *Journal of the American Medical Association, 272,* 1749–1756.

Stevens, J., Ammerman, R. T., Putnam, F., & Van Ginkel, J. (2002). Depression and trauma history in first-time mothers receiving home visitation. *Journal of Community Psychology, 30,* 551–564.

Warner, R., Appleby, L., Whitton, A., & Faragher, B. (1997). Attitudes toward motherhood in postnatal depression: Development of the Maternal Attitudes Questionnaire. *Journal of Psychosomatic Research, 43,* 351–358.

Whitton, A., & Appleby, L. (1996). Maternal thinking and the treatment of postnatal depression. *International Review of Psychiatry, 8,* 73–78.

Zeskind, P. S., & Stephens, L. E. (2004). Maternal selective serotonin reuptake inhibitor use during pregnancy and newborn neurobehavior. *Pediatrics, 113,* 368–375.

## About the Authors

**Robert T. Ammerman**, PhD, ABPP, is Scientific Director, Every Child Succeeds, and professor of pediatrics, Cincinnati Children's Hospital Medical Center and University of Cincinnati College of Medicine. He received his doctorate in clinical psychology at the University of Pittsburgh and completed a psychology internship at Western Psychiatric Institute and Clinic, University of Pittsburgh School of Medicine. His research interests include child abuse prevention, optimizing the effectiveness of community-based prevention programs, and family violence.

**Amy L. Bodley**, MSSA, LISW, is Project Therapist for the Maternal Depression Treatment Program, Every Child Succeeds. She received a masters of science in social administration from Case Western Reserve University. Her interests include maternal depression and infant mental health. She is also a certified adoption assessor, conducting home studies for adoptive families.

**Frank W. Putnam**, MD, is Director of the Mayerson Center for Safe and Healthy Children, Associate Scientific Director, Every Child Succeeds, and Professor of Pediatrics and Psychiatry, Cincinnati Children's Hospital Medical Center and University of Cincinnati College of Medicine. He received his MD from Indiana University and completed a residency in psychiatry at Yale University and in child and adolescent psychiatry at George Washington University. His research interests include prevention and treatment of child abuse and dissemination of evidence-based programs to community providers.

**Wendi L. Lopez**, MS, PsyD, received a master's degree in physiology from Indiana University, Indianapolis, and a doctoral degree in clinical psychology from the University of Indianapolis. She is currently a Pediatric Psychology Fellow at the University of Oklahoma Health Sciences Center in Oklahoma City. Her research interests include childhood maltreatment and the psychological impact of chronic medical conditions in childhood.

*(Continued)*

(Continued)

**Lauren J. Holleb**, BA, received her bachelor's degree at Miami University in Ohio. She is currently a graduate student in the developmental-clinical psychology program at the University of Maine. Her current research interests include children's peer relationships and social cognition.

**Jack Stevens**, PhD, is a psychologist with Columbus Children's Hospital and Assistant Professor of Pediatrics at The Ohio State University College of Medicine and Public Health. He received his doctorate in clinical psychology from Indiana University. He completed his postdoctoral training at Cincinnati Children's Hospital Medical Center. His research interests include childhood disruptive behavior disorders and child abuse prevention.

**Judith B. Van Ginkel**, PhD, is President, Every Child Succeeds, and Professor of Pediatrics, Cincinnati Children's Hospital Medical Center and University of Cincinnati College of Medicine. She received her doctorate in political science at the University of Cincinnati. Her research interests include applying business models of quality assurance to early prevention programs.

# 4 Women and Generalized Anxiety Disorder

Marilyn is a homeless woman who is 34 years old and currently living with her three children in a homeless shelter where she is receiving meals, counseling, and a safe environment. She reports having been sexually abused as a child, and she indicates that this was previously disclosed to a social worker when she was in school. At that time, she was referred to a mental health center, where she discussed the abuse extensively. She tends to worry about events and problems over which she has no control. It is difficult for her to concentrate on what other families in the shelter are working on in group therapy because she is preoccupied with where the staff is at all times. Marilyn should be concerned about where and how she and her children will live in the future, but she is unable to make plans for the future. Instead, she seems to constantly be restless and irritable when making plans about living arrangements.

Generalized anxiety disorder (GAD) is one of the most common mental health problems in the United States and in the world (Grant et al., 2005). With this in mind, women are between two and three times more likely than men to have an anxiety disorder (Alexander, LaRosa, & Bader, 2001; Bekker & van Mens-Verhulst, 2007; Shear, Feske, & Greeno, 2000). Although approximately one third of women experience an anxiety disorder at some point in their lives, and anxiety is a risk factor for major depression and suicide, only about half of women with GAD receive treatment (Gwynn et al., 2008). In addition, research has shown that women may mask the disorder by using alcohol and other substances or by binge eating (Shear et al., 2000).

In the U.S., exposure to social adversity, specifically poverty and trauma, in the environment contributes to GAD in women who lack financial and social support (Corcoran, Danziger, & Tolman, 2003). The finding seems consistent with those in a recent study conducted in Belgium in which researchers found that GAD was significantly associated with living alone,

low level of education, and unemployment (Ansseau et al., 2008). The extent
to which women's anxiety is interpreted as a psychological problem depends
to an extent on cultural scripting (Friedman, 1997). Women's somatic
expressions of distress and anxiety may be perceived to be quite normative
and legitimate in some cultures. For example, in Newfoundland, the attack
of the Old Hag is a folk tale that explains both psychological and physical
symptoms in females (Ness, 1978).

## Definition of Generalized Anxiety Disorder

GAD is a persistent and common disorder that is characterized by at least
6 months of worry and anxiety that is not connected to recent stressful
events and may include feelings of threat, restlessness, irritability, sleep disturbance, and tension (Alastair, 2005; Tyrer & Baldwin, 2009). Moreover,
GAD is also characterized by an individual's sense of being unable to control
or predict events (Mineka & Zinbarg, 2006). Each of those characteristics
is actually a component of an anxiety syndrome that is often comorbid with
other disorders, particularly depression and substance abuse. Interestingly,
aspects of GAD syndrome are measurable in terms of palpitations, dry
mouth, and sweating (Tyrer & Baldwin, 2009). Typically, the course of GAD
is chronic, with symptoms that come and go; as a result, women who
experience GAD are likely to have ongoing impairment and disability
related to the disorder (Wittchen, 2002).

Alastair (2005) contended that "true" or "pure" GAD is somewhat rare
due to comorbidity with other disorders such as depression (Kendler,
Gardner, Gatz, & Pedersen, 2007). However, Ruscio et al. (2007) suggested
that the definition of GAD be broadened in order to capture the real picture
of this disorder (see Azid, 1999). Those researchers argue that the require-
ment of 6-month duration, excessive worry, and three associated symptoms
exclude many individuals who might be considered to have GAD. In fact,
when researchers used the United States National Comorbidity Survey data
and criteria in a time frame of less than 6 months, the prevalence of GAD
doubled. This is important in light of the possibility that lesser manifesta-
tions of GAD may predict the onset of other disorders, and this has particular implications for the possible prevention of depression among
adolescent females.

## Prevalence

In a study of 43,093 participants, the prevalence of 12-month and lifetime
GAD in the U.S. was 2.1% and 4.1% (Grant et al., 2005; see also Vesga-
Lopez et al, 2007). Grant and colleagues found that being female, middle-
aged, widowed, separated, divorced, and low-income presented the greatest

risk factors for GAD. By comparison, being Asian, Hispanic, or Black decreased the risk of GAD, which suggests that culture and ethnicity may play a role in protecting women from experiencing GAD or mediating its effects. The results of studies in Europe indicate that GAD is a significant mental health disorder there as well (Lieb, Becker, & Altamura, 2005; Munk-Jorgensen et al., 2006; Wittchen, 2002).

As noted in the introductory paragraph, most studies suggest that women experience anxiety disorder two to three times more often than males (Bekker & van Mens-Verhulst, 2007). Women who experience GAD are often seen in primary care, and due to worry, tend to use primary care more often than other patients (Kroenke, Spitzer, Williams, Monahan, & Lowe, 2007). Even so, researchers have found that approximately 40% of individuals who experience GAD receive no treatment for the disorder (Kroenke et al., 2007), which suggests that there are a considerable number of poor women who experience GAD, particularly those who have little access to services.

Several studies also address the impairment and disability that accompanies GAD. Revicki, Brandenburg, Matza, Hornbrook, and Feeny (2008) evaluated the effect of GAD, as well as anxiety severity, on the health-related quality of life (HRQL) among patients with GAD. As one might expect, the researchers found that anxiety symptoms resulted in impairment to HRQL and daily functioning, and the disability associated with GAD is greater for women than for men (Vesga-Lopez et al., 2007). Perhaps most important, GAD was found in one study to be predictive of suicide attempts and suicidal ideation, but not completions (Cougle, Keough, Riccardi, & Sachs-Ericcson, 2009).

Coelho, Cooper, and Murray (2007) noted the comorbidity of GAD and generalized social phobia (GSP). GSP is social phobia that occurs across a wide variety of situations. While both disorders seem to develop in families, one disorder does not appear to cause the other, and each is independent of the other. Low-income women (and their family members) may be especially vulnerable to developing both disorders within the context of stigmas associated with being economically disadvantaged and being female. It seems plausible that the stigmas attached to low-income women, particularly those on welfare, might result in considerable anxiety.

## Etiology

Genetic theory may explain as much as 25% of lifetime GAD, and it may provide the best explanation of GAD, especially when one considers the findings in twin studies. Hettema, Neale, and Kendler (2001) found in a meta-analysis of twin studies that the major source of GAD in families was genetic. Moffitt et al. (2007) examined the risk factors for GAD in a birth cohort followed through to 32 years of age and found that the antecedent risk factors for GAD and comorbid GAD and major depressive disorder (MDD) were similar. However, the researchers found that other risk factors in childhood, such as childhood sexual abuse (Borkovec, Alcaine, & Behar, 2004; Phillips, Hammen, Brennan, Najman, & Bor, 2005) and a history of depression in the family (Vesga-Lopez et al., 2007), may explain true GAD but not MDD. This finding indicates that GAD may exist apart from depression initially, depending on life experience.

Biochemical processes may also explain GAD in young females to some extent. Schiefelbein and Susman (2006) examined the relationship between anxiety type and change in cortisol levels in adolescents over time. Cortisol is often referred to as the stress hormone and as such, it is involved in one's response to stress and anxiety; cortisol plays a role in regulating blood pressure and immune/autoimmune responses. Specifically, the researchers examined the relationships between cortisol levels and GAD in youth between 9 and 14 years of age over an 18-month period of time. In testing for anxiety every 6 months, the major finding in the study was that greater changes in cortisol correlated with increased generalized and social anxiety in young females but not in young males.

Cognitive and learning theories also provide a context for better understanding GAD. One proposition is that metacognitive beliefs and meta-worry help to develop and maintain control over fear of events, though the relationship between meta-worry and GAD is contingent on the frequency of meta-worry (Wells, 2005). Along those lines, Mineka and Zinbarg (2006) contended that individuals (particularly women) who have a history of unpredictable lifestyles and trauma experiences, such as rape (Kilpatrick, Edmunds, & Seymour, 1992), are prone to GAD, and for those individuals, worry is a cognitive avoidance response that is reinforced by attention, which in turn, "suppresses legitimate emotional responding" (Mineka & Zinbarg, p. 20; see also Mohlman, 1999). Because this process may lead to more negative thoughts over the worry, and thus anxiety, it results in a vicious cycle. Likewise, a looming cognitive style, or style in which one constructs mental scenarios and appraisals of unfolding threat, may contribute to GAD (Riskind & Williams, 2005).

Psychosocial theories explain GAD in women relative to the broader environment, especially women's roles in society. Shear et al. (2000) emphasized that gender roles, gender-role stress, social relationships, and exposure to social adversity contribute to a higher prevalence of anxiety disorders among women than among men. While masculinity, or assertiveness and activity as contrasted with femininity and affiliation, appears to serve as women's protection against anxiety, this protection appears to be lost when women adhere strictly to masculine norms of behavior, such as in a workplace in which masculine norms set the context for behavior.

Family functioning may account for GAD as well. Ben-Noun (1998) found that the rate of dysfunctional families was higher among parents with GAD than among parents without GAD (see also Coelho et al., 2007). In marital relationships, women with GAD have lower emotional and intellectual intimacy satisfaction or experiences (Dutton, 2002; Minnen & Kampman, 2001). In addition, they tend to use an avoidant approach to solve problems, are ambivalent in expressing emotions, and feel unaccepted by spouses (Dutton, 2002). This may explain why the perception of parental alienation is more closely correlated with high GAD symptom scores among females in midadolescence than among males in either early or midadolescence (Hale, Engels, & Meeus, 2006).

# Screening and Assessment Measures

Many social workers are employed in settings wherein they have opportunities to screen women for GAD. We identify rapid screening measures that focus on the key components of GAD at points in the lifespan of women, specifically in terms of worry, the distinction between depression and anxiety, and self-control and emotional regulation. Due to the possibility that GAD predicts suicidal behavior and ideation, we have included a measure of suicidal ideation in adult and elderly women for use if it seems warranted. Based on a review of literature, we have included a measure of cognition for elderly women in light of the likelihood of the presence of developmental cognitive impairment in responding to measures.

## Prepubescent and Adolescent Females

Screening prepubescent and pubescent females seems warranted in light of the finding that early anxious and withdrawn behaviors predict later internalizing behavior or withdrawal or rumination (Goodwin, Fergusson, & Horwood, 2004; Masi et al., 2004). Unfortunately, anxiety may go undiagnosed in females because internalizing behaviors receive less attention in social environments than the externalizing behaviors of their male counterparts. In this regard, the evidence indicates that generalized anxiety in females may be associated with other factors, including attention-deficit/hyperactivity disorder, as well as learning disabilities (Quinn, 2005), early adverse stressors, such as maternal partner changes and childhood sexual abuse (Borkovec, Alcaine, & Behar, 2004; Phillips, Hammen, Brennan, Najman, & Bor, 2005), and parental alienation (Hale et al., 2006). In addition, the lack of attention to this group of females may also be due to the fact that adolescent females tend to worry as a function of development, making it difficult to know the extent to which worry is a primary symptom of GAD. With this in mind, we recommend instruments that social workers in various settings can use to screen both prepubescent and pubescent females for GAD.

> Beck Anxiety Inventory (BAI)
>
> State-Trait Anxiety Inventory for Children (STAIC)
>
> Columbia Suicide Screen (CSS)

The BAI is a 21-item inventory designed to discriminate anxiety from depression in adults, but it can be used with most adolescents, depending on their cognitive abilities (Beck, Epstein, Brown, & Steer, 1988). Each item describes a common symptom of anxiety. The respondent is asked to rate how much he or she has been bothered by each symptom over the past week on a 4-point scale ranging from 0 to 3. The items are summed to obtain a total score that can range from 0 to 63. Reliability coefficients range from .30 to .71 (median = .60). A subsample of patients (n=83) completed the BAI after 1 week, and the correlation between intake and 1-week BAI scores was .75. The correlations of the BAI with a set of self-report and clinician-rated scales were all significant. Women tend to score 4 points higher than men do, indicating that on average women in the sample may experience more anxiety than males.

The STAIC is a 20-item instrument used for screening children between 9 and 12 years of age for anxiety (Spielberger, Gorsuch, Lushene, Vagg, & Jacobs, 1983) The STAIC was developed to distinguish between anxiety as a function of a personality trait and anxiety as a fleeting feeling state. The instrument can be administered verbally to younger children and is easy to read. Respondents are asked to give two ratings for each item on a 3-point Likert-type scale; one rating concerns how relaxed they feel at the moment and the other concerns how they usually feel.

The CSS is a rapid 11-point self-report questionnaire to screen for suicidal behaviors in teens (Shaffer et al., 2004) The CTSS includes four stem items that address current and past suicidal ideation and attempts, depression, and alcohol and substance abuse. If the respondent answers *yes* to questions about suicidal behavior, he or she is asked *yes/no* questions about the seriousness of the problem, whether the respondent is receiving help for this problem, and whether the respondent would like to have help with this problem. The stem questions for depression and substance abuse are answered using a 5-point Likert-type scale (*1 = no problem; 5 = very bad problem*). If the problem is rated as a bad problem or a very bad problem, respondents are then asked about their concern regarding the problem, including whether they have seen a professional or have made an appointment to see a professional. The CSS is a new brief screening instrument that has excellent concurrent validity and that seems to predict the risk of suicidal ideation and attempts.

## Young Adult and Middle-Aged Women

Recipients of welfare, most of whom are women, experience GAD at a higher rate than women in the general population (Corcoran et al., 2003). In their study of 503 African American and White single women with children on welfare, the authors found that women in the sample, whose mean age was 29 years, experienced GAD at a higher rate than their counterparts in the general population of women (see Corcoran et al., 2003). Although the rate of GAD rose from 6.4% to 19% among women who participated in all four interviews, the rates for African American women were significantly lower than those for White women in two of three interviews in which they reported symptoms that met the criteria for GAD. This result suggests that ethnicity may be a protective factor against GAD (see also Grant et al., 2005); for example, it may be that African American single women with children are able to cope more effectively than White women with stress that is due to lack of financial resources or lack of social supports.

Anxiety disorders are prevalent during the perinatal period as well (Ross & McLean, 2006; Wenzel, Haugen, Jackson, & Brendle, 2005), and we assume that they are especially prevalent among women with few resources, based on the prevalence among women on welfare (Corcoran et al., 2003). We do know that the rates of both GAD and obsessive-compulsive disorder are higher for women in the perinatal period than for women in the general population (Ross & McLean, 2006). Heron, O'Connor, Evans, Golding, and Glover (2004) found that antenatal anxiety occurs frequently and contributes to intense postpartum depression (see also Sutter-Dallay, Giaconne-Marcesche, Glatigny-Dallay, & Verdoux, 2004). GAD during the perinatal period warrants attention in order to understand more completely how it may affect maternal quality of life and child development.

Interestingly, in a large representative sample, researchers also found a subsequent higher rate of GAD in younger women (under 20 years of age) whose pregnancies ended in abortion compared to the rate of GAD in their counterparts whose pregnancies resulted in childbirth (Cougle, Reardon, & Coleman, 2005). If antenatal and postpartum GAD is mitigated by mothers' contact with their infants postpartum (Lonstein, 2007; Wenzel et al., 2005), then it may be that the lack of infant contact among women who end pregnancies in abortion explains subsequent GAD. Another possible explanation of this phenomenon is that abortions may be more stressful and anxiety-provoking for younger women than for older women (Cougle et al., 2005).

Penn State Worry Questionnaire (PSWQ)

Generalized Anxiety Disorder-7 (GAD-7)

Beck Anxiety Inventory (BAI; see reference and discussion in previous section)

Acceptance and Action Questionnaire-II (AAQ-II)

Anxiety Screening Questionnaire (ASQ 15)

The PSWQ (Meyer, Miller, Metzger, & Borkovec, 1990) is a 16-item measure that asks adult respondents to rate how typical specific worry-related feelings are (1 = Not at all typical; 5 = Very typical of me). Examples of items include *If I do not have enough time to do everything, I do not worry about it*; *My worries overwhelm me*; *I do not tend to worry about things*; *Many situations make me worry*; and *I know I should not worry about things, but I just cannot help it*. The psychometric properties of the PSWQ have been well documented.

The GAD-7 is a 7-item scale that can be used to screen for GAD (Spitzer, Kroenke, Williams, & Lowe, 2006). Respondents are asked to rate on a 4-point Likert-type scale how often they were bothered by the following problems in the previous 2 weeks (0 = *not at all sure*; 3 = *nearly every day*): feeling nervous, anxious, or on edge; not being able to stop or control worrying; worrying too much about different things; trouble relaxing; being so restless that it's hard to sit still; becoming easily annoyed or irritable; and feeling afraid as if something awful might happen. The scores in each column are summed and a score of 10 (or more) is a cut point for GAD. The sensitivity at the cut point was 89%, and the specificity was 82%, which is acceptable. Cut points of 5, 10, and 15 may be interpreted as representing mild, moderate, and severe levels of anxiety respectively. This measure can be found at http://www.healthandage.com/Are-You-Over-Anxious.

The AAQ-II is a 10-item self-report measure that assesses emotional avoidance and emotion-focused inaction or lack thereof (Bond & Bunce, 2003). It includes items such as *Emotions cause problems in my life* and *Worries get in the way of my success*. The AAQ-II shows a significant correlation with other measures of anxiety and phobic avoidance in both clinical and nonclinical samples, and is moderately and negatively correlated with measures of depression and stress. Alpha coefficients range between .81 and .87.

The ASQ-15 is a 15-item brief anxiety disorder screening instrument designed for use in primary care settings, and as such, clinicians in other disciplines may use this measure as well (Wittchen & Boyer, 1998). It consists of stem questions for MDD, panic disorder, social phobia, agoraphobia, PTSD, and GAD. The ASQ was studied in a large, primary care-based sample size, is brief, and is in the public domain. It has demonstrated acceptable use as a measure of GAD, and its measures of sensitivity and specificity have been estimated at .89 and .82 respectively.

## Elderly Women

Weissman and Levine (2007) noted concern about GAD and other anxiety disorders in elderly women, even though some researchers posit that GAD may be a protective factor against mortality in elderly women (Holwerda et al., 2007). For example, worry may lead many elderly women with GAD to seek medical care early, and thus, GAD may play a preventive role in the diagnostic process. In fact, Wittchen (2002) found that the rate of GAD in primary care (8%) is significantly higher than in the general population (1%), but more important, the rate of GAD is higher for women in midlife (10%). Although Alastair (2005) suggests that late-life anxiety is often symptomatic of depression, this may be difficult to determine given the cognitive errors that may accompany GAD (Caudle et al., 2007).

Penn State Worry Questionnaire (PSWQ; see reference and discussion in previous section)

Hospital Anxiety and Depression Scale (HADS)

Beck Anxiety Inventory (BAI; see reference and discussion in adolescent section)

Anxiety Screening Questionnaire (ASQ-15; see reference and discussion in previous section)

Cognitive Somatic Anxiety Questionnaire (CSAQ)

The HADS is a 14-item measure used to screen for depression and anxiety in nonpsychiatric, medically ill nursing home patients (Zigmond & Snaith, 1983). The HADS-A is a 7-item anxiety subscale used to assess anxious mood, restlessness, and anxious thoughts, and HADS-D assesses symptoms that reflect the lack of interest in activities. Respondents are asked to use a 4-point Likert-type scale to indicate the extent to which they have experienced each symptom in the past week. Scores are summed, and for both scales, 0–7 is normal, 8–10 indicates a mild problem, and 15–21 is a severe problem. The HADS has excellent internal consistency (ranges from .89 to .93), and correlates positively with other measures of depression and anxiety.

The CSAQ is a 14-item self-report measure developed to screen for cognitive and somatic components of trait anxiety (Schwartz, Davidson, & Goleman, 1978). The measure has two subscales, each of which is associated with self-regulation techniques. Examples of the cognitive and somatic components, respectively, are *I worry too much over something that doesn't really matter* and *I feel jittery in my body*. This instrument provides insight into the extent to which cognitive and somatic aspects contribute to generalized anxiety.

## Cultural Nuances in Screening Women for Generalized Anxiety Disorder

Clinicians should be mindful that symptoms of anxiety may vary by ethnicity and culture (Azid, 1999). For example, Awaritefe reports that

African patients may complain of "worms or parasites in the head" or "heat in the head" (Friedman, 2001, 39). These are nondelusional descriptions of anxiety that one would likely hear in Nigeria. Antony, Orsillo, and Roemer (2001) pointed out that there are culture-bound syndromes as well, such as the Japanese *taijin kyōfushō* (see Mezzich, Kleinman, Fabrega, & Parron, 1996) and the Hispanic *ataques de nervios* (Guarnaccia & Rogler, 1999). In the first syndrome, the individual may have social phobia that presents as anxiety due to fear of making another person uncomfortable (the opposite of social phobia in western culture). In the second syndrome, the symptoms of anxiety may be "screaming uncontrollably, as well as attacks of anger" (Antony et al., 2001).

## Evidence-Based Practice

In this section, we highlight evidence-based psychological therapies that are categorized as cognitive-behavioral therapy (CBT) and psychodynamic supportive therapy and compare them to treatment as usual and wait list, as well as to each other. Hunot, Churchill, Teixeira, and Silva de Lima (2009) conducted a systematic review that focused on nonpharmacological evidence-based treatment of GAD in individuals between 18 and 75 years of age. This review relied on searches of the Cochrane Depression, Anxiety & Neurosis Group and the Cochrane Central Register of Controlled Trials, as well as results from supplemental searches of Medline, PsycInfo, and EMBASE (Hunot et al, 2009). We remind the reader that more women than men experience GAD, as well as utilize available services, so we believe the results of the review are applicable to women. In addition, we draw on more recent studies in the Cochrane Central Register of Controlled Trials to identify evidence-based practices that can be used for intervention and prevention with preadolescent and adolescent females and with women older than 75 years of age.

Hunot et al. (2009) included 22 randomized and quasirandomized controlled studies in outpatient settings between 1981 and 2003 that involved 1,060 participants whose primary diagnosis was GAD. Only the data from 13 studies were used, 8 of which recruited adult participants and 5 of which were limited to elderly participants. The authors concluded that the review provided robust evidence that psychological therapy using a CBT approach is effective in addressing GAD. While this review does not demonstrate that non-CBT approaches are effective, it does not imply that they are ineffective. CBT was compared against supportive therapy (nondirective therapy and placebo conditions) in 6 studies, but no significant differences were found, a finding that is likely due to the heterogeneity in the studies, especially the variance in number of therapy sessions. Subsequent to the collection in 2006 of the data used for the Hunot et al. review, several recent studies in the Cochrane Central Register of Controlled Trials have importance for the current treatment of GAD in adolescents, young and middle adults, and elderly women. Those are highlighted in the following sections.

## Adolescence

It is noteworthy that studies of adolescents address multiple types of anxiety disorders, including GAD. Based on teacher, parent, and self-reports, Bernstein, Layne, Egan, and Tennison (2005) found that group CBT with students between 7 and 11 years of age was more effective than no treatment and that group CBT with parent training was more effective than group CBT only. Similarly and based on teacher reports, Kendall, Hudson, Gosch, Flannery-Schroeder, and Suveg (2008) found that family CBT and individual CBT were more effective than family education among students between students 7 and 14 years of age who experienced either seasonal affective disorder (SAD), GAD, or social phobia. These studies could be replicated by social workers, especially by school social workers in a school district.

## Young and Middle Adulthood

The results in recent studies support the notion that CBT is the most effective practice in treating GAD in adults (Fava et al., 2005; Kehle, 2008; Stanley et al., 2009). The Kehle and Stanley et al. studies were conducted in agency and primary care settings, demonstrating that persons who present with GAD in nonpsychiatric settings can be treated effectively. Interestingly, Fava et al. (2005) found that adding well-being therapy to CBT was more effective than CBT alone. Well-being therapy focuses on an individual's autonomy, personal growth, environmental mastery, purpose in life, positive relations, and self-acceptance (Ryff, 1989), all aspects of life that warrant emphasis in the lives of women, especially those who are economically disadvantaged.

Additional studies show promise in the areas of family functioning, acupuncture, computer use, and acceptance-based therapy. When GAD patients receiving CBT with partners received nonhostile criticism, their relationships improved to a greater degree than GAD patients who had not received nonhostile criticism (Zinbarg, Lee, & Yoon, 2007). Individuals taking medications to address GAD experienced fewer adverse effects when they received acupuncture (Luo, Liu, & Mei, 2007). Computer-assisted retraining of persons with GAD to pay less attention to threats that cause them worry resulted in significantly reduced attention to threat compared to persons who received a control treatment (Hazen, Vasey, & Schmidt, 2009). In this case, individuals in the experimental group used the computer to see varied types of threats (some of which caused more anxiety than others), whereas those in the sham group used the computer to see a consistent type of threat more frequently.

By comparison, individuals with GAD who received immediate (versus delayed) behavioral therapy to accept internal fears and worries showed reduced GAD symptoms that were maintained at 3 and 9-month assessments (Roemer, Orsillo, & Salters-Pedneault, 2008).

### Late Adulthood

As with depression, stepped or collaborative care is recommended for anxiety disorders in elderly women, who tend to be poorer and live longer than their male counterparts. For example, collaborative care that first involves education about anxiety, monitoring, and then selecting a treatment modality (CBT, medication, or both) is recommended (Sullivan et al., 2007). Implementing this approach may be very useful in preventing the overuse and misuse of prescription medications by elderly women, especially after they experience the death of spouses or partners.

## Summary _____

In sum, social workers must be especially cognizant of the likelihood that females may be biologically and genetically predisposed to GAD. Within that context, it seems plausible that GAD is a function of learned behavior that reinforces worry as a means of avoiding emotional responding to threats in their social environments, and this may be particularly debilitating for low-income women. Social workers might also anticipate that perceived threats may actually be interpreted differently in the cultural scripts of women, particularly the scripts of poor White women, compared to the scripts of women from racial or ethnic minority groups. Worry may be a learned aspect of the script and a means of maintaining control over unpredictable events; in turn, the lack of emotion that allows women with GAD to avoid responding emotionally might explain why being single, widowed, or divorced are risk factors for the disorder.

It is important that social workers screen for GAD in light of the possibility that it may precede depression and may predict suicidal ideation and suicide attempts. In screening women for GAD, clinicians should pay particular attention to the components of GAD, specifically worry, the differentiation between depression and anxiety, cognition, and emotional regulation. In the process, it is important for social workers to give appropriate weight to each component relative to what might be most important at each point in the lifespan of women. Last, social workers must be culturally competent and use clinical judgment in identifying symptoms of anxiety among women from nonwestern cultures. Finally, social workers in a variety of settings can provide CBT if they have appropriate training or make referral to clinicians who have expertise in using CBT, as this method has been shown to be effective practice for adults suffering from GAD.

## Discussion Topics

1. Discuss the underlying issues related to the definition and prevalence of GAD.

2. Identify the various correlates of GAD among women, and how those correlates relate to low-income women.

3. Explain the etiological issues social workers must consider with respect to GAD.

4. Consider the possible role of coping in GAD, and how social workers can address this in assessing and treating low-income women.

5. Explore how screening differs by age, ethnicity, and lifespan issues among low-income women.

---

### CASE STUDY 4.1

Casey is a 38-year-old white female and the mother of three boys ages 9, 8, and 7. She has never been married and currently lives with her male partner. She completed high school, but is currently unemployed and dependent on her partner for income. She has never held steady employment, and she quit the job in a factory she held the longest (2 months) because she just could not handle being around people. She lives in a small, rural town and reports having no interests, religion, or spirituality. She was raised primarily by foster parents and institutionalized caretakers because her biological mother was distant and her father was both mentally and physically abusive. She has no siblings. Casey worries excessively about a number of activities, and the worry has been out of control for most of the last year. It causes her poor concentration, irritability, and sleep disturbance. Past traumatic events, such as child abuse, and stressors in her life are some of the causes of this, but she worries about whether or not it will rain. She is socially isolated, has poor socialization skills, and is constantly tense.

### Case Questions

What is your preliminary screening/assessment of the aspects associated with Casey's anxiety?

What role, if any, did her family history play in setting the context for current symptoms?

What screening and assessment measures might you implement to effectively understand the treatment needs that might best help Casey?

To what extent does depression precede GAD or vice versa in this situation?

Would your treatment plan for Casey be different if she were a member of a racial or ethnic minority group?

## Illustrative Reading

# Cognitive Behavior Therapy and Worry Reduction in an Outpatient With Generalized Anxiety Disorder

Siamak Khodarahimi

*Islamic Azad University-Eghlid Branch*

Nnamdi Pole

*Smith College, Northampton, MA*

**Corresponding Author:** Siamak Khodarahimi, Islamic Azad University-Eghlid Branch, Eghlid, Fars, Iran, e-mail: Khodarahimi@yahoo.com

This article describes the treatment of a 27-year-old female with a particularly challenging manifestation of generalized anxiety disorder (GAD) with prominent worry. A manualized cognitive–behavioral therapy (CBT) protocol, including problem-solving training, cognitive restructuring, and relaxation training techniques, was tailored to the patient's presenting profile. Several self-report measures administered during the pretreatment, posttreatment, and follow-up periods, including: the Penn State Worry Questionnaire (PSWQ), the Why Worry-II (WW-II), the Ahwaz Worry Inventory (AWI), and the Intolerance of Uncertainty Scale (IUS), indicated significant worry reduction following treatment. Many difficulties were encountered, most notably designing and monitoring homework. Treatment implications are discussed.

**Keywords:** GAD, cognitive-behavioral therapy, problem solving training, cognitive restructuring, relaxation training, worry

## Theoretical and Research Basis

Anxiety includes pervasive feelings of tension, dread, apprehension, and impending disaster, as well as unpleasant feelings of stress, uneasiness, tension, and worry (Salm et al., 2004). Among these, worry has often been singled out as a basic component of anxiety (Barlow, 2002). Worry can be explained as feeling uneasy, concerned, or troubled about something replaying in one's mind. It initiates a chain of thoughts and images that may be excessive and uncontrollable (Brosschot, Gerin, & Thayer, 2006). Worry is usually centered on real-life problems, but may not be realistic (Van Rijsoort, Emmelkamp, & Vervaeke, 2001). It can involve rumination about past, present, or anticipated problems. Clark and Claybourn (1997) found that individuals who worry often selectively focus on the possible negative consequences of events.

While worry is something that most people experience, it can reach pathological levels in certain individuals. Evidence suggests that pathological worry may emerge from subjective feelings of vulnerability, perceptions of uncontrollability, and intolerance of uncertainty (Buhr & Dugas, 2006; Dugas, Marchand, & Ladouceur, 2005; Van Rijsoort et al., 2001). Worry is believed to be a dimension of many anxiety disorders, including generalized anxiety disorder (GAD; Van Rijsoort, Emmelkamp, & Vervaeke, 1999;

Van Rijsoort et al., 2001). Indeed, beginning with the *Diagnostic and Statistical Manual of Mental Disorders 3rd edition, Revised* (*DSM-III-R;* American Psychiatric Association [APA], 1987) and continuing through the current *DSM-IV-TR* (APA, 2000), excessive worry has been delineated as the primary diagnostic criterion for GAD. In GAD, worry has been characterized by uncontrollable negative thoughts and images about future events (Borkovec, Robinson, Pruzinsky, & Dupree, 1983).

Cognitive behavioral theories suggest that anxiety disorders may be associated with a distorted perception of danger-related information, and empirical research has shown that anxiety is associated with systematic cognitive biases (Khodarahimi, 2005). For example, *interruption theory* (Mandler, 1984) highlights a process whereby ongoing cognitive activity is interrupted by an event, which produces diffuse autonomic arousal. The source of interruption is then evaluated either positively or negatively. If arousal is very high and the appraisal suggests that threat is involved, then fear and anxiety will result. Other research has shown that anxious individuals, including those with GAD (Mogg, Mathews, & Weinman, 1989), can show a pattern of selective information processing that favors the encoding of threatening information (Dalgleish & Watts, 1990; Mathews & Macleod, 1994; Mathews, Mogg, Kentish, & Eysenck, 1995; Williams, Watts, MacLeod, & Mathews, 1988).

Dugas et al. (2005) identified four main variables in conceptualizing anxiety within a cognitive–behavioral framework: (a) intolerance of uncertainty, which promotes "what if" thinking and compensatory worry, (b) positive beliefs about the usefulness of worry, (c) negative problem orientation (e.g., low problem-solving confidence which leads to catastrophic worrying), and (d) cognitive avoidance (internal strategies aimed at curtailing distressing thoughts and threatening images). Riskind and Williams (2005) argued that a fifth variable should be included in a cognitive–behavioral model for anxiety: looming cognitive style (LCS). LCS is characterized by a perception of constant impending danger. Individuals with LCS experience anxiety and worry in response to their appraisal that danger is unfolding (Riskind & Williams, 2005). Thus, LCS is theorized to be both a cognitive vulnerability factor and a maintaining factor in anxiety-related disorders. In addition, adverse early life events may influence these five cognitive–behavioral therapy (CBT) components and thereby also serve as a predisposing factor in development of anxiety disorders (Hattema, Prescott, Myers, Neale, & Kendler, 2005).

As originally formulated by Clark and Fairburn (1997), the CBT model for GAD mostly emphasized techniques for identifying and modifying thoughts and beliefs that prevent GAD patients from engaging in or benefiting from exposure treatment (Alford & Beck, 1997; Zinbarg, Barlow, Brown, & Hertz, 1992). GAD patients report greater frequency and intensity of worry, more difficulty controlling worry, and increased levels of impairment and depression compared to control groups (Mennin, Heimberg, & Turk, 2004). In addition, Dugas et al. (2005) found that intolerance of uncertainty is more characteristic of patients with GAD as compared to patients with panic disorder. Dugas and Robichaud (2006) examined the predictive value of the cognitive–behavioral model for severity of GAD diagnoses. Utilizing a clinical sample, they demonstrated that all components of the cognitive–behavioral model accurately predicted severity of GAD diagnosis, with intolerance of uncertainty again showing the strongest predictive value of the components. In sum, several

*(Continued)*

(Continued)

strands of evidence suggest that worry is an integral part of GAD and that CBT may be a useful method of reducing worry. Despite the aforementioned, there is a lack of systematic evidence that specific CBT techniques contribute to ameliorating the worry component in GAD. Thus, our case study examined the efficacy of the CBT techniques for worry reduction in an outpatient with GAD.

## Case Presentation

Sahar (a pseudonym) was 27 years old and referred for outpatient psychological services in Shiraz city, Fars province, Iran. She was married, had two children, and belonged to an upper social class. She had been feeling tense since her teens. She reported excessive worry, was self-conscious, tended to have sweaty palms, and perspired profusely when tense. She described her symptoms as follows: "my heart is shaken with overwhelming worry about threatening events but without any obvious danger." She and her family experienced significant distress as a result of her symptoms. For example, her spouse stated that she became easily and frequently worried about everyday life, particularly if she was slightly delayed in returning home. The family also experienced apprehension at the prospects of traveling, shopping, and working with her.

## Presenting Complaints

The patient's primary complaints were global worrying thoughts, beliefs, and images about herself or her family. She was aggressive in coping with stressful situations and also over-conscientious. She reported palpitations, breathing difficulties, sweaty palms, increased muscular tension, tension headaches, butterflies in her stomach, nausea, abdominal cramps in her right lower quadrant, and frequent loose bowel movements. When she became highly anxious, her face became flushed or pale, she exhibited tremor, and her hands became cold. She had difficulty falling asleep (initial insomnia) and frequently awoke from sleep after 2 to 3 hours with chaotic dreams of failure and breakdowns. Her condition was usually chronic and mild, but became worse when she encountered interpersonal stressors. For example, exacerbation of her problems during the 2 years prior to treatment was coincident with difficulty adjusting to her first newborn and sexual problems with her husband. She also had increased premenstrual tension and painful menstruation.

## History

Sahar's mother also suffered from chronic anxiety. Her father died when she was an adolescent. Sahar showed signs of anxiety in her young infancy. Though she was a shy girl, her early childhood and school adjustment were satisfactory until high school, when she become self-conscious about her weight. At the age of 16, she developed a peptic ulcer and was treated with Librium for her high stress. She performed normally in academic tasks in her university years but suffered from behavioral, emotional, physical, and cognitive symptoms of anxiety. These symptoms were partly related to disturbed interpersonal relationships with her peers at school. In sum, she exhibited anxiety and worry symptoms throughout adolescence, college, and her later adulthood. At the age of 22, she met full diagnostic criteria for GAD.

## Assessment

Sahar was screened and evaluated by clinical interview to determine whether she met *DSM-IV-TR* (APA, 2000) diagnostic criteria for GAD and/or other Axis I disorders. She also completed the self-report measures described below.

*Penn State Worry Questionnaire* (*PSWQ;* Meyer, Miller, Metzger, & Borkovec, 1990). The PSWQ is a 16-item self-report measure of the tendency, intensity, and uncontrollability of excessive and uncontrollable worry in adults. Example items include, "My worries really bother me" and "I know I shouldn't worry but I just can't help it." All items are rated on a 5-point Likert-type scale ranging from 1 (*not at all typical of me*) to 5 (*very typical of me*), and its scores range from 16 to 80 with higher scores reflecting greater levels of worry. The PSWQ has shown good internal consistency, a= .86-.95, test–retest reliability, $r = .74$-.93, and good convergent and divergent validity in prior research (Molina & Borkovec, 1994).

*Why Worry-II* (*WW-II;* Holowka, Dugas, Francis, & Laugesen, 2000). The WW-II is a 25-item questionnaire of positive beliefs about worry (e.g., "By worrying, I can find a better way to do things"). All items are rated on a 5-point Likert-type scale from 1 (*strongly disagree*) to 5 (*strongly agree*) yielding total scores ranging from 25 to 125. Five factors have emerged from the WW-II suggesting five subscales characterizing worry as: (a) an aid to problem solving, (b) a source of motivation, (c) a way of preventing negative emotion, (d) a way of preventing negative outcomes, or (e) a positive personality trait. However, only the WW-II total scale score was examined in the present study. The WW-II has demonstrated high internal consistency and adequate validity and reliability in prior studies (Dugas, Letarte, Rheaume, Freeston, & Ladouceur, 1995; Freeston, Rheaume, Letarte, Dugas, & Ladouceur, 1994).

*Ahwaz Worry Inventory* (*AWI;* Taghvaee, 1997). The AWI assesses economic worry, self-esteem worry, future worry, vocational worry, worry about relations with others, cognitive worry, worry from insecurity, and worry about details. It consists of 20 items (e.g., "I feel insecure") with four possible answers: "always," "often," "sometimes," and "never" coded 3, 2, 1, and 0 respectively. AWI total scores range from 0 to 60. In previous research, the AWI has demonstrated good test–retest reliability, $r = .71$ (Taghvaee, 1997) and construct validity, that is, positive correlations with the somatic complaints subscale of SCL–90–R (Derogatis, 1977) and the *Emotional Control Questionnaire* (*ECQ;* Roger & Nesshoever, 1987).

*Intolerance of Uncertainty Scale* (*IUS;* Freeston et al., 1994). The IUS is a 27-item self-report instrument assessing the general idea that uncertainty in life is unacceptable, bad, or frustrating. Sample items include, "I can't stand being undecided about my future" and "One should always look ahead so as to avoid surprises." All items are rated on a 5-point Likert-type scale from 1 (*not at all characteristic of me*) to 5 (*entirely characteristic of me*). IUS total scores range from 27 to 135. The IUS has shown excellent internal consistency (a = .91), good test–retest reliability ($r = .78$) (Dugas, Freeston, & Ladouceur, 1997), and acceptable convergent and divergent validity (e.g., stronger correlations with other measures of worry than measures of obsessions or panic; Dugas, Gosselin, & Ladouceur, 2001).

*(Continued)*

(Continued)

## Case Conceptualization

Interview and rating-scale data indicated that Sahar met diagnostic criteria for GAD at the beginning of treatment. Based on information gleaned from the patient and her spouse, she experienced above average levels of pathological worry since the time she was 23 years old and exhibited clear symptoms for GAD with prominent worry. Specifically, Sahar developed a chain of worries about future events in a range of domains including: financial, familial, and interpersonal dimensions of her life. She was very agitated, restless, impulsive, irritable, excessively worried, embarrassed, upset, and self-conscious.

## Course of Treatment and Assessment of Progress

Sahar was treated with individual CBT for GAD. CBT emphasizes the connection between thoughts, feelings, and behavior (Allen, MacKenzie, & Hickman, 2000; Dugas & Robichaud, 2006; Flores, Russell, Latessa, & Travis, 2005; Grant, Mills, Mulhern, & Short, 2004; McGuire, 1996) and focuses on providing practical, short-term, and present-centered techniques that can be implemented by the client in a variety of situations (Corey, 2005; Ryckman, 2004). The concepts and techniques of cognitive–behavioral treatment have received ample empirical support (Bourne, 1995; Corey, 2005; Craske, Barlow, & O'Leary, 1992; Dugas & Robichaud, 2006; McGuire, 1996). Clinicians are also free to choose from a variety of CBT techniques, leading to great flexibility in treatment (Clark & Fairburn, 1997; Corey, 2005).

Sahar was prescribed the typical regimen of CBT for GAD, which is one session weekly for 16 weeks. The cognitive component of her treatment consisted of problem-solving training (PST) and cognitive restructuring (CR; Craske et al., 1992), and the behavioral component consisted of relaxation training (RT) readily available through self-help books (Bourne, 1995; Dobson, 2001; Otto, Smits, & Reese, 2004; Zinbarg et al., 1992). In Craske et al. (1992) GAD treatment protocol, PST is first introduced to the client using psychoeducation. Clients are told that many people with GAD tend to view problems in vague and catastrophic terms and that many fail to generate solutions to problems (Meichenbaum & Jaremko, 1983). Clients are instructed as to how to break problems into more manageable segments and multiple "brainstorming" sessions teach clients how to generate productive solutions.

CR was developed as a means of addressing negative cognitive representations, such as expectations, beliefs, or self-statements. There are various types of CR, but all variations involve first helping the client become aware of self-statements, expectations, or beliefs that reflect unhelpful ways of thinking about the self, the world, or the future (Arciero & Guidano, 2000; Bryant, Moulds, Guthrie, & Nixon, 2005; Dudley, 1997; Khodarahimi, 2005). Cook and Heath (1999) provided a four stage process for CR of cognitive distortions in cognitive–behavior therapy: (a) elicit automatic thoughts, (b) identify underlying irrational beliefs, (c) challenge the irrational beliefs, and (d) replace the irrational beliefs with suitable alternatives.

### Sessions 1 and 2: Psychoeducation

The first and second sessions are designated for introducing patients to the philosophy and rationale of PST, CR, and RT. Sahar was provided with education about the CBT view of GAD and the rationale for the CBT techniques. She was also told that successful treatment would require considerable effort on her part including practicing techniques in and out of sessions.

### Sessions 3 Through 6: CBT Training and Practice of GAD

The second phase of treatment included training and practicing cognitive and relaxation techniques for coping with GAD and outlining Sahar's specific symptom pattern. CBT techniques including effective problem solving and cognitive restructuring techniques were addressed carefully. She monitored her performance and recorded her progress in a daily notebook. She discussed these records in each session with her therapist.

### Sessions 7 Through 15: Problem-Solving Training, Cognitive Restructuring, and Relaxation Training

In this stage, Sahar was encouraged to engage in various in-session and out-session worry evoking situations. Each in-session situation was scripted, read, and closely observed by the therapist following the patient's hierarchy of worrying situations from least to most worrying. Complete mastery of each step was required before the patient moved to more anxiety-provoking steps on her hierarchy. Toward the most severe end of the hierarchy, the scripted content included imagining that a worrying situation was occurring in the room, and that the patient encountered it using problem solving, cognitive restructuring, and/or relaxation during 20 minute intervals without activating worry, upset, or other GAD symptoms. Several sessions lasted longer than the traditional one hour appointment time to accommodate the imaginal exposure.

### Session 16: Relapse Prevention and Termination

The final treatment session involved a review of Sahar's progress, completion of her CBT guided tasks, generalization of her gains to other problematic symptoms, and a discussion of how to prevent relapse. In addition, she was asked to discuss ways to use what she learned in therapy to confront other GAD and worry symptoms that were not specifically targeted in treatment. Finally, the majority of the last session was devoted to creating a written document to summarize her progress and achievements for future reference. She completed the self-report outcome measures on the day following her final session and then again 2 months later (to assess the stability of her gains).

## Complicating Factors

A few challenges were encountered in the treatment. Consistent with her cultural context, Sahar voiced an initial preference for receiving pharmacologic treatment for her GAD. She required additional psychoeducation in Stage 1 to become persuaded by the CBT rationale and approach to treating GAD. In addition, extra effort was required to motivate Sahar to prioritize completing the psychotherapy homework, which she perceived to be in competition with her household responsibilities and the needs of her spouse and children. To assist with this, the anxiety hierarchy was prepared and the homework was assigned in collaboration with her spouse. The actual implementation of the CBT homework was arranged and supervised by an experienced assistant in her home. A final complicating factor emerged when Sahar reported that she might have a physical illness that would interfere with her treatment. However, after referral to a university medical center, she was deemed to be physically healthy and able to complete the CBT treatment.

*(Continued)*

(Continued)

**Follow-Up**

Two months after the final treatment session, Sahar and her spouse attended a follow-up session. The session involved: (a) posttreatment assessment, (b) celebration of accomplishments, and (c) review of relapse prevention strategies. In this session, Sahar completed the self-report measures described above and was assessed for *DSM-IV-TR* diagnostic criteria for GAD. Results indicated that she maintained a substantial decrease in GAD symptoms, including worry (see Figure 1).

**Treatment Implications of the Case**

The present case has implications for tailoring cognitive behavior therapy interventions to individual clients in outpatient settings. First, in general agreement with CBT models for GAD (Clark & Fairburn, 1997), the techniques employed in the case emphasized identifying and modifying the thoughts and beliefs that prevented Sahar from engaging in accurate thinking (Alford & Beck, 1997; Zinbarg et al., 1992). The specific components, that is, problem-solving training, cognitive restructuring and the relaxation training techniques were apparently useful in this outpatient situation, as anticipated by earlier work (Bourne, 1995; Cook & Heath, 1999; Dobson, 2001; Otto et al., 2004; Zinbarg et al., 1992). The treatment was effective in increasing certainty and worries tolerance and thus was able to improve problem solving and reduce cognitive distortions (Dugas et al., 2005). The therapy also reduced worries about the future, family, interpersonal, emotional, and physical

**Figure 1**   CBT Effects on Worry and GAD

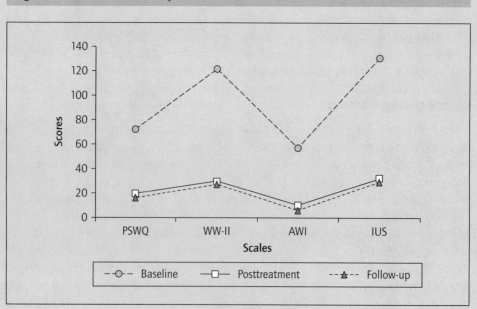

contexts. Finally, the present case study documents one way of addressing cultural concerns and other barriers to participating in CBT for GAD.

## Recommendations to Clinicians and Students

Enacting CBT techniques and procedures requires both rigorous theoretical and practical training, and attention to detail. For example, patients should be assessed for education, intelligence, and cognitive capabilities to determine whether they are capable of understanding and implementing CBT. Clinicians should also be sure to apply a comprehensive manualized CBT protocol for treating GAD in outpatient settings. Similarly, careful, progressive and ongoing assessment of GAD symptoms, including differential and complementary diagnosis, self-report scales, assessment of comorbidity, and an analysis of correspondence between treatment components and outcome should be taken into consideration by the clinician throughout therapy. Similarly, in agreement with CBT models, the worry construct and its vicious cycle in GAD treatment may require personalized tailored intervention in clinical practice. Finally, future research and theory development may be directed to refining these CBT techniques for implementation in outpatient cross-cultural settings.

### Declaration of Conflicting Interests

The authors declared that they had no conflicts of interests with respect to their authorship or the publication of this article.

### Funding

The authors received no financial support for the research and/or authorship of this article.

## References

Alford, B. A., & Beck, A. T. (1997). *The integrative power of cognitive therapy.* New York: Guilford.

Allen, L. C., MacKenzie, D. L., & Hickman, L. J. (2000). The effectiveness of cognitive behavioral treatment for adult offenders: A methodological, quality-based review. *International Journal of Offender Therapy and Comparative Criminology, 45,* 498–514.

American Psychiatric Association. (1987). *Diagnostic and statistical manual of mental disorders* (3rd ed., rev.). Washington, DC: Author.

American Psychiatric Association. (2000). *Diagnostic and statistical manual of mental disorders* (4th ed., rev.). Washington, DC: Author.

Arciero, G., & Guidano, V. F. (2000). Experience, explanation and the quest for coherence. In R. A. Niemeyer & J. D. Raskin (Eds.). *Constructions of disorders: Meaning making frameworks for psychotherapy.* Washington, DC: American Psychological Association.

Barlow, D. H. (2002). *Anxiety and its disorders: The nature and treatment of anxiety and panic* (2nd ed.). New York: Guildford.

Borkovec, T. D., Robinson, E., Pruzinsky, T., & Dupree, J. A. (1983). Preliminary exploration of worry: Some characteristics and processes. *Behaviour Research and Therapy, 21,* 9–16.

*(Continued)*

(Continued)

Bourne, E. J. (1995). *The anxiety and phobia workbook.* Oakland, CA: New Harbinger Publications.

Brosschot, J. G., Gerin, W., & Thayer, J. F. (2006). The perseverative cognition hypothesis: A review of worry, prolonged stress-related physiological activation, and health. *Journal of Psychosomatic Research, 60,* 113–124.

Bryant, R. A., Moulds, M. L., Guthrie, R. M., & Nixon, R. D. (2005). The additive benefit of hypnosis and cognitive-behavioral therapy in treating acute stress disorder. *Journal of Consulting and Clinical Psychology. 73,* 334–340.

Buhr, K., & Dugas, M. J. (2006). Investigating the construct validity of intolerance of uncertainty and its unique relationship with worry. *Journal of Anxiety Disorders, 20,* 222–236.

Clark, D. A., & Claybourn, M. (1997). Process characteristics of worry and obsessive intrusive thoughts. *Behaviour Research and Therapy, 34,* 163–173.

Clark, D. M., & Fairburn, C. G. (1997). *Science and practice of cognitive-behavior therapy.* London: Oxford University Press.

Cook, J. R., & Heath, D. H. (1999). *Cognitive behavioral therapy: Components of treatment.* Paper presented at Awareness, the 8th Biennial Conference on EFAPs, Vancouver, British Columbia: Canada.

Corey, G. (2005). *Theory and practice of counseling & psychotherapy* (7th ed.). Belmont, CA: Brooks/Cole-Thompson Learning.

Craske, M. G., Barlow, D. H., & O'Leary, T. A. (1992). *Mastery of your anxiety and worry.* Albany, NY: Graywind Publications.

Dalgleish, T., & Watts, F. N. (1990). Biases of attention and memory in disorders of anxiety and depression. *Clinical Psychology Review, 10,* 589–604.

Derogatis, L. R. (1977). *SCL-90-R: Administration, scoring and procedures manual for the revised version.* Baltimore, MD: Johns Hopkins University Press.

Dobson, K. S. (2001). *Handbook of cognitive-behavior therapies* (2nd ed). New York: Guilford.

Dudley, C. D. (1997). *Treating depressed children: A therapeutic manual of cognitive behavioral interventions.* Oakland, CA: New Harbinger Publications.

Dugas, M. J., Freeston, M. H., & Ladouceur, R. (1997). Intolerance of uncertainty and problem orientation in worry. *Cognitive Therapy and Research, 21,* 593–606.

Dugas, M. J., Gosselin, P., & Ladouceur, R. (2001). Intolerance of uncertainty and worry: Investigating specificity in a nonclinical sample. *Cognitive Therapy and Research, 25,* 551–558.

Dugas, M. J., Letarte, H., Rheaume, J. E., Freeston, M. H., & Ladouceur, R. (1995). Worry and problem solving: Evidence of a specific relationship. *Cognitive Therapy and Research, 19,* 109–120.

Dugas, M. J., Marchand, A., & Ladouceur, R. (2005). Further validation of a cognitive- behavioural model of generalized anxiety disorder: Diagnostic and symptom specificity. *Anxiety Disorders, 19,* 329–343.

Dugas, M. J., & Robichaud, M. (2006). *Cognitive-behavioral treatment for generalized anxiety disorder: From science to practice.* New York: Routledge.

Flores, A. W., Russell, A. L., Latessa, E. J., & Travis, L. F. (2005). Evidence of professionalism or quackery: Measuring practitioner awareness of risk/need factors and effective treatment strategies. *Federal Probation, 69,* 9–14.

Freeston, M. H., Rheaume, J. E., Letarte, H., Dugas, M. J., & Ladouceur, R. (1994). Why do people worry? *Personality and Individual Differences, 17,* 791–802.

Grant, A., Mills, J., Mulhern, R., & Short, N. (2004). *Cognitive behavioural therapy in mental health care.* London: SAGE.

Hattema, J. M., Prescott, C. A., Myers, J. M., Neale, M. C., & Kendler, K. S. (2005). The structure of genetic and environmental risk factors for anxiety disorders in men and women. *Archives of General Psychiatry, 62,* 182–189.

Holowka, D. W., Dugas, M. J., Francis, K., & Laugesen, N. (2000). *Measuring beliefs about worry: A psychometric evaluation of the Why Worry-II Questionnaire.* Poster presented at the annual convention of the Association for Advancement of Behavior Therapy, New Orleans, LA.

Khodarahimi, S. (2005). *The effects of psychotherapy on personality structure among outpatients with anxiety disorders.* Unpublished doctoral dissertation, Atlantic International University, U.S.

Mandler, G. (1984). *Mind and body: Psychology of emotion and stress.* New York: Norton.

Mathews, A., & Macleod, C. (1994). Cognitive approaches to emotion and emotional disorders. *Annual Review of Psychology, 45,* 25–50.

Mathews, A., Mogg, K., Kentish, J., & Eysenck, M. (1995). Effect of psychological treatment on cognitive bias in generalized anxiety disorder. *Behavior Research and Therapy, 33,* 293–303.

McGuire, J. (1996). *Cognitive behavioral approaches: An introductory course on theory and research.* Liverpool, UK: Department of Clinical Psychology, University of Liverpool.

Meichenbaum, D. S., & Jaremko, M. E. (1983). *Stress reduction and prevention.* New York: Plenum.

Mennin, D. S., Heimberg, R. G., & Turk, C. L. (2004). Clinical presentation and diagnostic features. In R. G. Heimberg, C. L. Turk., & D. S. Mennin (Eds.), *Generalized anxiety disorder: Advances in research and practice* (pp. 3–28). New York: Guilford.

Meyer, T. J., Miller, M. L., Metzger, R. L., & Borkovec, T. D. (1990). Development and validation of the Penn State Worry Questionnaire. *Behaviour Research and Therapy, 28,* 487–495.

Mogg, K., Mathews, A., & Weinman, J. (1989). Selective processing of threat cues in anxiety states: A replication. *Behavior Research and Therapy, 27,* 317–323.

Molina, S., & Borkovec, T. D. (1994). *The Penn State Worry Questionnaire: Psychometric properties and associated characteristics.* In G. C. L. Davey & F. Tallis (Eds.), *Worrying: Perspective on theory, assessment, and treatment* (pp. 265–283). Oxford, England: John Wiley & Sons.

Otto, M. W., Smits, J. A. J., & Reese, H. E. (2004). Cognitive behavior therapy for anxiety disorders. *Journal of Clinical Psychiatry, 65,* 34–41.

Riskind, J. H., & Williams, N. L. (2005). The looming cognitive style and generalized anxiety disorder: Distinctive danger schemas and cognitive phenomenology. *Cognitive Therapy and Research, 29,* 7–27.

Roger, D., & Nesshoever, W. (1987). The construction and preliminary validation of a scale for measuring emotional control. *Personality and Individual Differences, 8,* 527–534.

Ryckman, R. M. (2004). *Theories of personality.* Belmont, CA: Wadsworth.

Salm, A. K., Pavelko, M., Krouse, E. M., Webster, W., Kraszpulski, M., & Birkle, D. L. (2004). Lateral amygdaloid nucleus expansion in adult rats is associated with exposure to prenatal stress. *Developmental Brain Research, 148,* 159–167.

Taghvaee, D. (1997). *Construction and validation of worry measurement scale and its relation with anxiety, depression and educational performance among university students in Islamic Azad University.* Unpublished master's thesis, Islamic Azad University Arak Branch, Iran.

Van Rijsoort, S., Emmelkamp, P. M. G., & Vervaeke, G. (1999). Assessment: The Penn State Worry Questionnaire and the Worry Domains Questionnaire: Structure, reliability and validity. *Clinical Psychology and Psychotherapy, 6,* 297–307.

Van Rijsoort, S., Emmelkamp, P. M. G., & Vervaeke, G. (2001). Assessment of worry and OCD: How are they related? *Personality and Individual Differences, 31,* 247–258.

Williams, J. M. G., Watts, F. N., MacLeod, C., & Mathews, A. (1988). *Cognitive psychology and emotional disorders.* Chichester, UK: Wiley.

Zinbarg, R. E., Barlow, D. H., Brown, T. A., & Hertz, R. M. (1992). Cognitive-behavioral approaches to the nature and treatment of anxiety disorders. *Annual Review of Psychology, 43,* 235–267.

*(Continued)*

(Continued)

## About the Authors

**Siamak Khodarahimi,** Clinical Psychologist PhD, and member of faculty staff at Islamic Azad University, Fars province, Iran. He has been involved in the translating, co-editing and writing of several books and research projects in clinical psychology. He has presented at conferences and published articles in journals. He has been a member of several psychology organizations, and reviewer of some international psychology journals. He is currently starting his Post-doctorate Fellowship of Psychology at University Sains Malaysia (USM), Penang, Malaysia.

**Nnamdi Pole,** PhD is an Associate Professor of Clinical Psychology at Smith College and a licensed psychotherapist. He is also an Associate Editor of *Psychological Bulletin* and a member of the editorial boards of the *Journal of Anxiety Disorders* and *Psychological Trauma: Theory, Research, Practice, and Policy*.

# 5

# Income and Substance Use Among Women

At the request of school personnel, you visit Jane, age 29 years, the mother of 9-year-old John, the child who is the focus of the school intervention. John is having difficulties attending school and is disruptive in the classroom when he is present. The family lives in a small rural community where the neighbors know each other and about each other. When Jane opens the door she appears to be intoxicated; she slurs her speech and seems to be in a stupor. When she walks away from the door, her gait is unsteady. In addition to John, Jane has two daughters who are 5 and 3 years of age. All three children live with Jane and her boyfriend Jack, who apparently financially supports Jane and the children. John has told his teacher that his mother and Jack drink heavily and that he and his sisters often have to get their own meals and prepare for bed by themselves.

Practitioners are especially challenged to address substance use disorders (SUDs) among economically disadvantaged women. Understanding substance use among low-income women takes on importance in this book because it co-occurs with post-traumatic stress disorder (PTSD), generalized anxiety disorder (GAD), and depression. While substance use may involve abuse or dependence, it may also involve substance misuse, or the use of a drug for a purpose other than that for which it is intended (Alexander, LaRosa, & Bader, 2001). Moreover, as with PTSD, GAD, and depression, substance use is more prevalent among low-income women than among women in the general population, even though it is less prevalent than among men in the general population.

# Substance Abuse and Substance Dependence _____

Substance abuse is defined as a "maladaptive pattern of substance use leading to clinically significant impairment or distress as manifested by one or more occurrences in a 12-month period of time" (American Psychiatric Association, 1994, pp. 181–183). Those occurrences include: (a) recurrent substance use that results in failure to fulfill major role obligations at work, school, or home; (b) recurrent substance use in situations in which it is physically hazardous, such as driving an automobile when impaired by SU; (c) recurrent substance-related legal problems; and continued substance use despite having persistent or recurrent social or interpersonal problems caused or exacerbated by the effects of the substance. As one can see, abuse of a substance results in negative social consequences for an individual and may lead to substance dependence. Therefore, one can assume that abuse is subsumed under the dependence diagnosis (American Psychiatric Association, 1994).

By comparison, substance dependence is defined as a "maladaptive pattern of substance use leading to clinically significant impairment or distress, as manifested by three or more occurrences in the same 12-month period of time" (American Psychiatric Association, 1994, pp. 181–183). The occurrences include: (a) tolerance, as defined by either a need for markedly increased amounts of the substance to achieve intoxication/desired effect or markedly diminished effect with continued use of the same amount of the substance; (b) withdrawal, as manifested by either the characteristic withdrawal syndrome for the substance, or the same or a similar substance being taken to relieve or avoid withdrawal symptoms; (c) the substance is often taken in larger amounts or over a longer period of time than intended; (d) there is a persistent desire or unsuccessful effort to cut down or control substance use; (e) a great deal of time is spent in activities necessary to obtain the substance, use the substance, or recover from its effects; (f) important social, occupational, and recreational activities are given up or reduced because of SU; and (g) the substance use is continued despite knowledge of having a persistent physical or psychological problem that is likely to have been caused or exacerbated by the substance, such as increased depression.

A critical feature of SUD is the route of administration an individual uses to administer the substance, particularly when the route determines that large amounts of a substance are delivered to the brain quickly, as in intravenous injection (American Psychiatric Association, 1994). The speed of the onset, duration of the effects, and use of multiple substances are also very important features to consider. These features provide insight into gender differences that characterize SU, and how men and women may experience particular substances in unique, significant ways, as well as how poor women may be at greater risk of SUDs than women in the general population.

# Prevalence

Based on national data collected in 2008, several trends emerge with regard to the use of substances among females (Substance Abuse and Mental Health Services Administration [SAMHSA], 2009). The use of illicit drugs among females 12 years and older increased from 5.8% in 2007 to 6.3% in 2008, with the greatest increase in the use of marijuana. By comparison, the use of illicit drugs and marijuana among males 12 years and older decreased slightly from 2007 to 2008 by .5% and .1%, respectively. Within the context that females now have more access to alcohol than ever before, 15% of females between 12 and17 years identified themselves as current drinkers in 2008, compared to 14.2% of males (SAMHSA, 2009b).

## Pregnancy

The literature examining the use and misuse of alcohol and other drugs in pregnant women suggest that substance abuse during pregnancy has been increasing. Specifically, recent data on alcohol use in the U.S. shows that the rate of first-trimester binge drinking by pregnant females between 15 and 44 years of age increased from 4.6% in 2005–2006 to 10.3% in 2007–2008 (SAMHSA, 2009b). The data also showed that 21.6% of pregnant adolescents between the ages of 15 and 17 used illicit drugs in 2008, compared to 12.9% of adolescents who were not pregnant. Even though first-time pregnant teens between 15 and 18 years can modify substance use (Kaiser & Hays, 2005), many single mothers on welfare use substances (Cook et al., 2009).

In a large multisite study of 1,632 women in the United States, researchers explored the prevalence and correlates of the use of alcohol, tobacco, and other substances, including methamphetamine (Arria et al., 2006). The self-reports of users and nonusers, as well as a positive meconium screen (earliest stools of an infant in which maternal substance use can be detected in utero), were used to determine the use of substances during pregnancy. The findings were as follows: tobacco (28%), alcohol (22.8%), marijuana (6.0%), methamphetamine (5.2%), barbiturates (1.3%), and other (<1% heroin, benzodiazepines, hallucinogens). Women who smoked and used illicit drugs were more likely to be single and less educated, and to utilize public financial assistance (Arria et al., 2006).

## Women on Welfare

Cook and colleagues (2009) surveyed urban single mothers nearing the end of their welfare eligibility regarding their mental health vulnerabilities. A total of 29.1% of the women had lifetime SUDs and 9% had SUDs in the past twelve months; by comparison, Bassuk, Buckner, Perloff, and Bassuk (1998) found that among single mothers receiving Aid to Families with Dependent

Children (AFDC) between 1992 and 1995 (before the Temporary Assistance for Needy Families [TANF] was implemented), 38.1% of mothers had a SUD, compared to 20.3% of the general female population. When one considers that all rates reported were much higher than rates for women in the general population, the use of substances may also negatively influence the ability of young single mothers on welfare to manage the multiple demands placed upon them necessary to comply with agency requirements (Seefeldt & Orzol, 2005).

## Chronically Disconnected Women

Illicit drug use or meeting criteria for alcohol dependence is significantly correlated with substance use among another group of women, the *chronically disconnected* (Turner, Danziger, & Seefeldt, 2006). This group of women includes those who expect to move from welfare to work but who are likely to be sanctioned for failure to meet the work requirements and time limits of TANF. For example, this may occur to a woman whose child is too old for her to declare him or her as a dependent or is no longer in the home for other reasons, such as child abuse or neglect. Turner and colleagues examined the plight of chronically disconnected women, 55% of whom were African American, and found that this group of women had gone without employment or welfare benefits for 1 month prior to an interview with researchers and for at least one quarter of the months during the 79-month study period. While this group of women comprised 9% of the welfare recipients in the study (Turner et al., 2006), it is likely that this number will increase as economic conditions in the United States worsen.

## Women Without Children Seeking Assistance

Drug and alcohol problems are also prevalent among childless women who are without resources and who have access only to general assistance (GA; Lown, Schmidt, & Wiley, 2006; Schmidt, Dohan, Wiley, & Zabkiewicz, 2002). GA is a mechanism of local welfare funding that evolved historically, but it is not available in all states. In addition to having drug and alcohol problems, Lown and colleagues found that many of these women, who accounted for nearly half of GA applicants in a California county, had experienced exposure to severe violence, family distress, and/or homelessness. The needs of women without children for substance use treatment, as well as for shelter and financial support, are neglected in society.

## Older Women

Although substance use diminishes with age, and older men use substances at a rate five times that of older women (Han, Gfroerer, Colliver, &

Penne, 2009), the use of prescription drugs by older women is important to consider in this chapter. Among older adults, the use and misuse of prescription medication has the potential for abuse (Pharm, Simoni-Wastila, & Yang, 2006). Within the context that the US population is aging, one estimate is that 11% of older women (over 50 years) misuse prescription drugs. In fact, drug abuse among older adults is associated with being female, being socially isolated, having a history of substance use or mental health disorders, and being medically exposed to prescription drugs, especially medicines used to treat depression and anxiety, as well as those used to treat sleep problems.

# Etiology

The etiology of substance use reflects a complex, dynamic process that involves relationships among genetic, biochemical, environmental, and developmental factors. In this section, we examine the extent to which genetic factors might influence women's use of substances across the lifespan, with a particular focus on the adolescent period, as well as how biochemical processes may affect women's SU. Last, evidence suggests that environmental factors play a key role in SU, and for women there are particular environmental factors that contribute to their use of substances.

## Genetic Contribution

Researchers have found that there is a genetic component to substance use at various points in lifespan development, specifically during adolescence (Dick et al., 2007). In Finnish twin studies, the genetic influence on drinking increases from adolescence into young adulthood. At age 14, genetics account for 18% of variance in first time drinking, and this *was significant for females but not males* (Rose, Dick, Viken, Pulkkinen & Kaprio, 2001). At 16 years, genetic factors explained one third of variance in patterns of drinking for both sexes; by 18 years, genetic factors explained half the variance (Rose, Dick, Viken, & Kaprio, 2001). It is noteworthy that there may be no change at all in genetic contributions to particular types of substance use across development, such as is the case with genetic contributions to smoking patterns (Agrawal & Lynskey, 2006; Dick et al., 2007).

## Biochemical Contribution

Physiological and hormonal differences by gender may influence the direct effects of a particular drug, as well as the progression from use to abuse or dependence (Lucas & Weatherington, 2005). For example, when men and women use equal doses of alcohol, women reach a higher peak of blood level alcohol concentration than men, due to the fact that men have higher levels of alcohol dehydrogenase (ADH) in their gastric mucosa than do women (Smith & Seymour, 2001). ADH is the enzyme responsible for initiating the metabolism of alcohol, and with age the amount of this enzyme decreases. Likewise, several researchers have also found that the rate of absorption, distribution, and metabolism of particular drugs, specifically crack cocaine, may vary with hormonal changes during the menstrual cycle (see Ersche, Clark, London, Robbins, & Sahakian, 2006; Lex, 1991; Strickland, 2001).

## Environmental Influences

Environmental factors mediate or amplify the genetic and biochemical processes that contribute to substance use. For example, although the contributions of genetic factors to alcohol use increase from early adolescence to young adulthood, the contributions of environmental factors to alcohol use decrease from adolescence into adulthood (Rose, Dick, Viken, & Kaprio, 2001) However, researchers found that alcohol use very early in adolescence is explained mostly by family, school, and neighborhood influences (Rose, Viken, Dick, Bates, Pulkkinen, & Kaprio, 2003). While tobacco, alcohol, and marijuana use are mediated by similar genetic influences, shared environmental influences such as inadequate parenting may be more specific to each substance (Young, Rhee, Stallings, Corley, & Hewitt, 2006). We focus here on interpersonal violence, employment, HIV/AIDS, and homelessness as environmental influences associated with the use of substances by poor and low-income women.

### Interpersonal Violence

The findings in studies of welfare and nonwelfare populations of women show a connection between SUD and victimization, including physical and sexual abuse in both childhood and adulthood (Golding, 1999). On average, between one fifth and one third of women in samples of poor and welfare poor women are exposed to partner violence (Cook et al., 2009; Tolman, Danziger, & Rosen, 2001; Tolman & Raphael, 2000). Among these women, violence occurs at a rate two to three times the rate of women in the general population (Tjaden & Thoennes, 2000). The results in one study show that TANF recipients in Michigan who reported domestic violence had five times the risk of substance dependence as did women who reported no domestic violence (Tolman et al., 2001; see also Cook et al., 2009). Among chronically disconnected women, nearly 40% had used illegal drugs or were dependent on alcohol, compared to 22.5% of other women on welfare (Turner et al., 2006). Likewise, single women applying for GA in California had very high rates of severe violence and were likely to have a drinking problem (Lown et al., 2006).

*Employment*

The reform of welfare in 1996 required women on welfare to work, and employment has had both a positive and a negative influence on the outcomes of women on welfare who have SUDs. The findings in one study indicate that women on welfare who have SUDs have benefitted in terms of earnings and employment, though the benefits have been less for them than for women on welfare who have no SUDs (Meara, 2006). In another study, researchers found no differences in the benefits of employment for women on welfare with and without SUDs (Schmidt, Zabkiewiscz, Jacobs, & Wiley, 2007). Even though women on welfare with SUDs may have improved employment outcomes, the number of women on welfare has decreased—at least while the economy allowed for the realistic hope of employment—albeit the jobs were low paying and in the secondary labor market. With the decrease in the number of women on welfare, Pollack and Reuter (2006) emphasized concern about the ability to recruit women on welfare into substance abuse treatment, given that a disproportionate number of women with SUDs in the general population do not seek treatment for SUDs (Greenfield et al., 2007).

*HIV/AIDS*

The Centers for Disease Control and Prevention (CDC, 2008) estimate that 1 in 5 cases of women diagnosed with HIV are associated with injection drug use. While women may contract HIV via needles or other injection equipment, women who use crack cocaine or other drugs may contract HIV in the process of exchanging sex for drugs. In the United States, women from ethnic minority groups are at particular risk of HIV infection, and the risk is disproportionately higher for Black and Hispanic women (Centers for Disease Control and Prevention, 2008). In particular, Black women with a diagnosis of HIV were more likely than women not infected to be unemployed; to use crack cocaine; to exchange sex for money, shelter, or drugs; and to receive public assistance.

*Homelessness or Lack of Shelter*

As noted earlier, interpersonal violence, HIV/AIDS, and SUDs are associated with homelessness or lack of shelter among women, and this is also true for women without children who seek GA. In a prospective study, researchers examined psychosocial, behavioral, and economic predictors of alcohol use to intoxication, the use of crack cocaine, and marijuana use among 402 women living in temporary shelters in a metropolitan county in the western United States and found that 92% had a history of homelessness (Tucker et al., 2005). Depressive symptoms and risky sexual behaviors predicted all three forms of SU, though additional risk factors for intoxication included the inability to cope effectively with stress, presence of depressive symptoms, and feeling susceptible to HIV. By comparison, additional significant risk factors for the use of crack cocaine included the competing needs for shelter and food, the inability to cope effectively with stress, experiencing depressive symptoms, and having a partner who drinks to intoxication. Similarly, additional risk factors for women who used marijuana were presence of depressive symptoms and a partner who drank to intoxication. Across substances, protective factors were the ability to cope effectively with stress and to have social support.

## Screening and Assessment Measures

According to SAMHSA, the goal of screening is to identify individuals who are at risk of developing a SUD or may have one at the time of screening, in order to refer them for additional assessment and possible treatment. It may be quite helpful for clinicians to build rapport with women and ask questions regarding the context of their lives prior to mentioning SU, primarily due to perceptions held by many women that substance use is inappropriate for women, particularly for those with children. For example, most individuals drink, so it may be helpful to begin by inquiring about drinking, such as "Please tell me about your drinking." If the answer is negative, then one might ask, "What made you decide not to drink?" in order to determine if the woman is a lifelong nondrinker or a more recent nondrinker. We describe several instruments that can be used for screening in the following sections. When possible, we have selected instruments that require no formal training to administer, as well as those available for free online or with permission from the author or publisher.

### Adolescents

---

Substance Abuse Subtle Screening Inventory-Adolescent Version (SASSI-A)

Tolerance-Angry/Annoyed, Cut down or quit (using), Eye-opener (modified CAGE for pregnant women) (T-ACE)

---

#### SASSI-A

The SASSI-A is designed to identify both substance abuse and dependency. We have included this instrument because it is recommended for focusing on substance abuse and for use with adolescents who may have emotional or behavioral disorders as well. It takes 15 minutes to administer and 10 minutes to score, and requires no special training (www.sassi.com).

*T-ACE*

The T-ACE is a 4-item questionnaire developed to identify alcohol use among pregnant women (http://pubs.niaaa.nih.gov/publications/arh 28-2/78-79.htm). It takes less than a minute and requires no training to administer. In fact, nonprofessionals can use this instrument. It can be downloaded from the Internet, but we recommend that users notify Elsevier at www.us.elsevierhealth.com.

# Adults

> Alcohol, Smoking and Substance Involvement Screening Test (ASSIST)
>
> Alcohol Use Disorders Screening Test (AUDIT)
>
> Tolerance, Worried, Eye-opener, Amnesia, K/Cut down (TWEAK)

*ASSIST*

The ASSIST was developed by the World Health Organization (WHO) to elicit information about the substances individuals have used in their lifetime and in the past 3 months. It also identifies problems associated with substance use, the risk in the present and future, dependence, and injection drug use. The ASSIST can be used with pregnant women as well. It can be administered in 10 minutes and scored in 5 minutes. While training is recommended, it is not required; it is available in several languages. It is available online at http://www.who.int/substance_abuse/activities/assist/en/index.html.

*AUDIT*

The AUDIT is a 10-item WHO questionnaire developed to identify adults whose alcohol use has resulted in health problems. Although it can be used alone for screening, it is linked to a brief intervention for use with heavy drinkers or referral to specialized treatment. It takes less than 2 minutes to administer, and it is intended for use by trained professionals, including social workers, and is available online at http://www.whqlibdoc.who.int/hq/2001/WHO_MSB_01.6a.pdf.

*TWEAK*

The TWEAK is a 5-item scale originally developed to screen for drinking during pregnancy, so it is most useful in identifying drinking problems in women. However, it has utility for screening drinking problems in men as well. It can be administered in 2 minutes, scored in 1 minute, and requires no special training to administer. It can be used as either a self-report or interview screen, and is available online at http://adai.washington.edu/instruments/pdf/TWEAK_252.pdf.

## Older Adults

Cut-down, Annoyed, Guilty, Eye-Opener (CAGE)

CAGE Adapted to Include Drugs (CAGE-AID)

### CAGE

The CAGE is a 4-item nonconfrontational questionnaire developed to identify alcoholism. Although it can be used with older men and women, clinicians should be cautious in interpreting results when it is used with older women, primarily because alcoholism may be less evident in older women. No special training is required, and the CAGE can be administered in less than a minute without additional probing questions. It is available online at http://pubs.niaaa.nih.gov/publications/inscage.htm.

### CAGE-AID

The CAGE-AID modifies the CAGE questions to include screening for drug use as well as alcohol use. We have included this instrument due to greater prevalence of prescription drug use among older women than among older men. It is noteworthy as well that the rate of alcohol use by older men is higher than the rate of use by older women. It is available online at http://www.associatedneurologists.com/cage.html.

# Evidence-Based Treatment

Greenfield et al. (2007) conducted a review of literature on substance abuse treatment entry, retention, and outcome in women with SUD. The review included 280 relevant articles published between 1975 and 2005 and found in the PsycInfo and Medline databases. Of the 280 articles, 90% were published after 1990, and of those, 40% were published after 2000. However, only 11.8% of the studies were randomized clinical trials. Using the findings from the review, we discuss what we know about women and entry into, retention in, and outcomes of treatment for SUDs. With this information, we highlight studies that have particular utility in working with economically disadvantaged women.

However, prior to examining the findings from the review, it is important to note that the National Institute on Drug Abuse identified the following approaches for treating substance abuse: (a) medications that can be used to address withdrawal, as well as the abuse or dependence itself; and (b) behavioral interventions that include treatment that focuses on behaviors and attitudes related to substance abuse. Behavioral treatment occurs in outpatient settings and may be in the form of cognitive-behavioral therapy (CBT), multidimensional family therapy (particularly for adolescents), motivational interviewing, and the provision of motivational incentives. By comparison, residential treatment often involves the use of therapeutic communities wherein patients use staff and other peers in the community to make changes on a daily basis and become resocialized into a drug-free lifestyle.

## Women and Treatment Entry

Given the number of women who have SUDs, few actually receive treatment (Brady & Ashley, 2005; Pelissier & Jones, 2005). A possible explanation is that women define SUDs in terms of health and/or mental health, and as a result, they are more likely to seek help in mental health facilities or in primary care settings (Weisner, 1993). Entry into treatment is more likely to occur a short period of time following onset (Mojtabai, 2005), and even though both men and women have low rates of ever receiving treatment, women are less likely than men to seek help specifically for a SUD.

Given that barriers vary by population, there are five key barriers that prevent women from seeking help for SUDs (Greenfield et al., 2007). First, economic barriers may keep women from seeking help (Rosen, Tolman, & Warner, 2004). Second, women have a higher rate of co-occurring mental health disorders, and finding treatment for both disorders can be challenging in the absence of financial resources and time (Sonne, Back, Zuniga, Randall, & Brady, 2003). Third, substance abuse treatment programs are often mixed-gender, and for women who may have experienced or be experiencing sexual and physical assault and abuse, mixed-gender treatment may be undesirable or threatening (Kilpatrick, Resnick, & Saunders, 1998). Fourth, due to stigma placed on this problem among women, they may lack the support they need to seek treatment. Fifth, women, especially poor women, fear losing custody of their children if they enter treatment (Kail & Elberth, 2002).

## Women and Treatment Retention

In small clinical, nonrandomized studies that focus on gender differences in retention and completion of SA treatment, the results are inconclusive

(Greenfield et al., 2007). In studies that involve larger population-based samples, the results show few or no gender differences in treatment retention (Greenfield et al., 2007; see also King & Canada, 2006). For example, among 10,010 patients admitted to 96 programs that included outpatient drug abuse, long-term residential, and outpatient methadone programs in 11 U.S. cities, researchers found that men were less likely than women to stay in treatment 90 days or more (Simpson et al., 1997). In contrast, among 4,689 patients 18 years and older, including 1,239 women, gender was not associated with treatment completion (Brady & Ashley, 2005).

## Individual Characteristics

However, certain individual characteristics do predict women's retention and completion of SA treatment. Among mixed-gender groups of outpatients who were insured, predictors of women's retention included higher income, being married, and being unemployed (Mertens & Weisner, 2000). Alcohol and opiate dependence, as well as referral from legal or victims' agencies, explained the extent to which women were retained in treatment (Green, Polen, Dickinson, Lynch, & Bennett, 2002). In women-only groups, there were associations between retention and select patient characteristics including psychological function, personal stability, social support, anger levels, treatment beliefs, and referral source (Brown, Melchior, & Huba, 1995; Davis, 1994; Haller & Miles, 2004; Stahler et al., 2005). In one study, patient characteristics that predicted retention were having fewer children, higher levels of personal stability, less involvement with child protective services, and fewer family problems (Kelly, Blacksin, & Mason, 2001). In a large representative sample of women in treatment for SUD who were referred from noncriminal justice agencies, retention rates were lower among women who were members of ethnic minority groups (Brady & Ashley, 2005).

## Program Type

In addition to individual characteristics, Greenfield and colleagues found that program type is associated with women's completing treatment. For example, researchers found that women-only facilities or those that offer child care influence positively the length of time women stay in treatment, though this may not necessarily mean completing treatment (Brady & Ashley, 2005). Women who received both mental health and substance abuse treatment were more likely to complete treatment than those who received substance abuse treatment only (Brady & Ashley, 2005). Specifically, in studies that involved random assignment, randomized trials, and quasiexperimental designs, the results suggest that women have higher rates of retention in facilities where policies allow for children (see Hughes et al., 1995; Roberts & Nishimoto, 1996; Szuster, Rich, Chung, & Bisconer, 1996).

Haller and Miles (2004) examined retention rates for women in outpatient treatment, in women-focused day treatment, and in male-based treatment. The type of program contributed to retention rates, and day treatment contributed most positively to outcomes. In terms of characteristics, women who had engaged in drug treatment previously and married women had greater retention rates in outpatient treatment. The severity of women's drug problems and anxiety level were associated with retention in a residential treatment facility (Haller & Miles, 2004).

## Women and Treatment Outcomes

Research findings suggest that gender per se may not predict treatment outcomes for women, though certain characteristics of women actually do predict outcomes. In general, findings from selected studies suggest that the following factors predict treatment outcomes for women: (a) educational attainment (Greenfield et al., 2003); (b) self-efficacy (Greenfield et al., 2000); (c) co-occurring major depression (Greenfield et al., 1998); and (d) a history of sexual abuse (Greenfield et al., 2002). For example, women made greater gains than men in a methamphetamine abuse program when they were able to demonstrate self-efficacy in overcoming family and medical problems (Hser, Evans, & Huang, 2005; see also Henskens, Mulder, & Garretsen, 2005; Satre, Mertens, Arean, & Weisner, 2003).

Co-occurring psychiatric disorders, abuse history, treatment retention and completion, and matching counselor with patient are associated with substance abuse treatment outcomes in women. In general, when psychiatric disorders co-occur with SUDs, treatment is less effective (Greenfield et al., 2007), especially for women (Benishek, Bieschke, Stoffelmayr, Mavis, & Humphreys, 1992; Brown, 2000). It is not surprising that abuse history also predicted increased psychiatric hospitalizations and increased use of outpatient treatment services among 700 individuals with SUDs (Pirard, Estee, & Kang, 2005). In one large HMO study, women who completed treatment had higher rates of abstinence than noncompleters (Green, Polen, Lynch, Dickinson, & Bennett, 2004). Matching clients by gender and/or ethnicity may enhance outcomes for women in SA treatment (Fiorentine & Hillhouse, 1999; Sterling, Gottheil, Weinstein, & Serota, 2001).

In comparing women-only (WO) and mixed-gender (MG) programs, the results in one randomized controlled trial, two randomized studies, and one agency study provide insights into the outcomes of women who participate in the two types of programs. In a randomized controlled trial, the results indicated that both WO and MG programs that are of exceptional quality will result in positive outcomes for women (Kaskutas, Zhang, French, & Witbrodt, 2005). In randomized studies focused on retention and outcomes, there was no difference between WO and MG programs in one study (Condelli, Koch, & Fletcher, 2000); in another study, women with crack cocaine addiction had retention rates significantly higher in the WO program. In a nonrandomized study wherein the agency changed from MG to WO programs, there was no difference in either retention or completion for women (Bride, 2001).

In terms of outcomes, women's perceptions and attitudes toward treatment warrant attention. In particular, attention should be given to (a) importance of counselor fit, (b) fear of sexual harassment or intimidation in MG programs, (c) the need for child care, and (d) the possibility that MG groups might inhibit women's participation (Nelson-Zlupko, Dore, Kauffman, & Kaltenbach, 1996). In the end, WO treatment programs may need to address particular subgroups of women in order to be most effective (Greenfield et al., 2007).

## Evidence-Based Interventions With Poor Women

Since SUDs frequently co-occur with PTSD, GAD, and depression among poor women, we first examine programs that have used the Seeking Safety (SS) interventions that were initially developed to address the co-occurrence of SUDs and PTSD, as well as other mental health disorders. Although the interventions have been used with men as well, we describe the programs that have implemented SS to address SUDs in the population of women who have co-occurring mental health problems, especially as those problems are related to trauma, single parenthood, lack of resources, and homelessness. We also describe programs that have been implemented specifically to address SUDs among women on welfare, and we bring attention to the use of motivational interviewing in addressing SUDs, a therapeutic approach that has both process and product aspects.

### Cognitive-Behavioral Therapy and Dialectical Behavior Therapy in Seeking Safety Interventions

Seeking Safety is a twenty-five session CBT intervention that focuses on PTSD and SUDs and that can be adapted to a variety of settings (Najavits, 2002; www.seekingsafety.org). Initially, the intervention was implemented in eight substance abuse treatment agencies in the Tampa Bay, Florida, area that were part of the Tampa Practice Improvement Collaborative. The 202 female participants were 37 years old, on average, and included Caucasians (47%), African Americans (38%), Hispanics (9%), Native Americans (3%), and other ethnicities (3%). Ninety-one percent of the women were unmarried, 80% were mothers, and 35% of mothers reported having had parental rights terminated, primarily due to a SUD. Nearly three fourths of the women reported problems with multiple substances, 88% of participants had experienced trauma, and 27% reported receiving case management. Most important, the SUDs were associated with PTSD, depression, and anxiety disorders. Below is a synopsis of several studies of the effectiveness of SS that may have utility for treating poor and economically disadvantaged women, especially those women with these selected co-occurring mental health disorders.

*Substance Use Disorders and Post-Traumatic Stress Disorder.* In one study, 17 female outpatients who met the criteria for PTSD and substance dependence engaged in 25 sessions over a 3-month period of time. All women had five or more lifetime traumas with the average age of first trauma at 7 years, and 65% had one or more co-occurring personality disorders. Despite the absence of a control group, data suggest that women can improve when treatment is adapted to them (Najavits, Weiss, Shaw, & Muenz, 1998).

In another study, 17 women in a minimum-security correctional setting engaged in 25 sessions over a 3-month period of time. The women met the criteria for PTSD, substance dependence, and histories of physical abuse, sexual abuse, or a combination of both types of abuse. The most common drug of choice was cocaine, and all women who wanted treatment were offered treatment. While incarcerated, women made significant progress in eliminating symptoms of PTSD, and when released, the same women had reduced the use of drugs and alcohol at 6-week and 3-month follow-ups (Zlotnick, Najavits, & Rohsenow, 2003).

In yet another study, 107 women in an urban, low-income population who experience PTSD and SUD were randomly assigned to two kinds of CBT and standard community treatment. Forty-one women received SS, 34 received CBT relapse prevention therapy, and 32 received standard community treatment. At the end of 3-, 6-, and 9-month follow-ups, women in the CBT groups reduced substance use, PTSD, and other psychiatric symptoms while the participants in community care made no progress (Hien, Cohen, Litt, Miele, & Capstick, 2004).

In a controlled trial, 359 homeless women veterans were recruited as potential candidates to receive SS. Once staff was trained and certified to implement SS, 91 randomly selected women received the intervention; they were compared to women who received other types of services. The SS cohort had significantly better outcomes over 1 year in terms of employment, social support, symptoms of mental health disorders, and PTSD (Desai, Harpaz-Rotem, Najavits, & Rosenheck, 2008).

Another study had a pre-experimental, static-group comparison design, comparing persons who had and had not completed the SS program. Participants in the comparison group were five women who met the criteria for abuse of alcohol, cocaine, or marijuana and who either met the diagnosis for or exhibited symptoms of PTSD. Participants completed the SS program, and outcomes were positive when measures used were urine toxicology screens, a posttest for symptoms of PTSD, the Trauma Symptom Checklist (TSC-40), and a self-report posttest of coping skills used to manage substance abuse and PTSD (Mcnelis-Domingos, 2004).

*SUDS and Other Disorders.* In another randomized controlled trial, 33 adolescent females who were outpatients received either SS or treatment as usual (TAU). Outcome measures included SUD, trauma-related symptoms, cognitions, functioning, attendance, and treatment satisfaction, and at the completion of treatment, women in the SS group had significantly better outcomes than the women in the TAU group. At a 3-month follow-up, some gains were maintained, so SS may be a promising intervention for adolescent females with SUDs and co-occurring mental health problems (Najavits, Gallop, & Weiss, 2006).

A preliminary sample of 20 women received outpatient mental health and dual diagnosis treatment at Harborview Mental Health Services Women's Dual Diagnosis Program. The program used SS to meet the emotional needs of the women in the program, and the intervention integrated CBT, dialectical behavior therapy (DBT), and contingency management into a comprehensive program. DBT offers a focus on validation and change and increases women's confidence in their potential for change (Linehan, 1995). The results of the study show that the number of psychiatric hospitalizations was reduced and the length of sobriety increased. Participants also improved significantly with respect to housing sufficiency and work productivity (Holdcraft & Comtois, 2002).

In using an integrated trauma-informed approach to treating women with co-occurring disorders and histories of trauma, baseline and 12-month assessments were completed with 136 women in an experimental group and 177 women in a comparison group. The intervention group received SS while the comparison group received similar services but not trauma-specific group treatment. Women who received SS showed significantly better treatment retention over 3 months and greater improvement on post-traumatic stress symptoms and coping skills. On most outcomes, those who completed treatment improved more than those who discontinued treatment. Improvements on symptoms of distress and drug problem severity were partially mediated by gains in coping skills (Gatz et al., 2007).

In a pilot study, opioid-dependent women in a methadone maintenance treatment program received 12 sessions of therapy on the gender-based model in group format over 2 months. Using a pretest-posttest design, researchers found significant improvements in drug use (verified by urinalysis), impulsive-addictive behavior, global improvement, and knowledge of the treatment concepts. The program was characterized by a high attendance rate

(87% of available sessions) and strong treatment satisfaction (Najavits, Rosier, Nolan, & Freeman, 2007).

### Intensive Case Management and Temporary Assistance to Needy Families

Although many studies have shown the effectiveness of the SS intervention, Morgenstern et al. (2006) implemented a study specific to women receiving TANF. The researchers compared a long-term coordinated care strategy or intensive case management (ICM) with usual care (UC). For the study, they recruited 302 substance-dependent women who were receiving TANF, assigned them randomly to ICM and UC, and followed up at 3, 9, and 15 months. ICM clients had significantly higher levels of substance abuse treatment initiation, engagement, and retention than UC clients. The ICM clients had much better attendance, and their abstinence rate was 5 times that among UC clients (see also Morgenstern et al., 2009).

### Motivational Interviewing

Motivational interviewing (MI) is listed in SAMHSA's National Registry of Evidence-based Programs and Practices (SAMHSA, 2007). MI is a goal-directed, client-centered approach to practice with women who abuse substances. The assumption in using this approach to intervention is that the primary barrier to client change is ambivalent attitudes or lack of resolve. It has been found to be effective in treating SUDs, including alcohol, heroin, and cocaine use and abuse (Baer, Kivlahan, Blume, McKnight, & Marlatt, 2001; Bernstein et al., 2005; Carroll et al., 2006). It is noteworthy, however, that many of the studies were conducted with college students, and there is no evidence that there are gender differences in outcomes. The following elements are usually included in using MI (Miller & Rollnick, 2002):

- Establishing rapport
- Asking open-ended questions to explore the consumer's own motivation for change
- Eliciting recognition of the gap between current and desired goals
- Asking permission before providing information or advice
- Responding to resistance without direct confrontation; rather resistance informs the clinician to adjust the approach
- Encouraging the consumer's self-efficacy for change
- Developing an action plan to which the client is willing to commit.

# Summary

While genetic and biochemical processes contribute to the abuse of and dependence on substances, environmental influences such as exposure to interpersonal violence, homelessness, and lack of employment are greater influences on the use of substances by poor women. Given that social workers often practice with low-income women, it is important that they are knowledgeable about the quick and simple screening instruments that are available and can be easily used to screen women with whom they practice for SUDs as well as for mental health problems. Since women with SUDs are more likely to seek mental health services than substance use services, social workers must recognize that a disproportionate number of women, especially poor women, do not receive treatment for SUDs for a variety of reasons, including the fear of losing custody of children or lack of economic resources.

If women do enter treatment, they are less likely than men to complete the treatment program; when women complete treatment successfully, it depends on several factors, such as the type of treatment program, the women's personal characteristics, and the intended outcomes of the treatment program. Even though evidence is lacking to clearly inform social work practitioners whether or not women-only (WO) programs are better than mixed-gender (MG) programs, they can appreciate the possibility that any program for women should focus to some extent on mental health problems as well as SUDs. In this regard, numerous other factors, such as patient-counselor fit, contribute to women's success for SUDs.

In terms of evidence-based practice, the most successful programs for women are those that address mental health problems as well as SUDs, primarily by integrating CBT into a comprehensive treatment program. This finding has special meaning in light of the fact that CBT has been found to be the most effective intervention to address PTSD, GAD, and depression—the disorders that often co-occur with SUDs among low-income women. In one program, the use of CBT was also found to be beneficial as a means of reinforcing and validating women's potential for change. More important, it may be that these interventions must be integrated into an intensive case management approach that has been found to work with women on welfare.

## Discussion Topics

1. Delineate the difference between substance abuse and substance dependence.

2. Explain what is meant by the route of administration of a substance, and why this is important to consider in relation to gender.

3. Discuss substance abuse and misuse as they are related to particular groups of low-income women, such as age, regional, and ethnic groups.

4. Debate the etiological explanations of substance use among women, especially the environmental influences, and describe how social workers might introduce screening for substance abuse to low-income women.

5. Consider the complexity of measuring outcomes of substance abuse treatment among poor women.

## CASE STUDY 5.1

Susan is 18 years of age and 6 months pregnant. She lives with her boyfriend, who is 26 years of age. She is not in school, not employed, and plans to go on welfare after she has the baby. Even though Susan is pregnant, she is losing rather than gaining weight and appears malnourished, unkempt, and somewhat confused. Susan's relationships with others, such as friends, are based on their common use of substances. One of her male friends (who may be the father of the baby) is believed to be involved in making methamphetamine. A neighbor is concerned about what goes on in the home and called the police to report her concern. Susan herself seems unconcerned with her health, her future, or the baby she is carrying.

### Case Questions

Given Susan's age and health status, what would be your major concerns about Susan's probable abuse or misuse of substances?

How would you go about screening for the use of particular substances in Susan's case, and which instruments would be most appropriate to use in the screening process?

How problematic do you think it will be to motivate Susan to be actively engaged in addressing what seems to be a serious and debilitating substance abuse problem?

How would you prioritize Susan's physical and mental health needs for intervention?

What other community resources and support do you believe Susan would need to effectively address the challenges she faces?

## Illustrative Reading

**Research on Social Work Practice**

*A Meta-Analysis of Motivational Interviewing:*
*Twenty-Five Years of Empirical Studies*

Brad W. Lundahl

Chelsea Kunz

Cynthia Brownell

Derrik Tollefson

Brian L. Burke

### Abstract

**Objective:** The authors investigated the unique contribution motivational interviewing (MI) has on counseling outcomes and how MI compares with other interventions. **Method:** A total of 119 studies were subjected to a meta-analysis. Targeted outcomes included substance use (tobacco, alcohol, drugs, marijuana), health-related behaviors (diet, exercise, safe sex), gambling, and engagement in treatment variables. **Results:** Judged against weak comparison groups, MI produced statistically significant, durable results in the small effect range (average $g = 0.28$). Judged against specific treatments, MI produced nonsignificant results (average $g = 0.09$). MI was robust across many moderators, although feedback (Motivational Enhancement Therapy [MET]), delivery time, manualization, delivery mode (group vs. individual), and ethnicity moderated outcomes. **Conclusions:** MI contributes to counseling efforts, and results are influenced by participant and delivery factors.

**Keywords:** motivational interviewing; meta-analysis; review

**Corresponding Author:**

Brad W. Lundahl

395 South 1500 East

Salt Lake City, UT 84121

E-mail: BradLundahl@socwk.utah.edu

### Introduction

Motivational interviewing (MI), which originated in the early 1980s, has become a well-recognized brand of counseling. A simple literature search using the term "motivational interviewing" as the keyword in one database, PsycInfo, revealed three references during the 10-year span of 1980 to 1989, 35 references from 1990 to 1999, and 352 from 2000 to December of 2008. Interest in MI continues to grow at a rapid pace (Prochaska & Norcross, 2007), perhaps because it is short-term, teachable, and has a humanistic philosophy.

Only a brief definition of MI is given here as many other sources provide thorough explanations (e.g., Arkowitz, Westra, Miller, & Rollnick, 2008; Miller, & Rollnick, 2002; Rollnick, Miller, & Butler, 2008). MI is a counseling approach that is, at once, a philosophy and a broad collection of techniques employed to help people explore and resolve ambivalence about behavioral change. In brief, the philosophy of MI is that people approach change with varying levels of readiness; the role of helping professionals is thus to assist clients to become more aware of the implications of change and/or of not changing through a non-judgmental interview in which clients do most of the talking. A central tenet of MI is that helping interventions are collaborative in nature and defined by a strong rapport between the professional and the client. MI is unmistakably person-centered in nature (cf., Rogers, 1951), while also being directive in guiding clients toward behavioral change.

Professionals trained in MI generally gain knowledge and skills in four areas, consistent with the overall philosophy of MI: (a) expressing empathy, which serves many goals such as increasing rapport, helping clients feel understood, reducing the likelihood of resistance to change, and allowing clients to explore their inner thoughts and motivations; (b) developing discrepancy, which essentially means that clients argue, to themselves, reasons why they should change by seeing the gap between their values and their current problematic behaviors; (c) rolling with resistance, which means that clients' reluctance to make changes is respected, viewed as normal rather than pathological, and not furthered by defensive or aggressive counseling techniques; and (d) supporting clients' self-efficacy, which means that clients' confidence in their ability to change is acknowledged as critical to successful change efforts.

Through meta-analysis, the current article examines the degree to which MI is able to help clients change. Considerable research has been applied to the question of whether MI is effective or efficacious, including primary studies, literature reviews, and meta-analyses. Indeed, many gold-standard trials have examined the question of efficacy of MI (e.g., Project Match, 1997, 1998) and several previous meta-analyses on MI have been published (Burke, Arkowitz, & Menchola, 2003; Hettema, Steele, & Miller, 2005; Vasilaki, Hosier, & Cox, 2006). While we believe these efforts have done much to enhance our understanding of MI's efficacy, we believe further investigation through meta-analytic techniques is warranted for several reasons. First, we believe a different approach to conducting a meta-analysis may reveal a "cleaner" picture of the unique contribution of MI as we delineate further below. Second, many new primary studies bearing on the effectiveness of MI have been published since the last meta-analysis, and our search yielded several articles not included in previous reviews. (Note: Studies included in this meta-analysis included both efficacy and effectiveness trials; we use the term "effectiveness" here for consistency.)

Prior to reviewing previously published meta-analyses, we briefly review the goals and methods used to conduct these types of studies (see Cooper & Hedges, 1994; Lipsey & Wilson, 2001; Lundahl & Yaffe, 2007). Meta-analysis is a method for quantitatively combining and summarizing the quantitative results from independent primary studies that share a similar focus. As most primary studies vary in the number of people who participated and the measurement tools used to assess outcomes, a meta-analysis utilizes a metric that can standardize results onto a single scale: an effect size. An effect size refers

*(Continued)*

(Continued)

to the magnitude of the effect or the strength of the intervention. For the current meta-analysis, we used Hedge's $g$ (a nonbiased estimate of Cohen's (1988) $d$) as our effect size, which is a measure of group differences expressed in standard deviation units. For example, an effect size of $d = 1.00$ would suggest positive movement of a full standard deviation of clients in the treatment group relative to the comparison group, whereas an effect size of $d = 0.50$ would suggest positive movement of a half of a standard deviation. In meta-analyses, convention holds that an effect size around the "0.20" range is small, yet statistically significant, whereas effect sizes in the "0.50" and "0.80" are moderate and large, respectively (Cohen, 1988).

In a meta-analysis, effect sizes are calculated from primary studies and then statistically combined and analyzed. In addition to describing the basic characteristics of the empirical studies of MI interventions, our review attempts to answer three questions that are commonly explored via a meta-analysis (Johnson, Mullen, & Salas, 1995). First, meta-analysis investigates the central tendency of the combined effect sizes. Second, meta-analysis is interested in understanding variability around the overall effect size. If variability is low, then the overall effect size is considered a good estimate of the average magnitude of effect across studies. If variability is high, then the overall effect size is not considered a good estimate, which leads to the third common question in meta-analysis:

> what predicts the variability. To predict or understand high variability, two types of moderator analyses can be conducted: (a) an analog to the analysis of variance (ANOVA), wherein effect size differences are examined based on categorical variables within studies (e.g., treatment format, type of comparison group used), and (b) a weighted multiple regression, which uses continuous variables (e.g., treatment length) as potential predictors of the mean effect size (Borenstein, Hedges, Higgins, & Rothstein, 2005).

We now turn to a brief review of the three existing meta-analyses in the field of MI. Burke et al. (2003) published the first of these studies. These authors included 30 controlled clinical trials that focused primarily on the implementation of MI principles in face-to-face individual sessions. In terms of comparative efficacy. MI treatments were superior to no-treatment or placebo controls for problems involving alcohol, drugs, and diet and exercise, with effect sizes ranging from $d = 0.25$ to $0.57$. There was no support for the efficacy of adaptations of MI in the areas of smoking cessation and HIV-risk behaviors in the two studies available at that time. Results were near zero (0.02) in the seven studies that compared MI treatments to other active treatments, although the MI treatments were shorter than the alternative treatments by an average of 180 min (three or four sessions). Interestingly, MI effects were found to be durable across sustained evaluation periods. While only a few studies were included in the moderator analyses, Burke et al. (2003) found that higher doses of treatment and using MI as a prelude to further treatment were associated with better outcomes for MI in substance abuse studies.

Hettema el al. (2005) published the second meta-analysis that included 72 studies in which the singular impact of MI was assessed or in which MI was a component of another active treatment. Among groupings with three or more studies, effect sizes ranged from a low of $d = 0.11$ to a high of $d = 0.80$ (p. 97) across all studies, all outcomes (e.g., alcohol use, treatment compliance), and all time frames. While an overall effect sizes was provided, it may have been unduly influenced by a single outlier study that had an effect size that was more than 400% larger $(d = 3.40)$ than the next largest value $(d = 0.80)$. The authors also investigated several possible correlates or moderators of the outcomes, finding no relationship between outcomes and the following variables: methodological quality, time of follow-up assessment, comparison group type, counselor training, participants' age, gender composition, problem severity, or problem area. The only significant predictors of effect size for MI were as follows: manualized interventions yielded weaker effects and benefits from MI decreased significantly as follow-up times increased.

Vasilaki and colleagues (2006) published the third meta-analysis. Unlike the previous two meta-analyses that examined a wide range of behaviors, this study focused exclusively on studies of interventions that targeted excessive alcohol consumption. To be included, studies needed to claim that MI principles were adopted as well as include a comparison group and utilize random assignment. The aggregate effect size for the 15 included studies, when compared to other treatment-control groups, was $d = 0.18$ and, when compared to other treatment groups, it was $d = 0.43$, although this difference by comparison group was not statistically significant.

Considering the converging outcomes across these three previous meta-analyses, there is sufficient evidence to support MI as a viable and effective treatment method. In many respects, the three studies point to a similar picture: outcomes tend to be in the low-to-moderate range of effect sizes and are not homogeneous. Key differences between these three meta-analyses include the fading of MI effects over time (supported by only two of the three reviews) and the moderating variables that emerged, ranging from dose and format of the treatment to manual guidance and sample ethnicity.

In the current meta-analysis, we sought to address two common shortcomings in the previous meta-analyses: (a) they ran moderator analyses with small numbers of studies and (b) they included studies that could not specifically isolate the unique effect of MI without being confounded by other treatments or problem feedback. Thus, the primary goal of the current meta-analysis was to investigate the unique effect of MI compared with other treatments or control conditions. While it can be argued that "pure" MI is not possible, given the likelihood of including other components, some studies utilize designs that allow for isolation of the unique contribution of MI or provide a direct comparison of MI to other treatments. Our review only included such studies in an effort to overcome the potential confounds found in prior meta-analyses. Furthermore, our review sought to examine and clarify the possibility of moderator effects.

## Method

### Literature Search

Three basic strategies were used to identify possible studies. First, we utilized a bibliography of outcome research assessing MI that was compiled by the co-founder of MI, Dr. William Miller. At the time of the literature search (2007), 167 articles were cited in the bibliography, all of

*(Continued)*

(Continued)

which were secured and screened for eligibility. Second, we identified articles using the references cited in other meta-analyses and review studies. Third, we conducted a broad literature search using various article databases; this strategy had the most emphasis. Four search terms were used to identify articles reporting on MI. The two "brand names" most commonly used with MI were used, namely "motivational interviewing" and "motivational enhancement." To ensure that we did not miss other articles, we also included more generic terms that involve motivational interventions, even though such interventions may not have used MI proper, the other terms were "motivational intervention" and "motivation intervention." These four terms were entered using the connector "OR" so that any one of these terms would generate a hit.

The following 11 databases were searched: Psycinfo, PsyCARTICLES, Psychology and Behavior, Medline, CINHAL, ERIC, Business Source Premier, PubMed Academic Search Premier, Social Services Abstracts, and Sociological Abstracts.

We note that the other three meta-analyses, as far as we can discern, searched no more than four databases, which may account for the larger number of studies included in the current study.

In total, this strategy yielded 5,931 potential articles. These references were exported using Endnote software. In this process, references were categorized by author and 861 duplicates were identified and discarded. Using Endnote, the remaining 5,070 articles were screened and discarded if they were pubished before 1984 or were dissertations. Articles before 1984 were discarded because MI was not introduced until this date. This step removed 85 articles. We then used Endnote to search within the remaining articles. Articles were excluded if they did not have the terms "motivational interviewing" or "motivational enhancement" in the keywords, leaving 1,288 articles. We then cross-referenced the 167 articles previously ordered from the bibliography with the articles retrieved in the basic literature search, which produced 1,128 articles that were screened for inclusion.

## Screening Articles for Inclusion

The 1,128 articles were screened by their source and abstracts. Articles were retained if the abstract indicated that (a) the main principles of Motivational Enhancement Therapy (MET; see next page for description) or MI were used; (b) a treatment group and a comparison group were included; (c) the intervention was delivered by humans; (d) the study was published in a peer-reviewed journal (Note: This was done to establish a more homogenous sample of studies, to facilitate potential replication by other researchers, and because searching the "gray" literature can introduce systematic sampling error); and (e) the study was reported in English. This screening strategy yielded 183 articles that were then retrieved and combined with the 167 articles taken from Miller's bibliography.

Once the articles were obtained, they were subjected to a more rigorous screening using two criteria. First, the study design had to isolate the impact of MI on client behavior change or to provide a clear head-to-head comparison of MI to another intervention. A study was therefore included if (a) there was a comparison with waitlist or control groups, even when the effects of attention (talk time) were not controlled for (such as by mere dissemination of written materials); (b) an intervention used MI as an additive component and the comparison group also used the same intervention minus MI; (c) MI was compared to a "treatment as usual" (TAU) condition as this represents a head-to-head comparison of MI and other treatments even though the design cannot precisely isolate the impact of MI; (d) the intervention was MET, even though this subdivision of MI includes feedback from standardized assessment measures (we used this subdivision as a possible moderator; see page 135); or (e) the comparison group included the dissemination of written materials, such as an information pamphlet, as we reasoned that this type of comparison group is likely a hybrid between a waitlist and a TAU comparison group. Studies were excluded from this review if MI was specifically combined with another, identified intervention and the comparison group was only a waitlist or control group. Finally, studies originating from the Project MATCH Research Group (1997, 1998) were excluded from this review, even though they represented head-to-head comparisons, because the result sections of these reports most consistently reported interaction effects whereas our meta-analysis required reporting of main effects. Thus, if we were to extract effect sizes, they would not be representative of the entire sample across all Project MATCH sites and participants resulting in systematic sampling bias.

## Coding Studies: Reliability

Following the screening process, all articles were independently coded for participant characteristics and for study characteristics. Coding was conducted by graduate-level research assistants (CK and CB) under the supervision of the primary author. Average inter-rater reliability was high $r = .89$ for continuous variables and for categorical variables $k = .86$ (Landis & Koch, 1977).

## Dependent Variables: Outcomes Assessed

MI interventions have targeted a wide range of behaviors and, as expected, a wide range of measurement tools have been used to assess outcomes. Among the studies included in our review, we identified eight broad outcomes related to health. Of these, seven addressed observable behaviors: alcohol use, marijuana use, tobacco use, miscellaneous drug use (e.g., cocaine, heroin), increases in physically healthy behavior (e.g., exercise, eating patterns), reductions in risk-taking behavior (e.g., unprotected sex), and gambling. The other category included indicators of emotional or psychological well-being (e.g., depression or stress). Three other outcomes were also assessed that related more directly to client motivation: engagement in treatment (e.g., keeping appointments, participation in treatment), self-reported intention to change (e.g., movement in the Stages of Change model; Prochaska & Norcross, 2007), and self-reported confidence in one's ability to change. Finally, three other outcome groups were identified but not included beyond initial results because fewer than three studies contributed to each of the outcome groups: eating disorder behavior (binging/purging), parenting practices, and drinking potable water.

Within each broad category above, the specific dependent measures we identified were multifaceted. For example, indicators related to alcohol use include, but are not limited to, abstinence rates, relapse rates, number of drinking days per week, number of drinks

*(Continued)*

(Continued)

consumed, number of binging episodes, blood alcohol concentration, dependency on alcohol, and/or problems arising from alcohol consumption (e.g., drinking and driving). Each indicator provides a nuanced perspective of alcohol use patterns, and different measurement tools may examine slightly different aspects of each perspective. In our review, we grouped the multifaceted aspects of a particular outcome into its broader category (e.g., alcohol use) so that the reader will have a general understanding of the value of MI.

## Potential Moderators

We examined eight categorical variables and seven continuous variables as potential moderators to the effects of MI across these studies. The seven categorical variables were coded as follows.

*Comparison group.* Coded as one of five types: (a) waitlist/control groups that did not receive any treatment while MI was being delivered; (b) treatment as usual (TAU) without a specific treatment mentioned (e.g., groups received the typical intervention used in an agency); (c) TAU with a defined or specifically named program (e.g., 12-step program or cognitive-behavioral therapy); (d) written materials given to the comparison group (e.g., pamphlet discussing the risks of unprotected sex, drug use, etc.); or (e) an attention control group wherein the comparison group received nonspecific attention.

*Clients' level of distress.* In an effort to estimate the degree to which MI works with populations with varying levels of distress, studies were coded into three groups: (a) significant levels of distress or impairment, which meant that most of the sample (i.e., above 50%) would qualify for a diagnosis (e.g., alcohol dependency) in a system such as the *Diagnostic and Statistical Manual of Mental Disorders (DSM)* or the *International Classification of Disease (ICD);* (b) moderate levels of distress, when a problematic behavior was targeted even though the behavior probably had not caused significant impairment in everyday functioning (e.g., occasional marijuana use, overweight college students); or (c) community sample, when the targeted behaviors were important, but the sample likely functioned well (e.g., increasing adherence to a medicine or exercise regime or increasing fruit and vegetable intake in an otherwise healthy sample of participants).

*MI type.* MI is usually delivered in one of two methods. First, "standard" or "pure" MI involves helping clients change through skills basic to MI as described above. A second way to deliver MI is one in which the client (often alcohol or drug addicted) is given feedback based on individual results from standardized assessment measures, such as the Drinker's Check Up (Miller, Sovereign, & Krege, 1988) or a modification of it; this approach is sometimes termed MET (Miller & Rollnick, 2002).

*Use of a manual.* Hettema et al. (2005) found that outcomes tended to be weaker when studies used a manual-guided process. If the study explicitly stated that a manual was used, above and beyond basic training in MI or MET, then it was coded as such; otherwise, studies were coded as not having used a manual.

*Role in treatment.* MI has been used in a variety of roles/formats in the treatment process, three of which were coded for this study as follows: (a) additive, when MI was integrated with another treatment to provide an additive component. Again, if used in an additive fashion, the study design needed to be such that the role of MI could be isolated. For example, additive would be coded if two comparison groups examined the value of a nicotine patch and only one group used MI: (b) prelude, when MI was used as a prelude to another treatment. The format of prelude treatments was conceptually similar to an additive model, except that the MI component came before another intervention: or (c) stand-alone, when MI was used as the only treatment for that group of participants.

*Fidelity to MI.* Confidence that an intervention is linked to outcomes is increased when adherence or fidelity to the intervention can be established. Research teams have developed tools to measure fidelity to key principles of MI (e.g., Welch et al., 2003). Among the studies included in our meta-analyses, three levels of fidelity assessment were coded: (a) no assessment of fidelity; (b) fidelity was assessed or monitored, often through some form of taping or recording, with a qualitative system that did not produce a standardized score; (c) fidelity was assessed, often through some form of recording, using a standardized system (e.g., the MI skill code, MISC; Miller, 2002) that produced a numeric score.

*Who delivered MI.* As MI is being used by a variety of professional groups, we investigated whether educational background influenced outcomes. The following groups were coded whenever sufficient information was provided: (a) medical doctor; (b) registered nurse or registered dietician; (c) mental health provider with either a master's degree or a PhD; (d) mental health counselor with a bachelor's degree; or (e) student status, which generally indicates that the student was being supervised by someone with a master's or PhD degree.

*Delivery mode.* MI is traditionally delivered via individual counseling, though it is occasionally delivered via group format.

*Continuous variables.* The seven continuous variables we coded as potential moderators of MI effects can be divided into two broad categories: sample characteristics and study characteristics. Most of the continuous moderators need little explanation. Three different characteristics of the sample were coded: participants' average age, percentage of participants who were male or female, and the percentage of the sample who were White, African American, or Hispanic. (Note that we also coded for other racial groups but too little information existed to support analyses).

For study characteristics, we coded the number of sessions in which MI was delivered, the total dosage of MI in minutes, and durability by listing the longest time period in which post-treatment measures were administered. Finally, study rigor was also coded using an 18-point methodological quality scale (see Appendix for details).

## Effect Size Calculation

Effect sizes were calculated and analyzed through Comprehensive Meta-Analysis, a software package that was produced by Borenstein, Hedges, Higgins, and Rothstein (2005). We used *Hedge's g* as our main measure of effect size, the standardized mean difference that uses an unbiased pooled standard deviation similar to *Cohen's d* but corrects for bias through calculating the pooled standard deviation in a different manner (Cooper & Hedges, 1994; Lipsey & Wilson, 2001). A random effects model was used for all analyses, which is more conservative than fixed effects models and assumes that effect sizes are likely to vary across samples and populations (Hunter & Schmidt, 2000). Effect size extraction and calculation were

*(Continued)*

(Continued)

performed by the primary and secondary authors. Thirty-one percent of the effect sizes were double coded, with interrater reliability being very high (98% agreement).

## Results

### Study Characteristics

In total, 119 studies met the inclusionary criteria for this review. Of these, 10 compared two conditions of MI or two different comparison groups within the same study, and one study compared four MI groups to a single comparison group. Thus, a total of 132 MI groups were contrasted. Across these 132 group comparisons, a total of 842 effect sizes were computed because almost all of the studies reported on multiple outcomes, multiple indictors of an outcome, or multiple measurements of an outcome across time. With the exception of the meta-regression analyses (see below), multiple measures of a particular construct were averaged within studies to prevent violations of independence.

As we expected, this large body of literature varied in populations of focus, outcomes of interest, and how MI was presented to clients. Table 1 details some of the variability found in the studies, including the number of participants in the study, outcomes assessed, type of MI delivered, and the effect size for each individual study. Effect sizes in Table 1 are collapsed across dependent variables and moderators.

### Overall Findings

We organized our results around the three goals of meta-analytic inquiries: central tendency, variability, and prediction (Johnson, Mullen, & Salas, 1995).

*What is the overall magnitude of effect of MI interventions?* The average effect size across the 132 comparisons and all outcomes was $g = 0.22$ (confidence interval [CI] 0.17-0.27), which was statistically significant, $z = 8.75$, $p < .001$. This value is consistent with Cohen's classification of a small but statistically meaningful effect. The lowest effect size for MI was -1.40 and the highest was 2.06, neither of which were outliers. To gain a more complete picture of the distribution of effect sizes, percentile ranks are reported. The effect size at the 25th percentile was 0.00, at the 50th percentile the effect size was 0.22, and at the 75th percentile the effect size was 0.50. Thus, 25% of the effect sizes were either neutral or negative, 50% of the effect sizes were greater than Cohen's classification of a small effect size, and 25% were larger than a medium effect size.

Given the wide variability of outcomes examined, populations targeted, and methods used to deliver and study MI, the overall effect size is likely too broad to guide clinical or administrative decision making. For that, we need to examine effect size variability.

How representative or homogeneous is the overall MI effect size? The overall effect size contained significant heterogeneity as evidenced by the within-class goodness of fit statistic, $Q_w(131) = 228.71$, $p < .001$. The presence of heterogeneity suggests that the findings vary based on features of participants and/or study characteristics, which can be further studied via moderator analyses.

What variables can account for the observed differences in MI effect sizes across these studies?

**Table 1** Selected Study Characteristics and Average Effect Sizes

| Study Name | N: Tx/ Comp | Compare Group | MI or MET | Session/ Minutes | Longest Follow-up (Months) | Targeted Behavior Change | Effect Size | CI |
|---|---|---|---|---|---|---|---|---|
| Ahluwalia et al. (2006) | 189/189 | Strong | MI | 6/120 | 7–9 | Cig | –0.35 | –0.66–0.06 |
| Anton et al. (2005) | 39/41 | Strong | MET | 4/– | 1–3 | AI, Eng | –0.15 | –0.70/0.41 |
| Baer, Kivlahan, Blume, MacKnight, and Marlatt (2001) | 164/164 | Weak | MET | 1/– | 4 years | AI | 0.31 | 0.06/0.56 |
| Baker et al. (2002) | 11/8 | Weak | MET | 1/– | 10–12 | AI, Mar, OD | 0.01 | –0.56/0.57 |
| Baker, Heather, Wodak, Dixon, and Holt (1993) | 25/27 | Weak | MI | 1/75 | 4–6 | Risks | –0.01 | –0.55/0.52 |
| Ball et al. (2007) | 34/25 | Strong | MET | 3/– | IM | AI | 0.09 | –0.37/0.56 |
| Ball et al. (2007) | 34/29 | Weak | MET | 3/– | IM | AI | 0.21 | –0.28/0.70 |
| Baros, Latham, Moak, Voronin, and Anton (2007) | 80/80 | Strong | MET | 4/– | 1–3 | AI | –0.16 | –0.47/0.15 |
| Beckham (2007) | 12/13 | Weak | MET | 1/52.5 | 1–3 | AI | 0.86 | 0.06/1.65 |
| Bennett et al. (2005) | 66/45 | Weak | MI | 1/60 | 7–9 | Health | 0.18 | –0.20/0.56 |
| Bernstein et al. (2005) | 70/48 | Weak | MI | 1/20 | 4–6 | OD | 0–13 | –0.19/0.45 |
| Bien, Miller, and Boroughs (1993) | 9/12 | Weak | MI | 1/60 | 4–6 | AI | 0.45 | –0.34/1.24 |
| Booth, Kwiatkowski, Iguchi, Pinto, and John (1998) | 95/97 | Strong | MI | 4/– | IM | Eng | –0.07 | –0.38/0.25 |
| Booth, Corsi, and Mikulich-Gilbertson (2004) | 283/294 | Strong | MI | 4/– | 1–3 | Eng | –0.03 | –0.26/0.19 |
| Borrelli et al. (2005) | 76/96 | Strong | MET | 4/80 | 10/12 | Cig | 0.28 | –0.32/0.89 |
| Bowen et al. (2002) | 82/82 | Strong | MI | 3/– | 10–12 | Eng | 0.40 | –0.04/0.85 |
| Brodie and Inoue (2005) | 22/18 | Strong | MI | 8/480 | 4–6 | Health | 0.49 | –0.14/1.11 |

*(Continued)*

**Table 1** (Continued)

| Study Name | N: Tx/ Comp | Compare Group | MI or MET | Session/ Minutes | Longest Follow-up (Months) | Targeted Behavior Change | Effect Size | CI |
|---|---|---|---|---|---|---|---|---|
| Brown and Miller (1993) | 67/64 | Strong | MET | 1/– | 1–3 | AI | 1.19 | 0.36/2.03 |
| Brown et al. (2006) | 13/13 | Strong | MET | 4/– | 4–6 | AI, IC/SC, OD | –0.18 | –0.53/0.18 |
| Butler et al. (1999) | 202/210 | Weak | MI | 1/60 | 4–6 | Cig, IC/SC | 0.24 | –0.15/0.62 |
| Carey et al. (2000) | 24/22 | Weak | MET | 4/360 | 1–3 | IC/SC | 0.48 | 0.00/0.96 |
| Carroll et al. (2005) | 37/42 | Weak | MET | 1/60 | 1–3 | AI, Eng, IC/SC OD, Risks | 0.03 | –0.80/0.86 |
| Carroll, Libby, Sheehan, and Hyland (2001) | 31/29 | Weak | MI | 1/105 | 1–3 | Eng | 0.55 | –0.09/1.18 |
| Channon et al. (2007) | 27/20 | Weak | MI | 4/250 | 13–24 | Health | 0.63 | 0.05/1.21 |
| Colby et al. (2005) | 18/20 | Weak | MET | 2/47.5 | 4–6 | Cig | 0.37 | –0.16/0.91 |
| Colby et al. (1998) | 43/42 | Weak | MI | 2/52.5 | 4–6 | Cig, IC/SC | 0.48 | –0.43/1.38 |
| Connors, Walitzer, and Dermen (2002) | 38/38 | Strong | MET | 1/90 | IM | Eng | 0.23 | –0.22/0.67 |
| Connor et al. (2002) | 38/50 | Weak | MET | 1/90 | 10–12 | AI, Eng, GWB, OD | 0.44 | 0.02/0.87 |
| Curry et al. (2003) | 156/147 | Weak | MI | 5/– | 10–12 | Cig | 0.34 | –0.22/0.90 |
| Daley, Salloum, Zuckoff, Kirisci, and Thase (1998) | 11/12 | Weak | MET | 9/– | 1–3 | Eng | 1.82 | 0.38/3.26 |
| Davidson, Gulliver, Longabaugh, Wirtz, and Swift (2006) | 76/73 | Strong | MET | 4/180 | IM | AI | –0.09 | –0.41/0.23 |
| Davis, Baer, Saxon, and Kivlahan (2003) | Total = 73 | Weak | MET | 1/57 | 1–3 | AI, Eng, GWB | 0.14 | –0.33/0.60 |
| Dench and Bennett (2000) | 27/24 | Weak | MI | 2/67.5 | IM | Eng, IC/SC | 0.19 | –0.61/0.98 |
| Dunn, Neighbors, and Larimer (2006) | 45/45 | Weak | MET | 1/45 | IM | ED, Bx, Eng, IC/SC | 0.18 | –0.24/0.59 |

| Study | N/N | Quality | MI/MET | Ratio | Sessions | Outcome | ES | CI |
|---|---|---|---|---|---|---|---|---|
| Elliot et al. (2007) | 168/186 | Strong | MET | 4/12.5 | 10–12 | Health | −0.13 | −0.34/0.08 |
| Elliot et al. (2007) | 168/135 | Weak | MET | 4/12.5 | 10.12 | Health | 0.26 | 0.04/0.49 |
| Emmen, Schippers, Wollersheim, and Bleijenberg (2005) | 61/62 | Weak | MET | 2/150 | 4–6 | AI, IC/SC | 0.18 | −0.21/0.57 |
| Emmons et al. (2001) | 116/120 | Weak | MET | 1/37.2 | 4–6 | Cig | 0.30 | 0.04/0.55 |
| Galbraith (1989) | 12/12 | Strong | MI | 1/45 | 10–12 | A/C | 0.51 | −0.27/1.30 |
| Gentilello et al. (1999) | 66/307 | Weak | MET | 1/30 | 10–12 | AI, Risks | 0.15 | −0.02/0.32 |
| Golin et al. (2006) | 30/35 | Strong | MI | 2/– | 1–3 | A/C, AI, Mar., Eng OD | 0.19 | −0.28/0.66 |
| Graeber, Moyers, Griffith, Guajardo, and Tonigan (2003) | 15/13 | Strong | MI | 21/80 | 10–12 | AI | 0.02 | −0.71/−0.75 |
| Gray, McCambridge, and Strang (2005) | 90/48 | Weak | MI | 1/120 | 1–3 | Eng | 0.00 | −0.27/−0.27 |
| Grenard et al. (2007) | 11/7 | Weak | MI | 1/– | 1–3 | OD | 0.25 | −0.47/−0.98 |
| Handmaker, Miller, and Manicke (1999) | 7/7 | Weak | MET | 1/37.5 | 4–6 | AI | 0.45 | −0.01/−0.91 |
| Harland et al. (1999) | 88/89 | Weak | – | 4/– | 10–12 | AI | 0.54 | 0.12/0.96 |
| Haug, Svikis, and DiClemente (2004) | 30/23 | Weak | MET | 3/180 | 1–3 | Eng, OD | 0.15 | −0.89/1.20 |
| Helstrom, Hutchison, and Bryan (2007) | 38/29 | Strong | MET | 1/50 | 7–9 | AI | 0.78 | 0.00/1.57 |
| Hillsdon, Thorogood, White, and Foster (2002) | 302/285 | Weak | MET | 1/50 | 7–9 | AI | 0.94 | 0.18/1.71 |
| Hodgins, Currie, El-Guebaly, and Peden (2004) | 28/24 | Weak | MET | 4/240 | 1–3 | AI, Risks, Mar. | 0.41 | −0.14/0.96 |
| Hodgins, Currie, El-Guebaly (2001) | 31/34 | Weak | MET | 6/60 | IM | Eng | 0.45 | −0.01/0.91 |
| Hodgins et al. (2001) | 31/33 | Weak | MI | 3/135 | 1–3 | AI. Mar., OD | 0.01 | −0.32/0.34 |
| Hulse and Tait (2003) | 47/37 | Weak | MET | 1/105 | 1–3 | IC/SC, Risks | 0.27 | −0.14/0.69 |
| Hulse and Tait (2002) | 58/62 | Weak | MI | 2/65 | <1 | Cig | −0.89 | −1.88/0.09 |

*(Continued)*

**Table 1** (Continued)

| Study Name | N: Tx/ Comp | Compare Group | MI or MET | Session/ Minutes | Longest Follow-up (Months) | Targeted Behavior Change | Effect Size | CI |
|---|---|---|---|---|---|---|---|---|
| Humfress et al. (2002) | 45/45 | Weak | MET | 20/1800 | 4–6 | AI, OD | –0.14 | –0.42/0.15 |
| Ingersoll et al. (2005) | 94/105 | Weak | MET | 1/30 | 1–3 | AI, Eng | 0.10 | –0.17/0.37 |
| Jaworksi and Carey (2001) | 26/26 | Strong | MET | 1/60 | 4–6 | A/C, IC/SC, Eng, OD | 0.20 | –0.21/0.61 |
| Johnston, Rivara, Droesch, Dunn, and Copass (2007) | 82/92 | Weak | MI | 1/30 | 3 years | AI | 0.43 | –0.11/0.97 |
| Juarez, Walters, Daugherty, and Radi (2006) | 21/15 | Weak | MET | 1/45 | IM | IC/SC | 0.49 | –0.30/1.29 |
| Juarez et al. (2006) | 21/18 | Weak | MET | 1/60 | 4–6 | AI, OD | 0.02 | –0.46/0.51 |
| Juarez et al. (2006) | 20/15 | Strong | MET | 3/180 | 4–6 | Eng | 0.48 | –0.21/1.17 |
| Juarez et al. (2006) | 20/18 | Strong | MET | 4/– | 4–6 | AI, GWB | 0.29 | –0.22/0.79 |
| Kahler et al. (2004) | 24/24 | Weak | MET | 6/– | 4–6 | AI, GWB | 1.20 | 0.64/1.76 |
| Kelly and Lapworth (2006) | 28/22 | Weak | MI | 19/– | 4–6 | Eng, Health | 0.82 | –0.20/1.84 |
| Kidorf et al. (2005) | 98/96 | Strong | MI | 6/– | 10–12 | Cig | 0.09 | –0.48/0.65 |
| Kreman et al. (2006) | 12/12 | Weak | MI | 3/60 | 10–12 | Cig | 1.00 | 0.32/1.69 |
| Kuchipudi, Hobein, Flickinger, and Iber (1990) | 45/49 | Weak | MI | 1/40 | 10–12 | AI | 0.09 | –0.42/0.61 |
| Larimer et al. (2001) | 64/52 | Weak | MET | 1/60 | 1–3 | AI, Mar. | 0.22 | –0.37/0.79 |
| Litt, Kadden, and Stephens (2005) | 137/128 | Weak | MET | 2/100 | 4–6 | AI | 0.11 | –0.26/0.48 |
| Longabaugh et al. (2001) | 182/188 | Weak | MET | 2/150 | 1–3 | Eng | 0.21 | –0.14/0.55 |
| Longabaugh et al. (2001) | 169/188 | Weak | MET | 2/100 | 4–6 | AI, risks | 0.36 | –0.09/0.80 |
| Longshore and Grills (2000) | 40/41 | Weak | MI | 1/40 | 1–3 | Eng, IC/SC | 1.00 | –0.02/2.02 |

| Study | N | Quality | Intervention | Ratio | Dose | Outcome | ES | C.I. |
|---|---|---|---|---|---|---|---|---|
| Maisto et al. (2001) | 73/85 | Weak | MET | 2/180 | 4–6 | Mar. | 1.20 | 0.81/1.59 |
| Maisto et al. (2001) | 73/74 | Strong | MET | 2/180 | 13–24 | Mar. | -0.08 | -0.39/0.22 |
| Maltby and Tolin (2005) | 7/5 | Strong | MI | 2/120 | IM | Eng, IC/SC, OD | 0.30 | -0.24/0.83 |
| Marijuana tx project (2004) | 128/137 | Weak | MET | 4/– | IM | A/C, GWB, IC/SC | 0.66 | 0.02/1.30 |
| Marsden et al. (2006) | 166/176 | Weak | MET | 3/54.5 | 4–6 | Cig | 0.11 | -0.23/0.45 |
| Martino, Carroll, Nich, and Rounsaville (2006) | 24/20 | Strong | MET | 1/– | 1–3 | Cig | -0.12 | -0.88/0.63 |
| McCambridge and Strang (2004a) | 65/81 | Weak | MI | 4/150 | <1 | Cig | -0.32 | -1.17/0.53 |
| McCambridge and Strang (2004b) | 84/78 | Weak | MI | 3.5/105 | 1–3 | Cig | 0.08 | -0.27/0.43 |
| Mhurchu, Margetts, and Speller (1998), 165 | 47/50 | Weak | MI | | IM | WSDP | 0.73 | 0.31/1.15 |
| Michael, Curtin, Kirkley, and Jones (2006) | 47/44 | Weak | MI | 3/150 | 10–12 | Al, GWB | 0.04 | -0.13/0.20 |
| Miller, Benefield, and Tonigan (1993) | 14/14 | Weak | MET | – | 13–24 | Eng | 0.12 | -0.18/0.41 |
| Valanis et al. (2003) | 126/127 | Weak | MI | – | 13–24 | Eng | 0.34 | 0.05/0.62 |
| Walker, Roffman, Stephens, Berghuis, and (2006) | 47/50 | Weak | MET | 2/90 | 1–3 | Mar. | 0.31 | 0.11/0.74 |
| Watkins et al. (2007) | 167/172 | Weak | MI | 4/180 | 1–3 | A/C | -0.01 | -0.22/0.20 |
| Weinstein, Harrison, and Benton (2004) | 120/120 | Weak | MI | 7/– | 10–12 | Parenting | 0.31 | 0.05/0.56 |
| Westra and Dozois (2006) | 25/30 | Weak | MI | 3/180 | IM | A/C, Eng | 0.54 | -0.03/1.10 |
| Wilhelm, Stephans, Hertzog, Rodehorst, and Gardener (2006) | 20/20 | Weak | MI | | | | 0.21 | -0.41/0.83 |

*Note.* Within a single study, authors often assessed several outcomes and the number of participants in both the treatment and the comparison group. Strong indicates the comparison group was a specific intervention. Weak indicates the comparison group was one of the following: control, waitlist, reading materials, or TAU that was not specified. Effect sizes averaged across measures and outcomes within each study. A/C = ability or confidence to change: AI = alcohol: Cig = cigarettes and tobacco: Comp = comparison group: Ed Bx = eating disorder behavior: Eng = engagement or compliance: Gam = gambling: GWB = general well-being IC/SC = intention to change/stages of change: IM = immediately after treatment: Health = increase healthy behavior OD = other drugs: Risks = reduce risk taking behavior: WSDP - water-safe drinking practices. C.I. = Confidence Interval: Tx = treatment group.

*(Continued)*

(Continued)

### *Step I: Subdividing effect sizes using potential categorical moderators.*

Based on findings from previous MI meta-analyses, we systematically examined potential moderators until between-group variance was eliminated, leaving homogeneous effect sizes that can confidently be interpreted.

*Comparison group.* We first examined the effect comparison group had on outcomes as the meta-analysis by Burke et al. (2003) suggested results varied based on this variable. In fact, significant heterogeneity was found, $Q_w = 14.75$ (4), $p < .01$. Further analyses (see Table 2) revealed that when MI was compared to a TAU program that involved a specific program (e.g., 12-step or cognitive-behavioral) effects were significantly lower than when compared against a waitlist/comparison group ($Q_b = 18.95$, $p < .001$), a generic TAU without a specific program ($Q_b = 11.72$, $p < .005$), or written material groups ($Q_b = 4.90$, $p < .05$). Group difference analyses revealed no other significant differences among or between other types of comparison groups. Next, all the "weak" comparison groups were combined ($g = 0.28$, $k = 88$) and compared to those studies that pitted MI against a specific treatment or a "strong" comparison group ($g = .09$, $k = 39$). Studies that compared MI to a weak comparison showed significantly higher effect sizes, $Q_b = 13.58$, $p < .001$. In addition to being interesting in its own right, this finding suggests further analyses should be run separately for those that used a strong comparison group and those that used a weak comparison group.

*Dependent variable.* Next, we explored whether effect sizes would differ based on the dependent variable, as it has previously been shown that MI was not equally effective for all problem types (e.g.. Burke et al., 2003). Table 2 presents effect sizes organized across the 14 outcome groups with sub-divisions for strong and weak comparisons. The preponderance of studies examined outcomes related to substance use, where MI originated: alcohol ($k = 68$), miscellaneous drugs ($k = 27$), tobacco ($k = 24$), and marijuana ($k = 17$). Of the 14 outcome groups, all yielded statistically significant positive effects for MI with the exception of emotional or psychological well-being, eating problems, and confidence in being able to succeed in change. The test of heterogeneity across the 11 dependent variable groupings was nonsignificant, $Q_b = 11.34$ ($df = 10$), $p = 0.34$, suggesting that the outcomes across dependent variables were, on the whole, statistically homogenous. Exploratory between group analyses were conducted, and no significant group differences were found.

In line with the finding that comparison group type moderates outcomes. MI did not show significant advantage over strong comparison groups for any outcome. When positioned against a weak comparison group, outcomes for substance use-related outcomes ranged from a low of $g = 0.16$ for miscellaneous drugs to a high of $g = 0.35$ for tobacco. These values are in the small but significant range. Of the remaining health-related behavior outcomes, the strongest effect was for gambling ($g = 0.39$), though the small number of studies also made these variables the least stable as evidenced by wide confidence intervals. The effect for increases in healthy behaviors, which comprised outcomes related to diet, exercise, and compliance with medical recommendations, was in the small range ($g = 0.19$). The effect size for reducing risky behaviors, which most often comprised outcomes related to sexual behavior and drug use, was also small ($g = 0.15$). When positioned against a weak comparison group effect sizes for the three variables that concern clients engagement in treatment ranged from a low of $g = 0.15$ for confidence to a high of $g = 0.35$ for engagement.

As was mentioned, when compared to other active, specific treatments such as 12-step or cognitive-behavioral therapy MI did not produce significant nonzero effect sizes in any outcome. In the case of tobacco ($g = -0.21$) and miscellaneous drugs ($g = -0.12$), effect sizes were in the negative range, though nonsignificant. Among substance use outcomes, then, MI is certainly better than no treatment and not significantly different from other specific treatments with some effects being greater than nil and some being negative.

*Client distress level.* We next questioned whether client's level of distress or impairment would moderate MI effects. Among the three different levels of distress, between group heterogeneity was not significant, $Q_b> = 2.39$ (2), $p = .67$, meaning that distress did not moderate MI effectiveness. As can be seen in Table 2, the same pattern tended to hold where outcomes were not significant if the comparison was made against a specific treatment program.

*Moderators Among Studies Comparing MI to Weak Comparison Groups.* The next moderator analysis examined whether results for MI compared to weak comparison groups (i.e., nonspecific TAU, waitlist control, written materials) would depend on the method of delivery—that is, MI in its basic form versus MET, which adds specific problem feedback to MI as described above. Table 3 presents detailed information. MET ($g = 0.32$) was significantly more likely to produce positive change compared to typical MI ($g = 0.19$), $Q_b = 4.97$ (1), $p < .03$. Furthermore, between group comparisons were made by subdividing the groups that involved typical MI ($k = 33$) and those that involved MET ($k = 50$). Table 3 presents these results among MI studies with weak comparison groups.

**Table 2**  Effect Sizes for Overall Effect and Initial Moderators

| Variable | k | Effect Size | CI | z Value/ p Value | Heterogeneity Q Value (df)/ p Value |
|---|---|---|---|---|---|
| Overall effectiveness (across studies) | 132 | 0.22 | 0.17/0.27 | 8.75/.001* | 228.71 (131)/.001* |
| Moderator: comparison group type | | | | | |
| Attention | 1 | 0.48 | 0.01/0.96 | 1.97/.050* | 14.75 (4)/.01* |
| Treatment as usual-nonspecific | 42 | 0.24 | 0.17/0.31 | 6.40/.000* | |
| Treatment as usual-specific | 39 | 0.09 | −0.01/0.18 | 1.77/.080, ns | |
| Waitlist/control | 35 | 0.32 | 0.22/0.42 | 6.49/.000* | |
| Written material | 10 | 0.24 | 0.09/0.38 | 3.10/.002* | |

*(Continued)*

**Table 2** (Continued)

| Variable | k | Effect Size | CI | z Value/ p Value | Heterogeneity Q Value (df)/ p Value |
|---|---|---|---|---|---|
| Comparisons: combined weak | 88 | 0.28 | 0.22/0.34 | 9.85/.000* | |
| Comparisons: strong | 39 | 0.09* | −0.01/0.18 | 1.77/.080, ns | 13.58 (1)/.001* |
| Moderator: dependent variables | | | | | 18.58 (13)/.14, ns |
| Health-related behaviors | | | | | |
| Alcohol-related problems | 68 | 0.15 | 0.09/0.21 | 4.76/.001* | |
| Strong comparison | 21 | 0.03 | −0.08/0.13 | 0.53/.597,ns | |
| Weak comparison | 47 | 0.20 | 0.12/0.27 | 5.31/.000* | 6.90 (1)/.009* |
| Marijuana-related problems | 17 | 0.26 | 0.10/0.43 | 3.17/.002* | |
| Strong comparison | 3 | 0.07 | −0.15/0.29 | 0.64/.525, ns | |
| Weak comparison | 14 | 0.30 | 0.11/0.49 | 3.10/.002* | 2.35 (1)/.125, ns |
| Tobacco-related problems | 24 | 0.25 | 0.10/0.41 | 3.18/.002* | |
| Strong comparison | 5 | −0.21 | −0.53/0.11 | −1.29/.196, ns | |
| Weak comparison | 18 | 0.35 | 0.22/0.48 | 5.20/.000* | 10.60 (1)/.001* |
| Miscellaneous drug problems | 27 | 0.08 | −0.03/0.20 | 1.46/.145, ns | |
| Strong comparison | 7 | −0.12 | −0.27/0.04 | −1.45/.146, ns | |
| Weak comparison | 10 | 0.16 | 0.02/0.29 | 2.28/.023* | 6.70 (1)/.010* |
| Increase healthy behavior | 11 | 0.21 | 0.06/0.36 | 2.78/.006* | |
| Strong comparison | 4 | 0.30 | −0.19/0.79 | 1.20/.229, ns | |
| Weak comparison | 7 | 0.19 | 0.08/0.60 | 3.30/.001* | 0.20 (1)/.658, ns |
| Reduce risky behavior | 10 | 0.14 | 0.04/0.25 | 2.77/.005* | |
| Strong comparison | 1 | 0.10 | −0.44/0.64 | 0.36/.716, ns | |
| Weak comparison | 9 | 0.15 | 0.04/0.26 | 2.66/.008* | 0.03 (1)/.855, ns |
| Gambling | 3 | 0.39 | 0.06/0.71 | 2.33/.020* | |
| Strong comparison | | | Not applicable | | |
| Weak comparison | 3 | 0.39 | 0.06/0.71 | 2.33/.020* | Not applicable |
| Emotional/ psychological well-being | 7 | 0.14 | −0.02/0.30 | 1.67/.095, ns | |

| | | | | |
|---|---|---|---|---|
| Strong comparison | 3 | 0.05 | −0.07/0.16 | 0.83/.408, ns | |
| Weak comparison | 4 | 0.33 | −0.03/0.68 | 1.80/.072, ns | 2.11 (1)/.146, ns |
| Eating problems | 1 | 0.18 | −0.23/0.59 | 0.87/.390, ns | |
| Strong comparison | Not applicable | | | | |
| Weak comparison | 1 | 0.18 | −0.23/0.59 | 0.87/.390, ns | Not applicable |
| Parenting practices | 2 | 0.29 | 0.06/0.53 | 2.43/.015* | |
| Strong comparison | Not applicable | | | | |
| Weak comparison | 2 | 0.29 | 0.06/0.53 | 2.43/.015* | Not applicable |
| Drinking safe water | 1 | 0.73 | 0.31/1.15 | 3.39/.001** | |
| Strong comparison | Not applicable | | | | |
| Weak comparison | 1 | 0.73 | 0.31/1.15 | 3.39/.001** | Not applicable |
| Approach to treatment | | | | | |
| Engagement | 34 | 0.26 | 0.15/0.37 | 4.78/.001** | |
| Strong comparison | 14 | 0.12 | 0.00/0.25 | 1.94/.053, ns | |
| Weak comparison | 20 | 0.35 | 0.21/0.50 | 4.80/.000* | 5.56 (1)/.018* |
| Intention to change | 23 | 0.24 | 0.13/0.34 | 4.35/.001** | |
| Strong comparison | 6 | 0.23 | −0.09/0.55 | 1.40/.161, ns | |
| Weak comparison | 17 | 0.24 | 0.13/0.35 | 4.15/.000* | 0.01 (1)/.944, ns |
| Confidence/ability | 11 | 0.18 | −0.06/0.42 | 1.44/.149, ns | |
| Strong comparison | 2 | 0.33 | −0.08/0.74 | 1.50/.114, ns | |
| Weak comparison | 9 | 0.15 | −0.13/0.43 | 1.07/.286, ns | 0.51 (1)/.473, ns |
| Moderator: clients' level of distress | | | | | 2.39 (2)/.674, ns |
| Community sample | 19 | 0.19 | 0.06/0.37 | 2.87/.004** | |
| Strong comparison | 5 | −0.01 | −0.27/0.25 | −0.09/.927, ns | |
| Weak comparison | 14 | 0.28 | 0.17/0.39 | 5.12/.00* | 4.14 (1)/.042* |
| Moderate levels of distress | 50 | 0.21 | 0.14/0.27 | 5.83/.001* | |
| Strong comparison | 15 | 0.12 | −0.01/0.25 | 1.79/.073, ns | |
| Weak comparison | 35 | 0.24 | 0.15/0.32 | 5.55/.000* | 2.40 (1)/.302, ns |
| Significant levels of distress | 44 | 0.19 | 0.10/0.28 | 4.22/.001* | |
| Strong comparison | 14 | 0.03 | −0.12/0.17 | 0.35/.729, ns | |
| Weak comparison | 30 | 0.26 | 0.16/0.35 | 5.08/.000* | 6.47 (1)/.011* |

*Note:* Numbers of studies vary because not all studies examined certain outcomes or reported on certain moderators. CI = confidence interval; *df* = degrees of freedom; *k* = number of studies; ns = nonsignificant. *p < .05.

*(Continued)*

(Continued)

Four other potential moderators were examined: whether a manual was used, format/ role of MI in the treatment process, how fidelity to MI was assessed, and who delivered MI. Analyses revealed no significant heterogeneity in any of these four variables, suggesting that they did not moderate outcomes (all $ps > .05$). Because homogeneity was found within these four moderators, further between group comparisons were not conducted.

*Moderators Among Studies Comparing MI to Strong Comparison Groups (Specific TAU).* Moderator analyses for MI compared to specific TAU were run in the same order as those that did not involve a specific intervention above. Table 4 presents detailed data. Given the relatively smaller number of studies ($k = 40$), the power to detect moderators was reduced and the confidence intervals thus tended to be wider.

If the comparison group included a specific intervention, no significant difference was found whether MI was delivered via its typical format or MET, $Q_h (1) = 0.03$, *ns.* Thus, further moderator analyses were collapsed across these two groups. The use of a training manual ($k = 25$, $g = 0.00$) was associated with significantly smaller outcomes compared to when a manual was not used ($k = 11$, $g = 0.45$; $Q_b = 5.96$, $p < .05$), which is similar to the finding by Hettema et al. (2005). Given this difference, further moderator analyses were divided into those that did and did not use a manual. In both subgroups, the format of MI did not moderate outcomes nor did assessment of fidelity to MI or who delivered the MI intervention (all ps > .06).

### Step 2: Examining potential continuous moderators via meta-regression

Analyses of continuous moderators were subdivided into those studies that compared MI interventions to a weak versus a strong comparison condition, as with the categorical analyses above. These results can be viewed in Table 5. Five participant characteristics were submitted to meta-regression:

Participant's average age, the percent of male participants within a sample (and by converse female), and three indicators of ethnicity. With regard to ethnicity, we assessed the percentage of the sample who was White, African American, or Hispanic. Four study characteristics were submitted to meta-regression; overall study rigor, the number of sessions in which MI was delivered, the number of minutes MI was delivered to the sample, and durability (the longest length of time that a follow-up assessment was taken, which replicates the categorical analysis of time since treatment). Note that the meta-regression analyses involved all possible comparisons across studies and all moderator groups. Thus, each effect size drawn from a study was entered into the regression analyses; while this does not technically violate assumptions of independence because each effect size was compared independently, some studies contributed more data than other studies because they reported on more outcome indicators.

*Studies Comparing MI to Weak Comparison Groups.* Only one of the participant characteristics was significantly associated with MI outcomes: Studies that included a higher percentage of African American participants in their sample had significantly better outcomes with MI, $z = 2.90$, $q$ value $= 8.43$ (1, 226), $p < .01$. Average age, percentage of male participants, and percentage of White or Hispanic participants did not significantly influence MI outcomes. With regard to study characteristics, rigor, number of sessions, and durability (measurement interval beyond completion of treatment) were not related to outcomes. By contrast, the amount of services delivered was positively related to outcomes with a significant effect ($z = 4.23$) for the total number of minutes, $q$ value = 17.89 (1, 428), $p < .01$, such that longer treatments produced higher effect sizes for MI.

*Studies Comparing MI to Strong Comparison Groups (Specific TAU).* Three of the participant characteristics were significantly associated with higher effect sizes. Studies that included older participants were more likely to have positive outcomes, $q$ value = 6.22 (1, 152), $p < .01$. Contrary to the previous regression analyses, in studies that used a TAU with a specific program, a higher percentage of African American participants was negatively associated with outcomes ($q$ value = 29.70, $p < .001$). Moreover, a significant negative relationship was found for the percentage of White participants ($q$ value = 6.27, $p < .01$). Thus, the higher the relative number of African American or White participants in the study (i.e., the lower the number of participants from other ethnic groups), the lower the overall mean MI effect sizes. Only one significant relationship emerged for the study characteristics in this subgroup. There was a significant negative relationship between study rigor and outcomes, $q$ value = 8.80 (1, 253), $p < .01$, such that studies with higher rigor ratings yielded lower effect sizes for MI.

*Step 3: Three further questions-treatment length, durability, and group MI*

**Table 3** Moderators Among Studies Comparing MI to Weak Comparison Groups (Waitlist, Written Materials, Nonspecific Treatment as Usual)

| Variable | k | Effect Size | CI | z Value/ p Value | Heterogeneity Q Value (df)/p Value |
|---|---|---|---|---|---|
| Moderator: motivational interviewing (MI) or | | | | | 4.97 (1)/.032* |
| Motivational Enhancement Therapy (MET) | | | | | |
| MI | 33 | 0.19 | 0.11/0.27 | 4.76/.001* | |
| MET | 50 | 0.32 | 0.23/0.40 | 7.51/.001* | |
| Moderator: use of manual | | | | | |
| Motivational interviewing | | | | | 0.53 (1)/.459, ns |
| Manual not used | 10 | 0.24 | 0.08/0.40 | 2.94/.003* | |
| Manual used | 23 | 0.17 | 0.08/0.26 | 3.82/.001* | |
| Motivational Enhancement Therapy | | | | | |
| Manual not used | 10 | 0.34 | 0.16/0.51 | 3.81/.001* | 0.23 (1)/.891, ns |

*(Continued)*

**Table 3** (Continued)

| Variable | k | Effect Size | CI | z Value/ p Value | Heterogeneity Q Value (df)/p Value |
|---|---|---|---|---|---|
| Manual used | 39 | 0.32 | 0.22/0.41 | 6.26/.001* | |
| Moderator: role of MI in treatment | | | | | |
| Motivational interviewing | | | | | 3.07 (2)/.218, ns |
| Additive | 14 | 0.12 | 0.01/0.24 | 2.09/.040* | |
| Prelude | 3 | 0.43 | 0.03/0.83 | 2.10/.040* | |
| Head-to-head | 16 | 0.23 | 0.12/0.33 | 4.12/.001* | 3.69 (2)/.160, ns |
| Motivational Enhancement Therapy | | | | | |
| Additive | 13 | 0.36 | 0.17/0.55 | 3.65/.001* | |
| Prelude | 7 | 0.16 | −0.01/0.33 | 1.84/.070, ns | |
| Head-to-head | 31 | 0.34 | 0.23/0.45 | 6.11/.001* | |
| Moderator: fidelity to MI model examined | | | | | |
| Motivational interviewing | | | | | 5.02 (2)/.083, ns |
| No assessment | 22 | 0.24 | 0.14/0.35 | 4.47/.001* | |
| Assessed, not scored | 6 | 0.23 | 0.07/0.39 | 2.76/.010* | |
| Assessed, standardized score | 5 | 0.03 | −0.13/0.19 | 0.36/.720, ns | |
| Motivational Enhancement Therapy | | | | | 3.15 (2)/.256, ns |
| No assessment | 21 | 0.42 | 0.27/0.56 | 5.59/.001* | |
| Assessed, not scored | 16 | 0.28 | 0.12/0.43 | 3.53/.001* | |
| Assessed, standardized score | 12 | 0.25 | 0.14/0.37 | 4.38/.001* | |
| Moderator: Who Delivered MI | | | | | |
| Motivational interviewing | | | | | 3.09 (3)/.389, ns |
| Mental health: Bachelors | 1 | 0.19 | −0.21/0.58 | 0.92/.360, ns | |
| Mental health: Masters/PhD | 5 | 0.39 | 0.13/0.65 | 2.98/.001* | |
| Nurse | 4 | 0.10 | −0.11/0.31 | 0.93/.350, ns | |
| Student | 3 | 0.23 | −0.09/0.54 | 1.43/.150, ns | |
| Motivational Enhancement Therapy | | | | | 0.47 (3)/.933, ns |

| | | | | |
|---|---|---|---|---|
| Mental health: Bachelors | 7 | 0.27 | 0.07/0.46 | 2.67/.008* |
| Mental health: Masters/PhD | 7 | 0.39 | 0.06/0.72 | 2.29/.022* |
| Nurse | 1 | 0.30 | 0.04/0.55 | 2.28/.022* |
| Student | 3 | 0.23 | −0.13/0.59 | 1.25/.212, ns |

*Note.* Numbers of studies vary because not all studies examined certain outcomes or reported on certain moderators. CI = confidence interval; *df* = degrees of freedom; *k* = number of studies; *ns* = nonsignificant. *\*p* < .05.

**Time in treatment.** To investigate whether MI is efficient compared to specific TAU or strong comparison groups, we assessed the number of appointments and total amount of time (minutes) spent in treatment. With regard to number of appointments, MI groups (*M* = 3.70, *SD* = 3.82) did not significantly differ from specific TAU groups (M = 4.37, *SD* = 4.81), *t* (51) = 1.38, *ns.* With regard to total time spent with clients (measured in minutes), specific TAU groups *(M* = 308, *SD* = 447) tended to meet for a longer time than MI groups (*AY* = 207, *SD* = 332), *t* (30) = 1.84, *p* < .08, though this difference did not reach statistical significance.

**Table 4**    Moderator Analyses for Studies Compared to Treatment as Usual Group With a Specific Treatment Program

| Variable | K | Effect Size | CI | z Value/p Value | Heterogeneity Q Value (df)/p Value |
|---|---|---|---|---|---|
| Moderator: motivational interviewing (MI) or | | | | | 0.03 (1)/.867, ns |
| Motivational Enhancement Therapy | | | | | |
| Motivational interviewing | 15 | 0.05 | −0.10/0.19 | 0.64/.534, ns | |
| Motivational Enhancement Therapy | 23 | 0.06 | −0.04/0.17 | 1.16/.245, ns | |
| Moderator: use of training manual | | | | | 5.96 (1)/.049* |
| Manual used | 25 | 0.00 | −0.07/0.07 | −0.08/.931, ns | |
| Manual not used | 11 | 0.45 | 0.09/0.81 | 2.46/.024* | |
| Moderator: role of MI in treatment | | | | | 0.95 (1)/.624, ns |
| Manual used | | | | | |
| Additive | 11 | −0.03 | −0.16/0.10 | −0.43/.667, ns | |
| Prelude | 6 | 0.07 | −0.08/0.22 | 0.91/.362, ns | |

*(Continued)*

**Table 4** (Continued)

| Variable | K | Effect Size | CI | z Value/p Value | Heterogeneity Q Value (df)/p Value |
|---|---|---|---|---|---|
| Head-to-head | 8 | 0.02 | −0.10/0.14 | 0.27/.392, ns | |
| Manual not used | | | | | 5.75 (2)/.056, ns |
| Additive | 4 | 0.10 | −0.43/0.62 | 0.36/.721, ns | |
| Prelude | 3 | 1.06 | 0.47/1.66 | 3.52/.001* | |
| Head-to-head | 4 | 0.54 | 0.13/0.96 | 2.57/.014* | |
| Moderator: fidelity to MI model examined | | | | | |
| Manual used | | | | | 1.28 (2)/.533, ns |
| No assessment | 7 | 0.08 | −0.06/0.21 | 1.12/.261, ns | |
| Assessed, not scored | 7 | −0.03 | −0.22/0.17 | −0.29/.767, ns | |
| Assessed, standardized score | 11 | −0.01 | −0.11/0.09 | −0.24/.806, ns | |
| Manual not used | | | | | Not applicable |
| No assessment | 11 | 0.45 | 0.09/0.81 | 2.46/.013* | |
| Insufficient studies to make comparisons on: | | | | | |
| assessed, not scored and assessed, standardized score | | | | | |
| Moderator: who delivered MI | | | | | |
| Manual used | | | | | 3.76 (3)/.294, ns |
| Mental health: Bachelors | 5 | −0.00 | −0.21/0.21 | −0.01/.989, ns | |
| Mental health: Masters/PhD | 2 | −0.04 | −0.24/0.17 | −0.36/.721, ns | |
| Nurse | 2 | 0.36 | 0.01/0.72 | 1.98/.045* | |
| Student | 2 | 0.05 | −0.19/0.28 | 0.38/.715, ns | |
| Manual not used | | | | | 1.34 (2)/.511, ns |
| Mental health: Masters/PhD | 1 | 0.69 | −0.18/1.56 | 1.56/.115, ns | |
| Nurse | 1 | 0.52 | −0.27/1.30 | 1.28/.204, ns | |
| Student | 2 | 1.06 | 0.49/.62 | 3.66/.001* | |

*Note.* Numbers of studies vary because not all studies examined certain outcomes or reported on certain moderators. CI = confidence interval; *df* = degrees of freedom; *k* = number of studies; *ns* = non significant. *$p < .05$.

*Durability.* To support continuous analyses of durability, outcomes were grouped into five different time frames: immediately following treatment ($g = 0.15$, $k = 15$), 3 months beyond treatment ($g = 0.14$, $k = 45$), between 4 and 12 months beyond treatment ($g = 0.29$, $k = 32$), up to 2 years beyond treatment ($g = 0.24$, $k = 3$), and 25 months or more ($g = 0.24$, $k = 2$). No significant differences emerged between time frames, $Q_b = 5.27$ (4), $p = .38$, *ns.* With the exception of the longest time frame, all effect sizes were significantly greater than zero (all *ps* < .02).

*Delivery mode.* Interest in group-delivered MI exists, yet no meta-analysis has investigated delivery mode as a moderator. We found very few studies that delivered MI in a group format (see Table 6), so we ran this analysis separately from the other moderators. Whereas no statistically significant differences were found, visual inspection suggests that delivering MI through a group format only may dilute effects compared to when MI is also delivered individually. The small number of studies addressing this question certainly warrants caution when making inferences from these results.

## Discussion

From a broad perspective, a robust literature exists that examines the ability of MI to promote healthy behavior change across a wide variety of problem areas. That 119 studies met our inclusion criteria is remarkable and suggests MI is an approach that will be part of the treatment landscape for the foreseeable future. To guide practitioners and researchers, we now pose and answer several practical questions that flow from this meta-analysis below.

### Does MI Work?

To the degree that MI is rooted in health care, social work, and psychology settings, the question of "does it work" is relevant. Our analyses strongly suggest that MI does exert small though significant positive effects across a wide range of problem domains, although it is more potent in some situations compared to others, and it does not work in all cases. When examining all the effect sizes in this review, the bottom 25% included effect sizes that ranged from zero to highly negative outcomes, which means MI was either ineffective or less effective when compared to other interventions or groups about a quarter of the time. Remember, a negative effect size does not necessarily suggest that participants receiving MI were directly harmed—just that the comparison group either progressed more or regressed less. Conversely, a full 75% of participants gained some improvement from MI, with 50% gaining a small but meaningful effect and 25% gaining to a moderate or strong level. Our results resemble findings from other meta-analyses of treatment interventions. Specially, Lipsey and Wilson (1993) generated a distribution of mean effect sizes from 302 meta-analyses of psychological, behavioral, or educational interventions, reporting the mean and median effect sizes to be around 0.50 *(SD = 0.29)*. The results of our meta-analysis are generally within one standard deviation of this mean effect size, indicating that MI produces effects consistent with other human change interventions.

*(Continued)*

(Continued)

### Table 5   Meta-Regression: Continuous Moderator Analyses

|  | Slope | z Value | q Value (df) | p Value |
|---|---|---|---|---|
| Comparison groups: waitlist, TAU, and written materials |  |  |  |  |
| Participant characteristics |  |  |  |  |
| Average age | −0.001 | −0.63 | 0.41 (1, 234) | .53, ns |
| % Male | −0.001 | −0.89 | 0.80 (1, 224) | .37, ns |
| % White | 0.001 | 0.67 | 0.44 (1, 319) | .51, ns |
| % African American | 0.003 | 2.90 | 8.43 (1, 226) | .044* |
| % Hispanic | 0.002 | 0.76 | 0.58 (1, 186) | .45, ns |
| Study characteristics |  |  |  |  |
| Rigor | −0.010 | −1.50 | 2.26 (1, 485) | .13, ns |
| Dose: # of sessions | 0.015 | 1.30 | 1.68 (1, 516) | .20, ns |
| Dose: # of minutes | 0.001 | 3.85 | 14.82 (1, 403) | .001* |
| Durability: F/U time | 0.002 | 0.18 | 0.03 (1, 543) | .85, ns |
| Comparison groups: TAU with specific treatment |  |  |  |  |
| Participant characteristics |  |  |  |  |
| Average age | 0.006 | 2.49 | 6.22 (1, 152) | .01* |
| %Male | −0.000 | −0.19 | 0.05 (1, 133) | .85, ns |
| %White | −0.003 | −2.51 | 6.27 (0, 213) | .01* |
| %African American | −0.007 | −5.47 | 29.70 (1, 130) | .001* |
| %Hispanic | −0.001 | −0.39 | 0.15 (1, 80) | .70, ns |
| Study characteristics |  |  |  |  |
| Rigor | −0.028 | −2.97 | 8.80 (1, 253) | .01* |
| Dose: # of sessions | 0.003 | 0.30 | 0.09 (1, 260) | .77, ns |
| Dose: # of minutes | 0.000 | 0.07 | 0.01 (1, 177) | .94, ns |
| Durability: F/U time | −0.017 | −1.04 | 1.09 (1,278) | .30, ns |

*Note:* Degrees of freedom of studies vary because not all studies examined certain outcomes or reported on certain moderators. *$p < .05$.

**Table 6**   Mode of Delivery: Group, Individual, or Combined Delivery

|  | N | *Effect Size* | *CI* | z *Value/*p *Value* |
|---|---|---|---|---|
| Collapsed across weak and strong comparisons |  |  |  |  |
| Combined | 3 | 0.45 | −0.46/1.36 | 0.96 (.34, *ns*) |
| Group | 5 | 0.05 | −0.19/0.28 | 0.38 (0.38, *ns*) |
| Individual | 104 | 0.23 | 0.17/0.28 | 7.76 (.001*) |
| MI compared to weak comparison groups |  |  |  |  |
| Combined | 2 | 0.76 | −1.02/2.55 | 0.84 (.40, *ns*) |
| Group | 2 | 0.33 | 0.02/0.64 | 2.09 (0.04*) |
| Individual | 76 | 0.28 | 0.22/0.34 | 8.89 (.001*) |
| MI compared to strong comparison groups |  |  |  |  |
| Combined | 1 | 0.15 | 0.89/1.20 | 0.29 (.77, *ns*) |
| Group | 3 | 0.13 | 0.33/0.08 | 2.09 (0.23, *ns*) |
| Individual | 29 | 0.06 | 0.04/0.16 | 1.12 (.25, *ns*) |

*Note:* CI = confidence interval. Numbers of studies vary because not all studies examined certain outcomes or reported on certain moderators. * *p* < .05.

### Should I or My Agency Consider Learning or Adopting MI?

On the whole, the data suggest "yes." While we did not perform a cost-benefit analysis, adopting MI is very likely to produce a statistically significant and positive advantage for clients and may do so in less time. Note that, when compared to other active treatments such as 12-step and cognitive-behavioral therapy (CBT), the MI interventions took over 100 fewer minutes of treatment on average yet produced equal effects. This holds across a wide range of problem areas, including usage of alcohol, tobacco, and marijuana. Furthermore, MI is likely to lead to client improvement when directed at increasing healthy behaviors and/or decreasing risky or unhealthy behaviors as well increasing client engagement in the treatment process. Of course, in MI fashion, the decision to adopt or even consider adopting MI requires considerable thought and is ultimately an individual (or agency) choice.

### Is MI Only Indicated for Substance Use Problems?

No. Although MI originated in substance abuse fields, its effectiveness is currently much broader. While most of the studies included in this analysis were related to substance use problems, MI was also effective for other addictive problems such as gambling as well as for enhancing general health-promoting behaviors. Furthermore, MI was associated with positive gains in measures of general well-being (e.g., lower stress and depression levels), which is interesting because MI is geared toward motivating clients to make some form of

*(Continued)*

(Continued)

change and directly targets clients' engagement in the change process. Thus, it may be that MI increased client well-being indirectly, after they had made successful changes in certain areas of their life.

### Is MI Successful in Motivating Clients to Change?

Yes. MI significantly increased clients' engagement in treatment and their intention to change, the two variables most closely linked to motivation to change. MI certainly shows potential to enhance client change intentions and treatment engagement, as well as possibly boost their confidence in their ability to change.

### Is MI Only Successful With Very Troubled Clients?

No. Our results suggest MI is effective for individuals with high levels of distress as well as for individuals with relatively low levels of distress. In fact, a recent study comparing MI to CBT for generalized anxiety disorder revealed that receiving MI was substantively and specifically beneficial for those reporting high worry severity at baseline, compared to those reporting severity not receiving MI (Hal Arkowitz, personal communication, November 2008).

### Is MI as Successful as Other Interventions?

To begin, MI is certainly better than no treatment and weak treatment such as a written materials or nonspecific TAU groups as judged by the significant positive changes. Furthermore, MI mostly held its own with specific TAU groups. While MI was not significantly better than such groups, it was at least as successful except in the case of tobacco use and miscellaneous drug-use problems. This finding mirrors the general "Dodo bird verdict" from psychotherapy reviews and meta-analyses that no one intervention model or theory is clearly superior (see Prochaska & Norcross, 2007). If MI is as successful as other interventions, then decision making about whether to adopt MI rests more with practical and theoretical considerations. Ease of learning MI and costs are practical concerns, whereas theoretical issues pertain to whether the individual or agency can adopt a client-centered model that emphasizes collaboration with clients over directing and pushing people to change. Of interest, MI does not require more resources, such as number of sessions or amount of time, and may require less time to achieve results similar to other specific treatments.

### Are the Effects of MI Durable?

Our analyses suggest that they are. Results did not significantly differ when participants' improvements were measured immediately following treatment, 3 months beyond treatment, or up to a year following treatment completion. This finding comes from over 97 comparisons with a minimum of 15 for each time frame; furthermore, our regression analyses showed a nonsignificant relationship across 842 effect sizes where time could be classified. Our results also suggest MI was durable at the 2-year mark and beyond, though so few studies evaluated such long-term outcomes that confidence has to be tempered pending further research.

### Should Practitioners Learn "Basic MI' or "MET?'

The answer to this question depends on many factors, such as whether standardized assessment tools exist for the target problem area under consideration and whether another specific intervention is already being used. First, if the main goal of the practitioner is to combine MI with other psychotherapy techniques such as CBT (e.g., Anton et al., 2006) or use MI as in integrative framework throughout treatment for clinical problems like depression (e.g., Arkowitz & Burke, 2008), then basic MI is the best choice. If the goal is to target specific behavior changes, however, then our review suggests that if another specific program is not currently being used, employing MET will produce significantly better results than only using MI. This makes theoretical sense because MET is "MI plus," adding a problem feedback component to the MI paradigm that could constitute an effective treatment in its own right. Furthermore, if one considers the findings originating from Project MATCH (1997, 1998), where MET produced results equal to CBT and 12-step in considerably less time, adopting MET seems like the right choice to specifically target addictive or other problem behaviors. Finally, MET may be easier to learn/ train because it is more focused than basic MI.

### Is Manual-Guided MI Superior to the Alternative?

Our results suggest not. When MI was compared to a weak comparison group, the use of a manual did not matter, whereas when MI was compared to a specific TAU, the use of a manual was significantly less effective. Hettema et al. (2005) found the use of a manual detracted from outcomes: our results suggest that this may be the case only when MI is being compared to a specific TAU. On one hand, treatment manuals should encourage fidelity to the MI approach, although fidelity also showed no significant correlations with MI outcome. Yet, MI by definition strives toward a humanistic, client-centered approach where a manual may interfere with truly centering on the client by causing practitioners to focus unduly on the manual. To our knowledge, no primary study has explicitly tested this question in a MI context and we hope future research into the process of MI will do so.

### Does the Format or Role of MI Influence Outcomes?

MI is a versatile approach. It has been used as additive to other interventions, as a prelude to another treatment where the assumption is that MI will serve a preparatory role, and as a stand-alone intervention. Our data suggest that MI format does not matter as judged by homogenous effect sizes. However, visual inspection revealed a fair amount of variability across different conditions, suggesting that basic MI may work best as a prelude to further treatment (as in Burke et al., 2003), whereas MET may be optimal as an additive or stand-alone intervention.

The overall finding that format of MI does not significantly influence its outcome fits with its basic philosophy. MI aims to improve the working alliance with a client, to manage resistance, to express empathy, and to build motivation to change while addressing ambivalence about change. These targeted goals seem broadly acceptable to most change efforts and are likely useful at any stage of an intervention process. Thus, it appears that one of the strengths of MI lies in its portability across many different treatment formats or roles.

*(Continued)*

(Continued)

### Does Level of Training Influence Success of MI?

Our data suggest "no." However, very few studies contributed data to this question, and any inferences must be made tentatively. Of note, William Miller has stated (personal communication, December 2006) that what is most important is a helping professional's ability to empathize with clients and not their training background (e.g., nursing, social work, psychology). Moreover, research has often suggested that little difference can be attributed to professional training in psychological arenas (e.g., Berman & Norton, 1985).

### Does MI Dosage Matter?

Our answer is that it likely does. When MI conditions were compared to weak (and shorter) alternatives, a significant postitive relationship was found, suggesting a dose effect—i.e. more treatment time was related to better outcomes for MI. The data therefore suggest that it cannot hurt to provide more MI and that it is unreasonable to assume that a very short MI intervention will lead to lasting change. That said, our data cannot suggest minimum or maximum levels of Mi-related contact. Many MI practitioners anecdotally report that MI becomes integrated within much of their treatment, such that it cannot be separated from other interventions, which thereby makes the question of dosage less pertinent.

### Does MI Work for Most Clients?

We cannot provide a simple response to this important question based on our review, although our data do suggest a few insights in that regard. On the whole. MI appears broadly capable of helping across many problem domains ranging from addictive to health-promoting behaviors. We also looked at two participant characteristics: age and ethnicity. Regression analyses showed a significant relationship between participants' average age and outcomes only when MI was compared to specific TAU, where studies with older participants yielded better results for MI. Considering developmental issues, MI is conducted within a cognitive medium and requires some degree of abstract reasoning that should be present after the age of 12 years (based on Piaget's (1962) model) and thus may not be as helpful for preteen children.

Our data also provide a mixed picture with regard to race. When MI was compared with a weak alternative, a significant positive correlation was found between percentages of African American participants and, to a lesser degree, Hispanic Americans for MI outcomes. Furthermore, when MI was compared to a strong alternative (specific TAU), a lower percentage of Whites and a lower percentage of African Americans (i.e., a higher percentage of other minorities) was significantly related to better MI outcomes. Taken together, these findings suggest that MI may be particularly effective with clients from minority ethnic groups (but not necessarily African Americans), a pattern similar to that reported by Hettema et al. (2005). We conjecture that MI may be particularly attractive to groups who have experienced social rejection and societal pressure because MI adopts a humanistic approach that prizes self-determination, although why results would differ by comparison group type is not clear to us at this juncture.

## Does MI Work in Group Formats?

Limited data can be applied to this question because only eight studies used some form of group delivery: however, our interpretation of the data is that relying solely on group-delivered MI would be a mistake. While no statistically significant differences emerged based on delivery mode (individual, group, or combined), visual inspection of Table 6 seems to discourage group-only delivery and may favor a combined approach instead

In summary, the combined results of the present meta-analysis as well as those previously published meta-analyses suggest a relatively low risk in implementing MI because it works across a wide range of problem behaviors/types and is unlikely to harm clients. Compared to other active and specific treatments. MI was equally effective in our review and shorter in length. When compared to weaker alternatives-such as waitlist, control groups, nonspecific TAU, or written material-MI provides a small yet significant advantage for a diverse array of clients regardless of symptom severity, age, and gender, with possibly an even stronger advantage for minority clients.

It is our sense that MI enjoys a clear and articulate theoretical frame accompanied by specific techniques that can readily be learned (e.g., Arkowitz & Miller, 2008; Markland, Ryan, Tobin, & Rollnick, 2005; Miller & Rollnick, 2004; Vansteenkiste & Sheldon, 2006). Indeed, a rather large body of training materials and trainers for MI has emerged along with mounting research addressing training effectiveness (e.g., see Burke, Dunn, Atkins, & Phelps, 2004), resulting in a rather standardized training approach (see motivationalinter-viewing.org). Moreover, MI researchers are also investing much time and energy into best practices in training MI (Teresa Moyers, personal communication, November 2008) and efforts to assess fidelity to MI are well underway (e.g.. Miller, 2002). Furthermore, MI has been judged to be an evidenced-based practice by organizations such as SAMHSA (Substance Abuse and Mental Health Service Administration). In sum, 25 years of MI research has generated broad scientific inquiry and deep scrutiny, and the MI approach has clearly passed the initial test.

The results of our meta-analysis suggest several potentially fruitful avenues for future MI research. In this review, we made the point that MI may well be more cost-effective than viable alternative treatments even if they are not more clinically effective. While only a handful of MI studies have examined this important variable to date, cost-effectiveness research would certainly add significantly to the MI literature and would be of special interest to policy makers and clinical administrators alike.

Furthermore, although a substantial amount of thought, practice, and research has already been devoted to MI, we still do not understand the precise links between its processes and outcomes (Burke et al., 2002). MI may work via increasing a specific type of client change talk—what they say in session about their commitment to making behavioral changes—and decreasing client speech that defends the status quo (Amrhein, Miller, Yahne, Palmer, & Fulcher, 2003). Consistent with its client-centered background. MI may also work through therapist interpersonal skills (such as accurate empathy as measured by the MISC; Miller, 2002), which are positively associated with client involvement as defined by cooperation, disclosure, and expression of affect

*(Continued)*

(Continued)

(Moyers, Miller, & Hendrickson et al., 2005). Thus, there may be two specific active components underlying the MI mechanism: a relational component focused on empathy and the interpersonal spirit of MI, both of which minimize client resistance, and a technical component involving the differential evocation and reinforcement of client change talk (Miller & Rose, 2009).

Finally, a considerable body of theory and research suggests that MI may be effective for clinical areas beyond the addictions, such as for depression and anxiety disorders (Arkowitz et al., 2008). Our review is supportive of such an assertion because virtually anytime MI has been tested empirically in new areas (e.g., health-promoting behaviors); it has shown positive and significant effects. Thus, we have likely not yet found the limits of the types of problems and symptoms to which MI can be profitably applied.

## Authors' Note

The first and last authors are affiliated with the MINT group and may, therefore, be biased. To control for this bias we explicitly instructed our research team that positive and negative findings were welcomed and expected. Further, we consciously determined to present the results regardless of whether they supported or undermined MI's effectiveness. Lastly, we strove to clearly detail our methodology to be transparent and to encourage possible replication.

### Declaration of Conflicting Interests

The authors declared no potential conflicts of interests with respect to the authorship and/or publication of this article.

### Funding

The Utah Criminal Justice Center, housed within the University of Utah, funded two research assistants (CK, CB) for this project.

### Acknowledgments

Thanks to the Utah Criminal Center who paid for the RAs; thanks to the J. Willard Marriott Library.

## Appendix

### Rating Study Rigor

Studies received 1-point if they did the following: reported on three or more demographic indicators of the sample, collected data at a follow-up period beyond immediate completion of the study, included more than one site, reported data from all dependent variables they assessed, utilized coders who were "blind" to participants' group assignment, utilized objective measurement tools (e.g., records, physiological indicators) instead of relying solely on client self-report, utilized a manual to direct training or standardized delivery, reported on dropouts, and included more than 20 participants in the intervention and comparison groups. Studies earned up to 2 points if the data used to calculate effect sizes came from means, standard deviations, and/or numbers of participants (percentages), 1 point if an exact statistic was used (e.g., $t$ test), and no point if effect sizes were derived from $p$ values. Studies earned 2 points if measurement of outcomes came from al least two sources (e.g., participant and collateral source), 1 point if collateral only, and no point if participant only. Studies earned 2 points if fidelity was assessed and considered high, 1 point if fidelity was assessed but not scored, and no point if fidelity was not measured. Lastly, studies earned 3 points if true randomization was used, 2 points if matched groups were used, 1 point if the groups were tested for pretreatment equivalence, and no point if groups were not equivalent or equivalence could not be determined.

# References

References marked with an asterisk "*" indicate studies included in the meta-analysis.

*Ahluwalia, J. S., Okuyemi, K., Nollen, N., Choi, W. S., Kaur, H., Pulvers, K., et al. (2006). The effects of nicotine gum and counseling among African American light smokers: A 2 × 2 factorial design. *Addiction, 101*, 883–891.

Amrhein, P. C, Miller, W. R., Yahne, C. E., Palmer, M., & Fulcher, L. (2003). Client commitment language during motivational interviewing predicts drug use outcome. *Journal of Consulting and Clinical Psychology, 71*, 862–878.

*Anton, R. F., Moak, D. H., Latham, P., Waid, L. R., Myrick, H., Voronin, K., et al. (2005). Naltrexone combined with either cognitive behavioral or motivational enhancement therapy for alcohol dependence. *Journal of Clinical Psychopharmacology, 25*, 349–357.

Anton, R. F., O'Malley, S. S., Ciraulo, D. A., Cisler, R. A., Couper, D., Donovan, D. M., et al. (2006). Combined pharmacotherapies and behavioral interventions for alcohol dependence. The COMBINE study: A randomized controlled trial. *Journal of the American Medical Association, 295*, 2003–2017.

Arkowitz, H., & Burke, B. L. (2008). Motivational interviewing as an integrative framework for the treatment of depression. In H. Arkowitz, H. A. Westra, W. R. Miller, & S. Rollnick (Eds.), *Motivational interviewing in the treatment of psychological problems,* (pp. 145–172). New York: Guilford.

Arkowitz, H., & Miller, W. (2008). Learning, applying, and extending motivational interviewing. In H. Arkowitz, H. A. Westra, W. R. Miller, & S. Rollnick (Eds.), *Motivational interviewing in the treatment of psychological problems,* (pp. 1–25). New York: Guilford.

Arkowitz, H., Westra, H. A., Miller, W. R., & Rollnick, S. (2008). *Motivational* interviewing in the treatment of psychological problems. New York: Guilford.

*Baer, J. S., Kivlahan, D. R., Blume, A. W., MacKnight, P., & Marlatt, G. A. (2001). Brief intervention for heavy-drinking college students: 4-year follow up and natural history. *American Journal of Public Health, 91*, 1310–1316.

*Baker, A., Heather, N., Wodak, A., Dixon, J., & Holt, P. (1993). Evaluation of a cognitive-behavioral intervention for HIV prevention among injecting drug users. *AIDS, 7*, 247–256.

*Baker, A., Lewin, T., Reichler, H., Clancy, R., Carr, V., Garret, R., et al. (2002). Evaluation of a motivational interview for substance use within psychiatric in-patient services. *Addiction, 97*, 1329–1337.

*Ball, S. A., Todd, M., Tennen, H., Armeli, S., Mohr, C., Affleck, G., et al. (2007). Brief motivational enhancement and coping skills interventions for heavy drinking. *Addictive Behaviors, 32*, 1105–1118.

*Baros, A. M., Latham, P. K., Moak, D., Voronin, K., & Anton, R. F. (2007). What role does measuring medication compliance play in evaluating the efficacy of Naltrexone? *Alcoholism: Clinical and Experimental Research, 31*, 596–603.

*(Continued)*

(Continued)

*Beckham, N. (2007). Motivational interviewing with hazardous drinkers. *Journal of the American Academy of Nurse Practitioners, 19,* 103–110.

*Bennett, J. A., Perrin, N. A., Hanson, G., Bennett, D., Gaynor, W., Flaherty-Robb, M., et al. (2005). Healthy aging demonstration project: Nurse coaching for behavior change in older adults. *Research in Nursing and Health, 28,* 187–197.

Berman, J. S., & Norton, N. C. (1985). Does professional training make a therapist more effective? *Psychological Bulletin, 98,* 401–407.

*Bernstein, J., Bernstein, E., Tassiopoulus, K., Heeren, T., Levenson, S., & Hingson, R. (2005). Brief motivational intervention at a clinic visit reduces cocaine and heroin use. *Drug and Alcohol Dependence, 77,* 49–59.

*Bien, T. H., Miller, W. R., & Boroughs, J. M. (1993). Motivational interviewing with alcohol outpatients. *Behavioral and Cognitive Psychotherapy, 21,* 347–356.

*Booth, R. E., Corsi, K. F., & Mikulich-Gilbertson, S. K. (2004). Factors associated with methadone maintenance treatment retention among street-recruited injection drug users. *Drug and Alcohol Dependence, 74,* 177–185.

*Bien, T. H., Miller, W. R., & Boroughs, J. M. (1993). Motivational interviewing with alcohol outpatients. *Behavioral and Cognitive Psychotherapy, 21,* 347–356.

*Booth, R. E., Corsi, K. F., & Mikulich-Gilbertson, S. K. (2004). Factors associated with methadone maintenance treatment retention among street-recruited injection drug users. *Drug and Alcohol Dependence, 74,* 177–185.

*Booth, R. E., Kwiatkowski, C., Iguchi, M., Pinto, F., & John, D. (1998). Facilitating treatment entry among out-of-treatment injection drug users. *Public Health Reports, 113,* 117–129.

Borenstein, M., Hedges, L., Higgins, J., & Rothstein, H. (2005). Comprehensive Meta-Analysis (Version 2) [Computer software]. Englewood, NJ: Biostat.

*Borrelli, B., Novak, S., Hecht, J., Emmons, K., Papandonatos, G., & Abrams, D. (2005). Home health care nurses as a new channel for smoking cessation treatment: Outcomes from project CARES (Community-nurse Assisted Research and Education on Smoking). *Preventive Medicine, 41,* 815–821.

*Bowen, D., Ehret, C., Pedersen, M., Snetselaar, L. Johnson, M., Tinker, L., et al. (2002). Results of an adjunct dietary intervention program in the woman's health initiative. *Journal of the American Dietetic Association, 102,* 1631–1637.

*Brodie, D. A., & Inoue, A. (2005). Motivational interviewing to promote physical activity for people with chronic heart failure. *Journal of Advanced Nursing, 50,* 518–527.

*Brown, J. M., & Miller, W. R. (1993). Impact of motivational interviewing on participation and overcome in residential alcoholism treatment. *Psychology of Addictive Behavior, 7,*211–218.

*Brown, T. G., Dongier, M., Latimer, E., Legault, L., Seraganian, P., Kokin, M., et al. (2006). Group-delivered brief intervention versus standard care for mixed alcohol/other drug problems: A preliminary study. *Alcoholism Treatment Quarterly, 24,* 23–40.

Burke, B., Arkowitz, H., & Dunn, C. (2002). The efficacy of motivational interviewing. In W. R. Miller, & S. Rollnick (Eds.), *Motivational inteiviewing: Preparing people for change* (2nd ed. pp. 217–250). New York: Guilford.

Burke, B. L., Arkowitz, H., & Menchola, M. (2003). The efficacy of motivational interviewing: A meta-analysis of controlled clinical trials. *Journal of Consulting and Clinical Psychology, 71,* 843–861.

Burke, B. L., Dunn, C. W., Atkins, D., & Phelps, J. S. (2004). The emerging evidence base for motivational interviewing: A meta-analytic & qualitative inquiry. *Journal of Cognitive Psychotherapy, 18,* 309–322.

*Butler, C. C., Rollnick, S., Cohen, D., Bachman, M., Russell, I., & Stott, N. (1999). Motivational consulting versus brief advice for smokers in general practice: A randomized trial. *British Journal of General Practice, 49,* 611–616.

*Carey, M. P., Baaten, L. S., Maisto, S. A., Gleason, J. R., Forsyth, A. D., Durant, L. E., et al. (2000). Using information, motivational enhancement, and skills training, to reduce the risk of HIV infection for low-income urban women: A second randomized clinical trial. *Health Psychology, 19,* 3–11.

*Carroll, K. M., Ball, S. A., Nich, C., Martino, S., Frankforter, T. L, Farentinos, C., et al. (2005). Motivational interviewing to improve treatment engagement and outcome in individuals seeking treatment for substance abuse: a multisite effectiveness study. *Drug and Alcohol Dependence, 81,* 301–312.

*Carroll, K. M., Libby, B., Sheehan, J., & Hyland, N. (2001). Motivational interviewing to enhance treatment initiation in substance abusers: An effectiveness study. *The American Journal on Addictions, 10,* 335–339.

*Channon, S. J., Huws-Thomas, M. V., Rollnick, S., Hood, K., Cannings-John, R. L., Rogers, C., et al. (2007). A multicenter randomized controlled trial of motivational interviewing in teenagers with diabetes. *Diabetes Care, 30,* 1390–1395.

Cohen, J. (1988). *Statistical power analysis for the behavioral sciences* (2nd ed.). Hillsdale, NJ: Erlbaum.

*Colby, S. M., Monti, P. M., Barnett, N. P., Rosenhow, D. J., Weissman, K., & Spirito, A. et al. (1998). Brief motivational interviewing in a hospital setting for adolescent smoking: A preliminary study. *Journal of Consulting and Clinical Psychology, 66,* 574–578.

*Colby, S. M., Monti, P. M., Tevyaw, T. O., Barnett, N. P., Spirito, A., Rosenhow, D. J., et al. (2005). Brief motivational intervention for adolescent smokers in medical settings. *Addictive Behaviors, 30,* 865–874.

*Connors, G. J., Walitzer, K. S., & Dermen, K. H. (2002). Preparing clients for alcoholism treatment: Effects on treatment participation and outcomes. *Journal of Consulting and Clinical Psychology, 70,* 1161–1169.

Cooper, H., & Hedges, L. V. (1994). *The handbook of research synthesis.* New York: Russell SAGE.

*Curry, S. J., Ludman, E. J., Graham, E., Stout, J., Grothaus, L., & Lozano, P. (2003). Pediatric-based smoking cessation intervention for low-income based women. *Archives of Pediatrics and Adolescent Medicine, 157,* 295–302.

*Daley, D. C., Salloum, I. M., Zuckoff, A., Kirisci, L., & Thase, M. E. (1998). Increasing treatment adherence among outpatients with depression and cocaine dependence: Results of a pilot study. *American Journal of Psychiatry, 155,* 1611–1613.

*Davidson, D., Gulliver, S. B., Longabaugh, R., Wirtz, P. W., & Swift, R. (2006). Building better cognitive-behavioral therapy: Is broad-spectrum treatment more effective then motivational-enhancement therapy for alcohol-dependent patients treated with Naltrexone? *Journal of Studies on Alcohol and Drugs, 68,* 238–247.

*Davis, T. M., Baer, J. S., Saxon, A. J., & Kivlahan, D. R. (2003). Brief motivational feedback improves post-incarceration treatment contact among veterans with substance use disorders. *Drug and Alcohol Dependence, 69,* 197–203.

*Dench, S., & Bennett, G. (2000). The impact of brief motivational intervention at the start of an outpatient day programme for alcohol dependence. *Behavioral and Cognitive Psychotherapy, 28,* 121–130.

*Dunn, E. C., Neighbors, C., & Larimer, M. E. (2006). Motivational enhancement therapy and self-help treatment for binge eaters. *Psychology of Addictive Behaviors, 20,* 44–52.

*Elliot, D. L., Goldberg, L., Kuehl, K. S. Moe, E. L., Breger, R. K. R., & Pickering, M. A. (2007). The PHLAME (Promoting Healthy Lifestyles: Alternative Model's Effects) firefighter study: Outcomes of two models of behavior change. *Journal of Occupational and Environmental Medicine, 49,* 204–213.

*Emmen, M. J., Schippers, G. M., Wollersheim, H., & Bleijenberg, G. (2005). Adding psychologist's intervention to physician's advice to problem drinkers in the outpatient clinic. *Alcohol & Alcoholism, 40,* 219–226.

*(Continued)*

(Continued)

*Emmons, K. M., Hammond, K., Fava, J. L. Velicer, W. F., Evans, J. L., & Monroe, A. D. (2001). A randomized trial to reduce passive smoke exposure in low income households with young children. *Pediatrics, 108,* 18–24.

*Gailbraith, I. G. (1989). Minimal intervention with problem drinkers: A pilot study of the effect of two interview styles on perceived self-efficacy. *Health Bulletin, 47,* 311–314.

*Gentilello, L. M., Rivara, F. P., Donovan, D. M., Jurkovich, G. J., Daranciang, E., Dunn, C. W., et al. (1999). Alcohol interventions in a trauma center as a means of reducing the risk of injury recurrence. *Annals of Surgery, 250,* 473–483.

*Golin, C. E., Earp, J., Tien, H. C., Stewart, P., Porter, C., & Howie, L. (2006). A 2–arm, randomized, controlled trial of a motivational interviewing-based intervention to improve adherence to antiretroviral therapy (ART) among patients failing or initiating ART. *Journal of Acquired Immune Deficiency Syndromes, 42,* 42–51.

*Graeber, D. A., Moyers, T. B., Griffith, G., Guajardo, E., & Tonigan, S. (2003). A pilot study comparing motivational interviewing and an educational intervention in patients with schizophrenia and alcohol use disorders. *Community Mental Health Journal, 39,* 189–202.

*Gray, E., McCambridge, J., & Strang, J. (2005). The effectiveness of motivational interviewing delivered by youth workers in reducing drinking, cigarette and cannabis smoking among young people: Quasi-experimental pilot study. *Alcohol & Alcoholism, 40,* 535–539.

*Grenard, J. L., Ames, S. L., Wiers, R. W., Thush, C., Stacy, A. W., & Sussman, S. (2007). Brief intervention for substance use among at risk adolescents: A pilot study. *Journal of Adolescent Health, 40,* 188–191.

Handmaker, N. S., Miller, W. R., & Manicke, M. (1999). Findings of a pilot study of motivational interviewing with pregnant drinkers. *Journal of Studies on Alcohol, 60,* 285–287.

*Harland, J., White, M., Drinkwater, C., Chinn, D., Farr, L., & Howel, D. (1999). The Newcastle exercise project: a randomized controlled trial of methods to promote physical activity in primary care. *British Medical Journal, 319,* 828–832.

*Haug, N. A., Svikis, D. S., & DiClemente, C. (2004). Motivational enhancement therapy for nicotine dependence in methadone-maintained pregnant women. *Psychology of Addictive Behaviors, 18,* 298–292.

*Helstrom, A., Hutchison, K., & Bryan, A. (2007). Motivational enhancement therapy for high-risk adolescent smokers. *Addictive Behaviors, 32,* 2404–2410.

Hettema, J., Steele, J., & Miller, W. (2005). Motivational interviewing. *Annual Review of Clinical Psychology, 1,* 91–111.

*Hillsdon, M., Thorogood, M., White, I., & Foster, C. (2002). Advising people to take more exercise is ineffective: A randomized controlled trial of physical activity promotion in primary care. *International Journal of Epidemiology, 31,* 808–815.

*Hodgins, D. C. Currie, S. R., & El-Guebaly, N. (2001). Motivational enhancement and self-help treatments for problem gambling. *Journal of Consulting and Clinical Psychology, 69,* 50–57.

*Hodgins, D. C., Currie, S, El-Guebaly, N., & Peden, N. (2004). Brief motivational treatment for problem gambling: A 24–month follow-up. *Psychology of Addictive Behaviors, 18,* 293–296.

*Hulse, G. K., & Tait, R. J. (2002). Six month outcomes associated with a brief alcohol intervention for adult in-patients with psychiatric disorders. *Drug and Alcohol Review, 21,* 105–112.

*Hulse, G. K., & Tait, R. J. (2003). Five year outcomes of a brief alcohol intervention for adult inpatients with psychiatric disorders. *Addiction, 98,* 1061–1068.

*Humfress, H., Igel, V., Lamont, A., Tanner, M., Morgan, J., & Schmidt, U. (2002). The effect of a brief motivational intervention on community psychiatric patients' attitudes to their care, motivation to change, compliance and outcome: A case control study. *Journal of Mental Health, 11,* 155–166.

Hunter, J. E., & Schmidt, F. L. (2000). Fixed effects versus random effects meta-analysis models: Implications for cumulative research knowledge. *International Journal of Selection and Assessment, 8,* 275–292.

*Ingersoll, K. S., Ceperich, S. D., Nettleman, M. D., Karanda, K., Brocksen, S., & Johnson, B. A. (2005). Reducing alcohol-exposed pregnancy risk in college women: Initial outcomes of a clinical trial of a motivational intervention. *Journal of Substance Abuse Treatment, 29, 173–180.*

*Jaworski, B. C., & Carey, M. P. (2001). Effects of a brief, theory-based STD-prevention program for female college students. *Journal of Adolescent Health, 29,* 417–425.

Johnson, B. T., Mullen, B., & Salas, E. (1995). Comparison of three major meta-analytic approaches. *Journal of Applied Psychology, 80,* 94–106.

*Johnston, B. D., Rivara, F. P., Droesch, R. M., Dunn, C., & Copass, M. K. (2007). Behavior change counseling in the emergency department to reduce injury risk: A randomized controlled trial. *Pediatrics, 110,* 267–274.

*Juarez, P., Walters, S. T., Daugherty, M., & Radi, C. (2006). A randomized trial of motivational interviewing and feedback with heavy drinking college students. *Journal of Drug Education, 36,* 233–246.

*Kahler, C. W., Read, J. P., Ramsey, S. E., Stuart, G. L., McCrady, B. S., & Brown, R. A. (2004). Motivational enhancement for a 12–step involvement among patients undergoing alcohol detoxification. *Journal of Consulting and Clinical Psychology, 72,* 736–741.

*Kelly, A. B., & Lapworth, K. (2006). The HYP program- targeted motivational interviewing for adolescent violations of school tobacco policy. *Preventive Medicine, 43,* 466–471.

*Kidorf, M., Disney, E., King, V., Kolodner, K., Beilenson, P., & Brooner, R. K. (2005). Challenges in motivating treatment enrollment in community syringe exchange participants. *Journal of Urban Health, 82,* 457–465.

*Kreman, R., Yates, B. C., Agrawal, S., Fiandt, K., Briner, W., & Shurmur, S. (2006). The effects of motivational interviewing on physiological outcomes. *Applied Nursing Research, 19,* 167–170.

*Kuchipudi, V., Hobein, K., Flickinger, A., & Iber, F. L. (1990). Failure of a 2–hour motivational intervention to alter recurrent drinking behavior in alcoholics with gastrointestinal disease. *Journal of Studies on Alcohol, 51,* 356–360.

Landis, J. R., & Koch, G. G. (1977). The measurement of observer agreement for categorical data. *Biometrics, 33,* 159–174.

*Larimer, M. E., Turner, A. P., Anderson, B. K., Fader, J. S., Kilmer, J. R., Palmer, R. S., et al. (2001). Evaluating a brief alcohol intervention with fraternities. *Journal of Studies on Alcohol, 62,* 370–380.

Lipsey, M., & Wilson, D. (1993). The efficacy of psychological, educational, and behavioral treatment: Confirmation from meta-analysis. *American Psychologist, 48,* 1181–1209.

Lipsey, M. W., & Wilson, D. B. (2001). *Practical meta-analysis.* Applied Social Research Methods Series (Vol. 49). Thousand Oaks, CA: Sage.

*Litt, M. D., Kadden, R. M., & Stephens, R. S. (2005). Coping and self-efficacy in marijuana treatment: Results from the marijuana treatment project. *Journal of Consulting and Clinical Psychology, 73,* 1015–1025.

*Longabaugh, R., Woolard, R. F., Nirenberg, T. D., Minugh, A. P., Becker, B., Clifford, P. R., et al. (2001). Evaluating the effects of a brief motivational intervention for injured drinkers in the emergency department. *Journal of Studies on Alcohol, 62,* 806–817.

*Longshore, D., & Grills, C. (2000). Motivating illegal drug use recovery: Evidence for a culturally congruent intervention. *Journal of Black Psychology, 26,* 288–301.

Lundahl, B. W., & Yaffe, J. (2007). Use of meta-analysis in social work and allied disciplines. *Journal of Social Service Research, 33,* 1–11.

*(Continued)*

(Continued)

*Maisto, S. A., Conigliaro, J., McNeil, M., Kraemer, K., Conigliaro. R. L., & Kelley, M. E. (2001). Effects of two types of brief intervention and readiness to change on alcohol use in hazardous drinkers. *Journal of Studies on Alcohol, 62,* 605–614.

*Maltby, N., & Tolin, D. F. (2005). A brief motivational intervention for treatment-refusing OCD patients. *Cognitive Behavioral Therapy, 34,* 176–184.

*Marijuana Treatment Project Research Group. (2004). Brief treatments for cannabis dependence: Findings from a randomized multisite trial. *Journal of Consulting and Clinical Psychology, 72,* 455–466.

Markland, D., Ryan, R., Tobin, V., & Rollnick, S. (2005). Motivational interviewing and self-determination theory. *Journal of Social & Clinical Psychology, 24,* 811–831.

*Marsden, J., Stillwell, G., Barlow, H., Boys, A., Taylor, C., Hunt, N., et al. (2006). An evaluation of a brief motivational intervention among young ecstasy and cocaine users: No effect on substance and alcohol use outcomes. *Addiction, 101,* 1014–1026.

*Martino, S., Carroll, K. M., Nich, C., & Rounsaville, B. J. (2006). A randomized controlled pilot study of motivational interviewing for patients with psychotic and drug use disorders. *Addiction, 101,* 1479–1492.

*McCambridge, J., & Strang, J. (2004a). Deterioration over time in effect of motivational interviewing in reducing drug consumption and related risk among young people. *Addiction, 100,* 470–478.

*McCambridge, J., & Strang, J. (2004b). The efficacy of a single-session motivational interviewing in reducing drug consumption and perceptions of drug related risk and harm among young people: Results from a multi-site cluster randomized trial. *Addiction, 99,* 39–52.

Mhurchu, C. N., Margetts, B. M., & Speller, V. (1998). Randomized clinical trial comparing the effectiveness of two dietary interventions for patients with hyperlipidaemia. *Clinical Science, 95,* 479–487.

*Michael, K. D., Curtin, L., Kirkley, D. E., & Jones, D. L. (2006). Group-based motivational interviewing for alcohol use among college students: An exploratory study. *Professional Psychology: Research and Practice, 37,* 629–634.

Miller, W. R. (2002). *Motivational interviewing skill code (MISC) coder's manual.* Retrieved November 2, 2008, from http://motivationalmtemew.org/training/MISC2.pdf

*Miller, W. R., Benefield, G., & Tonigan, J. S. (1993). Enhancing motivation for change in problem drinking: A controlled comparison of two therapist styles. *Journal of Consulting and Clinical Psychology, 61,* 455–461.

Miller, W. R., & Rollnick, S. (2002). *Motivational interviewing: Preparing people for change* (2nd ed.). New York: Guilford.

Miller, W. R., & Rollnick, S. (2004). Talking oneself into change: Motivational interviewing, stages of change, and the therapeutic process. *Journal of Cognitive Psychotherapy, 18,* 299–308.

Miller, W. R., & Rose, G. S. (2009). Toward a theory of motivational interviewing. *American Psychologist, 64,* 527–537.

Miller, W. R., Sovereign, R. G., & Krege, B. (1988). Motivational interviewing with problem drinkers: II. The drinker's check-up as a preventive intervention. *Behavioural Psychotherapy, 16,* 251–268.

*Miller, W. R., Yahne, C. E., & Tonigan, S. (2003). Motivational interviewing in drug abuse services: A randomized clinical trial. *Journal of Counseling and Clinical Psychology, 71,* 754–763.

*Mitcheson, L., McCambridge, J., & Byrne, S. (2007). Pilot cluster-randomized trial of adjunctive motivational interviewing to reduce crack cocaine use in clients on methadone maintenance. *European Addiction Research, 13,* 6–10.

*Monti, P. M., Colby, S. M., Barnett, N. P., Spirito, A., Rohsenow, D. J., & Myers, M. et al. (1999). Brief intervention for harm reduction with alcohol-positive older adolescents in a hospital emergency department. *Journal of Consulting and Clinical Psychology, 67,* 989–994.

*Morgenstern, J., Parsons, J. T., Bux, D. A., Jr., Irwin, T. W., Wainberg, M. L., Muench, F., et al. (2007). A randomized controlled trial of goal choice interventions for alcohol use disorders among men who sex with men. *Journal of Counseling and Clinical Psychology, 75,* 72–84.

Moyers, T. B., Miller, W. R., & Hendrickson, S. M. L. (2005). How-does motivational interviewing work? Therapist interpersonal skill predicts client involvement within motivational interviewing sessions. *Journal of Consulting and Clinical Psychology, 73,* 590–598.

*Mullins, S. M., Suarez, M., Ondersma, S. J., & Page, M. C. (2004). The impact of motivational interviewing on substance abuse treatment retention: A randomized control trial of women involved with child welfare. *Journal of Substance Abuse Treatment, 27,* 51–58.

*Murphy, J. G., Duchnick, J. J., Vuchinich, R. E., Davison, J. W., Karg, J. W., Olson, A.M., et al. (2001). Relative efficacy of a brief motivational intervention for college student drinkers. *Psychology of Addictive Behaviors, 15,* 373–379.

*Naar-King, S., Wright, K., Parsons, J. T., Frey, M., Tempi in, T., Lam, P., et al. (2006). Healthy choices: Motivational enhancement therapy for health risk behaviors in HIV-positive youth. *AIDS Education and Prevention, 18,* 1–11.

*Nock, M. K., & Kazdin, A. E. (2005). Randomized controlled trial of a brief intervention for increasing participation in parent management training. *Journal of Consulting and Clinical Psychology, 73,* 872–879.

*Peterson, P. L., Baer, J. S., Wells, E. A., Ginzler, J. A., & Garrett, S. B. (2006). Short-term effects of a brief motivational intervention to reduce alcohol and drug risk among homeless adolescents. *Psychology of Addictive Behaviors, 20,* 254–264.

Piaget, J. (1962). The stages of the intellectual development of the child. *Bulletin of the Menninger Clinic, 26,* 120–128.

*Picciano, J. F., Roffman, R. A., Kalichman, S. C., Rutledge, S. E., & Berghuis, J. P. (2001). A telephone based brief intervention using motivational enhancement to facilitate HIV risk reduction among MSM: A pilot study. *AIDS and Behavior, 5,* 251–262.

Prochaska, J. O., & Norcross, J. C. (2007). *Systems of psychotherapy: A transtheoretical approach.* South Melbourne, Australia: Thomson Brooks/Cole.

Project MATCH Research Group. (1997). Matching alcoholism treatment to client heterogeneity: Project MATCH post treatment drinking outcomes. *Journal of Studies on Alcohol, 58,* 7–29.

Project MATCH Research Group. (1998). Matching alcoholism treatment to client heterogeneity: Project MATCH three-year drinking outcomes. *Alcoholism: Clinical and Experimental Research, 23,* 1300–1311.

Rogers, C. R. (1951). *Client centered therapy.* Boston: Houghton-Mifflin.

*Rohsenow, D. J., Monti, P. M., Colby, S. M., & Martin, R. A. (2002). Brief interventions for smoking cessation in alcoholic smokers. *Alcoholism: Clinical and Experimental Research, 26,* 1950–1951.

Rollnick, S., Miller, W. R., & Butler, C. C. (2008). *Motivational interviewing in health care: Helping patients change behavior.* New York: Guilford.

*Rosenblum, A., Cleland, C., Magura, S., Mahmood, D., & Kosanke, N. (2005). Moderators of effects of motivational enhancements to cognitive behavioral therapy. *The American Journal of Drug and Alcohol Abuse, 31,* 35–58.

*Saitz. R., Palfal, T. P., Cheng, D. M., Horton, N. J., Freedner, N., Dukes, K., et al. (2007). Brief intervention for medical inpatients with unhealthy alcohol use. *Annals of Internal Medicine, 146,* 167–176.

*Saunders, B., Wilkinson, C., & Phillips, M. (1995). The impact of a brief motivational intervention with opiate users attending a methadone programme. *Addiction, 90,* 415–424.

*Schermer, C. R., Moyers, T. B., Miller, T. B., Miller, W. R., & Bloomfield, L. A. (2006). Trauma center brief interventions for alcohol disorders decrease subsequent driving under the influence arrests. *The Journal of Trauma Injury, Infection, and Critical Care, 60,* 29–34.

*(Continued)*

(Continued)

*Schmaling, K. B., Blume, A. W., & Afari, N. (2001). A randomized controlled pilot study of motivational interviewing to change attitudes about adherence to medications for asthma. *Journal of Clinical Psychology in Medical Settings, 8,* 167–171.

*Schneider, R. J., Casey, J., & Kohn, R. (2000). Motivational versus confrontational interviewing: A comparison of substance abuse assessment practices at employee assistance programs. *The Journal of Behavioral Health Services and Research, 27,* 60–74.

*Secades-Villa, R., Femande-Hermida, J. R., & Amaez-Montaraz, C. (2004). Motivational interviewing and treatment retention among drug user patients: A pilot study. *Substance Use and Misuse, 39,* 1369–1378.

*Sellman, J. D., Sullivan, P. F., Dore, G. M., Adamson, S. I., & MacEwan, I. (2001). A randomized controlled trial of motivational enhancement therapy (MET) for mild to moderate alcohol dependence. *Journal of Studies on Alcohol, 62,* 389–396.

*Smith, D. E., Kratt, P. P., Heckenmeyer, C. M., & Mason, D. A. (1997). Motivational interviewing to improve adherence to a behavioral weight-control program for older obese women with NIDDM. *Diabetes Care, 20,* 52–53.

*Smith, S. S., Jorenby, D. E., Fiore, M. C., Anderson, J. E., Mielke, M. M., Beach, K. E., et al. (2001). Strike while the iron is hot: Can stepped-care treatments resurrect relapsing smokers? *Journal of Counseling and Clinical Psychology, 699,* 429–445.

*Soria, R., Legido, A., Escolano, C., Yeste, A. L., & Montoya, J. (2006). A randomised controlled trial of motivational interviewing for smoking cessation. *British Journal of General Practice, 56,* 768–774.

*Spirito, A., Monti, P. M., Barnett, N. P., Colby, S. M., Sindelar, H., & Rosenhow, D. J. (2004). A randomized clinical trial of a brief motivational intervention for alcohol-positive adolescents treated in an emergency department. *The Journal of Pediatrics, 145,* 396–402.

*Stein, M. D., Anderson, B., Charuvastra, A., Maksad, J., & Friedmann, P. D. (2002). A brief intervention for hazardous drinkers in a needle exchange program. *Journal of Substance Abuse Treatment, 22,* 23–31.

*Stein, M. D., Charuvastra, A., Maksad, J., & Anderson, B. J. (2002). A randomized trial of a brief alcohol intervention for needle exchangers (BRAINE). *Addiction, 97,* 691–700.

*Stein, L. A. R., Colby, S. M., Bamett, N. P., Monti, P. M., Golembeske, C., & Lebeau-Craven, R. (2006). Effects of motivational interviewing for incarcerated adolescents on driving under the influence after release. *The American Journal on Addictions, 15,* 50–57.

*Stein, L. A. R., Monti, P. M., Colby, S. M., Bamett, N. P. Golembeske, C., & Lebeau-Craven, R. (2006). Enhancing substance abuse treatment engagement in incarcerated adolescents. *Psychological Services, 3,* 25–34.

*Steinberg, M. L., Ziedonis, D. M., Krejci, J. A., & Brandon, T. H. (2004). Motivational interviewing with personalized feedback: A brief intervention for motivating smokers with schizophrenia to seek treatment for tobacco dependence. *Journal of Consulting and Clinical Psychology, 72,* 723–728.

*Stephens, R. S., Roffman, R. A., & Curtin, L. (2000). Comparison of extended versus brief treatments for marijuana use. *Journal of Consulting and Clinical Psychology, 68,* 898–908.

*Stotts, A. L., DeLaune, K. A., Schmitz, J. M., & Grabowski, J. (2004). Impact of a motivational intervention on mechanisms of change in low-income pregnant smokers. *Addictive Behaviors, 29,* 1649–1657.

*Stotts, A. L., DiClemente, C. C., & Dolan-Mullen, P. (2002). One-to-one: A motivational intervention for resistant pregnant smokers. *Addictive Behaviors, 27,* 275–292.

*Stotts, A. L., Potts, G. F., Ingersoll, G., George, M. R., & Martin, L. E. (2006). Preliminary feasibility and efficacy of a brief motivational intervention with psychophysiological feedback for cocaine abuse. *Substance Abuse, 27,* 9–20.

*Stotts, A. L., Schmitz, J. M., Rhoades, H. M., & Grabowski, J. (2001). Motivational interviewing with cocaine with cocaine-dependent patients: A pilot study. *Journal of Consulting and Clinical Psychology, 69*, 858–862.

*Tappin, D. M., Lumsden, M. A., Gilmour, W. H., Crawford, F., McIntyre, D., Stone, D. H., et al. (2005). Randomised controlled trial of home based motivational interviewing by midwives to help pregnant smokers quit or cut down. *British Medical Journals, 331*, 373–377.

*Tappin, D. M., Lumsden, M. A., McIntyre, D., McKay, C., Gilmour, W. H., Webber, R., et al. (2000). A pilot study to establish a randomized trial methodology to test the efficacy of a behavioural intervention. *Health Education Research: Theory and Practice, 15*, 491–502.

*Tappin, D. M., Lumsden, M. A., Mckay, C., McIntyre, D., Gilmour, H., Webber, R., et al. (2000). The effect of home-based motivational interviewing on the smoking behavior of pregnant women: A pilot randomized controlled efficacy study. *Ambulatory Child Health, 6*, 34–35.

*Thevos, A. K., Kaona, F. A. D., Siajunza, M. T., & Quick, R. E. (2000). Adoption of safe water behaviors in Zambia: Comparing educational and motivational approaches. *Education for Health, 13*, 366–376.

*UKAAT (United Kingdom Alcohol Treatment Trial) Research Team. (2005). effectiveness of treatment for alcohol problems: Findings of the randomised UK alcohol treatment trial. *British Medical Journal, 331*, 541–544.

*Valanis, B., Glasgow, R. E., Mullooly, J., Vogt, T., Whitlock, E. E., Boles, S. M., et al. (2002). Screening HMO women overdue for both mammograms and pap tests. *Preventive Medicine, 34*, 40–50.

*Valanis, B., Whitlock, E. E., Mullooly, J., Vogt, T., Smith, S., Chen, C., et al. (2003). Screening rarely screened women: Time-to-service and 24–month outcomes of tailored interventions. *Preventive Medicine, 37*, 442–450.

Vansteenkiste, M., & Sheldon, K. (2006). There's nothing more practical than a good theory: Integrating motivational interviewing and self-determination theory. *British Journal of Clinical Psychology, 45*, 63–82.

Vasilaki, E., Hosier, S., & Cox, W. (2006). The efficacy of motivational interviewing as a brief intervention for excessive drinking: A meta-analytic review. *Alcohol and Alcoholism, 41*, 328–335.

*Walker, D. D., Roffman, R. A., Stephens, R. S., Berghuis, J., & Kim, W. (2006). Motivational enhancement therapy for adolescent marijuana users: A preliminary randomized controlled trial. *Journal of Consulting and Clinical Psychology, 74*, 628–632.

*Watkins, C. L., Auton, M. F., Deans, C. F., Dickinson, H. A., Jack, C. I. A., Light body, E., et al. (2007). Motivational interviewing early after acute stroke: A randomized, controlled trial. *Stroke, 38*, 1004–1009.

*Weinstein, P., Harrison, R., & Benton, T. (2004). Motivating parents to prevent caries in their young children: One year findings. *Journal of the American Dental Association, 135*, 731–738.

Welch, G., Rose, G., Hanson, D., Lekarcyk, J., Smith-Ossman, S., Gordon, T., et al. (2003). Changes in Motivational Interviewing Skills Code (MISC) scores following motivational interviewing training for diabetes educators. *Diabetes, 52*, A421.

* Westra, H. A., & Dozois, D. J. A. (2006). Preparing clients for cognitive behavioral therapy: A randomized pilot study of motivational interviewing for anxiety. *Cognitive Therapy and Research, 30*, 481–498.

*Wilhelm, S. L., Stephans, M. B. F., Hertzog, M, Rodehorst, T. K. C., & Gardener, P. (2006). Motivational interviewing to promote sustained breastfeeding. *Journal of Obstetric, Gynecologic, & Neonatal Nursing, 35*, 340–348.

# 6

# Borderline Personality Disorder and Women

## *Comorbidity With Mood, Anxiety, and Substance Use Disorders*

> Jean is a 29-year-old Caucasian female who came in for a scheduled intake appointment following hospitalization for her second suicide attempt (an attempted overdose of prescription medication). During the interview, she was well-dressed, though her personal hygiene fell below standards, with her hair uncombed and dirt on her face and hands. Jean stated that she has felt suicidal since she turned 18. Jean explained that she wants to stay in bed most of the day and night, and when she is not in bed, she is often involved in intense relationships with friends and relatives. She explained that she often has periods of crying during the day. Jean stopped going to high school in her sophomore year, when her mother home-schooled her. She states that she feels "empty" and does not know who she is. Jean has a history of self-mutilation and admits to having been sexually abused by her father, who is currently in jail for assault.

We have included borderline personality disorder (BPD) in this book to reflect its comorbidity with the mental health disorders most prevalent among poor women. The co-occurrence of BPD with mood, anxiety, and substance use disorders (Bornovalova, Gratz, Delany-Brumsey, Paulson, & Lejuez, 2006) signals the need for social workers to better understand the prevalence and etiology of the disorder by gender, as well as how to screen and treat poor women with whom they practice for BPD. Given the high lethality associated with BPD, we believe this disorder warrants special attention, particularly in light of the finding that being female with less education and low income are key risk factors for BPD.

# Definition

The essential feature of BPD is a pervasive pattern of instability of inter-personal relationships, self-image, and affects (American Psychiatric Association, 2000). This feature is frequently marked by impulsivity that begins in early adulthood and is exhibited in numerous contexts. Identifying five of the following nine categorical criteria allows for the clinical diagnosis of BPD: (a) a sense of abandonment and/or attempt to avoid abandonment; (b) a pattern of unstable and intense relationships; (c) an unstable self-image and sense of self; (d) impulsivity in areas such as spending money irresponsibly or engaging in unsafe sex; (e) engagement in suicidal or self-injurious behaviors; (f) instability in affect, such as intense irritability that may last a few hours to a few days; (g) possible chronic feelings of emptiness; (h) boredom and restlessness, often including the inappropriate expression of anger; and (i) display of extreme sarcasm or anger, especially in a love relationship.

Currently, clinicians use the aforementioned nine criteria in diagnosing BPD. However, some experts believe that the categorical system with nine criteria has 256 different configurations or clusters with a BPD diagnosis, making the diagnosis less exact (Peele & Kadekar, 2007). In this regard, others believe that dimensional models might be more exact in diagnosing personality disorders than the categorical systems, and therefore should be considered for inclusion in the new *DSM-V*. For example, one dimensional model proposed includes the following five dimensions: (a) extraversion versus introversion; (b) antagonism versus compliance; (c) constraint versus impulsivity; (d) emotional dysregulation versus emotional stability; and (e) unconventionality versus being closed to experience (Widiger, Simonsen, Sirovatka, & Regier, 2007).

One diagnostic issue is the extent to which BPD should or should not be an Axis I diagnosis as opposed to an Axis II diagnosis. New, Triebwasser, and Charney (2008) argued that the severity of symptoms associated with BPD should be taken much more seriously, and as a result, consideration should be given to reclassifying the disorder to Axis I. The association of BPD with both major depressive disorder (MDD) and post-traumatic stress disorder (PTSD) suggest that BPD may actually be a bipolar spectrum illness. Historically, many experts have believed that Axis II disorders (personality disorders) result from environmental factors whereas Axis I disorders (mood, anxiety, and substance use disorders) result from biological or organic factors. In sum, the argument can be made that BPD might better be diagnosed on Axis I due primarily to the "affective dysregulation symptoms" (New et al., 2008, p. 657).

Yet another diagnostic issue relates to when a BPD diagnosis should be made. On the one hand, there are those researchers who believe that a diagnosis can be made more immediately using a structured interview schedule; on the other hand, there are clinicians who believe that the diagnosis should come over time (Zimmerman & Mattia, 1999). Individuals seen at a time when they are seeking treatment for BPD may be likely to present with symptoms of co-occurring disorders (Western, 1997), which suggests that BPD may not be the primary diagnosis. In the latter case, the clinical evaluation may lack the thoroughness necessary to identify co-occurring disorders (Widiger & Rogers, 1989). This issue seems to be salient in understanding the prevalence rate of BPD in epidemiological versus clinical studies.

## Prevalence and Onset

BPD seems to be more prevalent in the general population than researchers and clinicians have believed in the past. In 2004–2005, 34,653 adults participated in the National Epidemiological Survey on Alcohol and Related Conditions (NESARC), which relied on face-to-face interviews. Grant et al. (2008) used data from this survey to examine the prevalence of alcohol and specific drug use disorders and BPD, as well as data from the 2001–2002 NESARC survey to examine prevalence of mood and anxiety disorders. The researchers reported that the lifetime rates of BPD among women and men were 6.2% and 5.6%, respectively. In this epidemiological study, BPD was more prevalent among Native American men; among younger, separated, divorced or widowed adults; and among adults with lower incomes and less education. By comparison, the results of community surveys show that the prevalence of BPD is 1% (Paris, 2005). As one might expect, however, BPD was found to be associated with substantial mental and physical disability, especially among women, and often co-occurs with mood, anxiety, and substance use disorders.

Although there was little difference in the prevalence of BPD by gender in epidemiological studies (Grant et al., 2008), the results in clinical studies show a greater prevalence of BPD among women (Paris, 2005). This might be due to biases in BPD assessment (Zlotnik, Rothschild, & Zimmerman, 2002) or in the treatment-seeking behavior of women diagnosed with BPD (Skodal & Bender, 2003). Although the onset of BPD occurs at a mean age of 18 years, the rates of BPD seem to decrease with age, particularly after the age of 44 years (Zanarini, Frankenburg, Hennen, Reich, & Silk, 2005; Zanarini, Frankenburg, Hennen, Reich, & Silk, 2006; Zanarini, Frankenburg, Hennen, & Silk, 2003), which may mean that BPD is less chronic than experts have previously thought (Grant et al., 2008).

Little research has focused on the relationship between race or ethnicity and BPD, though results of the NESARC indicate that the rates of BPD are higher among Native American men and lower among Hispanic men and Asian women (Grant et al., 2008). Bornovalova et al. (2006) examined risk factors for BPD in a sample of patients in residential drug and alcohol treatment that was comprised of 93% African Americans, 44% of whom were females. The researchers found that the risk factors for BPD in this nonrepresentative sample were being female, having less education, having high stress reactivity, and having undergone emotional abuse.

In understanding why a chapter on BPD is included in this book, it is helpful to understand the extent to which this disorder co-occurs with PTSD, depression, generalized anxiety disorder (GAD), and substance use disorder (SUD; Grant et al., 2008). The percentages of women with 12-month rates of PTSD, MDD, GAD, or any SUD and who also have a 12-month rate of BPD are 27%, 18%, 32.2%, and 16.9%, respectively. Reciprocally, the percentages of women with a 12-month rate of BPD as the primary diagnosis and who also have 12-month rates of PTSD, MDD, GAD, and any SUD are 38.2%, 22.5%, 26.4%, 44.5%, respectively. These percentages show the extent to which women with BPD may have additional disorders, as well as the extent to which women, especially poor women, may be at risk of PTSD, depression, GAD, and SUD.

When one considers that 50.5% of women who have any drug dependence, 47.2% of women with bipolar I disorder, and 35.4% of women with bipolar II disorder also have a diagnosis of BPD, these percentages take on importance for poor women. Equally important, among women with BPD, 55.7% have some type of mood disorder, 67.6 have some type of anxiety disorder, especially PTSD (Herman, 1992), and 44.5% have some type of SUD (see Trull, Sher, Minks-Brown, Durbin, & Burr, 2000). One can see that BPD is likely to result in depression and anxiety among women, and one might also speculate that women with BPD use substances to mediate anxiety and depression. This may be especially true for poor women, who often lack access to mental health and substance abuse services.

The most dangerous aspect of BPD is lethality as it relates to suicidal behaviors and suicide completion. Because women with BPD are especially fragile in terms of emotional stability and self-image, they are at risk of suicide completion (Soloff, Fabio, Kelly, Malone, & Mann, 2005). Although suicide attempts by patients with BPD are considered communicative gestures, 9–10% of persons with BPD complete suicide (see Gunderson & Ridolfi, 2001; Linehan et al., 2006; Paris & Zweig-Frank, 2001). In fact, Linehan et al. (2006) noted that BPD is one of only two disorders that include suicidal behavior as a criterion for diagnosis as well as treatment. According to the Work Group on Borderline Personality Disorder (2001), the rate of suicide is 50 times greater among individuals with BPD than among the general population. It is noteworthy that suicidality peaks in the early 20s, but completed suicide most often occurs after the age of 30 (Paris, 2003).

# Etiology

There tends to be agreement among experts that the diathesis-stress model provides the best explanation of BPD. According to this model, predispositions or vulnerabilities are mediated or amplified by external stressors (Linehan, 1993; Paris, 1997). In this context, biochemical processes, genetic predispositions, and external stressors contribute to the symptoms that characterize BPD. Likewise, another way to think of BPD is to consider it as the result of biological vulnerability and environmental adversity (Bornovalova et al., 2006). In this section, we discuss the biochemical processes, genetic factors, and external stresses that contribute to BPD.

## Genetic Heritability and Biochemical Processes

The results in both twin and family studies indicate that heritability accounts for between 50% and 60% of variance in traits associated with BPD (Torgersen 2000; White, Gunderson, Zanarini, & Hudson, 2003), especially instability (Livesley, Jang, & Vernon, 1998) and impulsivity (Hinshaw, 2003). Based on meta-analyses of data on serotonin-related genes, researchers have found that a low level of serotonin is linked to the suicidal behavior of women with BPD, which seems to be due to a particular serotonin-related gene (Lyons-Ruth et al., 2007; see also Anguelova, Benkelfat, & Turecki, 2003; Stanley et al., 2000). Young adults with low socioeconomic status who carry the gene that results in low levels of serotonin have been found to be vulnerable to developing either antisocial traits, such as harming others, or borderline traits, such as harming themselves (Lyons-Ruth et al., 2007).

Neurobiological factors may also contribute to BPD. Oldham (2005) noted that women with BPD have deficits in cognitive functioning relative to decision-making (Bazanis et al., 2002), conflict resolution (Posner et al., 2002), and the ability to maintain control over emotions without effort (Lenzenweger, Clarkin, Fertuck, & Kernberg, 2004; Posner et al., 2002). Using structural magnetic resonance imaging, researchers found that BPD is related to small parietal cortex and hippocampal size (Irle, Lange, & Sachsse, 2005). As with PTSD, the size of the parietal cortex and hippocampus likely results in the person with borderline lacking control over emotions and behavior (Johnson, Hurley, Benkelfat, Herpertz, & Taber, 2003).

Results of additional studies provide evidence that neurobiological factors may contribute to BPD. For example, King-Casas et al. (2008) found that the inability of individuals with BPD to recognize norm violations (specifically, the inability to signal trustworthiness to partners) contributes to a lack of cooperation in interpersonal relationships. Similarly, researchers have found that individuals with BPD overread and misread emotional cues; for example, they overread anger in neutral faces (Blair, Colledge, Murray, & Mitchell, 2001; Lynch et al., 2006; Wagner & Linehan, 1999). Interestingly, a sample of treatment-seeking females with severe BPD symptomatology were found to have a history of childhood ADHD (Phillipsen et al., 2008), specifically the combination of inattention, hyperactivity, and impulsivity.

### Psychological and External Stressors

The gene-environment interaction is especially significant when one considers that stressful life events predict increased suicidal behaviors among those with the short serotonin-related gene but not among those with the long serotonin-related gene (Caspi et al., 2003). Interestingly, Bornovalova et al. (2006) found that stress reactivity was associated with BPD in a sample of mostly African American inpatients in a drug and alcohol abuse treatment center, even when the researchers controlled for gender, education, emotional abuse, and ability to have control over emotions. Although this finding may be unique to this sample, it brings into question the extent to which particular groups of individuals, especially poor women, may be vulnerable to BPD in light of an inability to cope with stressful life events in their lives.

For example, Sansone, Reddington, Sky, and Wiederman (2007) examined the relationship between a history of domestic violence and BPD or borderline personality symptomatology (BPS) among 52 primarily Caucasian, well-educated female patients seen in an outpatient internal medicine clinic. Even though the number of patients with BPS was small, the results show an association between BPS and increased likelihood of being a victim of intimate partner violence. This brings into question the extent to which impulsivity, anger, or inability to read cues place women with BPD at risk of intimate partner violence and abuse or exacerbates such abuse.

Numerous researchers have identified risk factors for BPD. In particular, researchers have identified childhood physical, emotional, or sexual abuse as external stressors and risk factors for BPD (Bandelow et al., 2005). Despite the evidence that supports this notion (Holm & Severinsson, 2008; Paris, 1997; Zanarini, 2000), others minimize the contribution of childhood abuse to BPD (New et al., 2008). In fact, Paris (2005) noted that many individuals report having had childhood problems as a result of poor functioning in their families of origin (see Paris, 1997). This brings into question the extent to which problems in the families of BPD women are a function of heritability, modeling, or both.

## Screening and Assessment Measures _____

Screening low-income women for BPD has utility when one considers that this disorder often co-occurs with PTSD, depression (MDD especially), GAD, and SUD. Given the finding that clinicians who treat individuals with BPD are reluctant to diagnose BPD during routine intake evaluations, it seems the best practice for social workers is to use caution in screening women for BPD. We recommend that social workers pay particular attention to identifying women who may have little or no access to services and for whom a referral might be especially beneficial in light of a diagnosis of PTSD, depression, GAD, or SUD, or who experience suicidal ideation and behavior. In screening female patients with a history of domestic violence for BPD in a primary care setting, Sansone et al. (2007) used two measures that seem appropriate for social workers to use in screening women for both the disorder, symptomatology of the disorder, and the risk of suicide often associated with the disorder.

Personality Diagnostic Questionnaire (PDQ-4)

Self-Harm Inventory (SHI)

## PDQ-4

Although the PDQ-4 (Hyler, 1994) is a 99-item, true-false, self-report measure that reflects the *DSM-IV* criteria for personality disorders, only 9 items of the measure reflect the criteria for BPD. A score of greater than 5 strongly indicates BPD. Earlier versions of the PDQ-4 have been found to have utility in screening for personality disorders in both clinical settings (Dubro, Wetzler, & Kahn, 1988; Hyler et al., 1990) and nonclinical settings (Johnson & Bornstein, 1992). When the 9-item BPD borderline scale was used, the Cronbach's alpha was .86 (see Patrick, Links, Van Reekum, & Mitton, 1995).

## SHI

The SHI is a 22-item, yes/no, self-report inventory survey that explores self-harming behavior (Sansone, Wiederman, & Sansone, 1998). For example, the items address the intentions of women to cut, burn, or overdose themselves. The total number of *yes* responses indicates the lethality, with a score of greater than 5 indicating a pathological direction. In comparison with the Diagnostic Interview for Borderline Patients (Gunderson, Kolb, & Austin, 1981), the SHI identified 84.7% of women as either meeting the BPD diagnosis or not (Sansone et al., 1998). In the Sansone study, the Cronbach's alpha was .89.

# Treatment and Intervention for Women With Borderline Personality Disorder

The evidence on treating BPD among women suggests that both psychotherapy and psychopharmacology have been proven to be effective interventions

(Paris, 2005), especially with respect to addressing suicidality or the lethality component of the disorder. In this book, we are concerned with the psychotherapeutic interventions that seem to work in treating females with BPD. According to the American Psychological Association's Society for Clinical Psychology, those include dialectical behavior therapy (Koons et al., 2001; Linehan et al., 2006; Verheul et al., 2003), schema-focused therapy (Giesen-Bloo et al., 2006; Young, Klosko, & Weishaar, 2003), and transference-focused therapy (Clarkin, Levy, Lenzenweger, & Kenberg, 2007; Giesen-Bloo et al., 2006). Of the three therapies, dialectical behavior therapy has the strongest research support for use with women.

---

Dialectical Behavior Therapy (DBT)

Schema-Focused Therapy (SFT)

Transference-Focused Psychotherapy (TFP)

---

## DBT

Linehan and colleagues developed DBT to address individuals who engage in suicidal and self-injurious behaviors such as self-mutilation (Linehan et al., 2006). As an intervention, DBT builds on behavioral and crisis interventions approaches, but it also relies on acceptance and tolerance inherent in both Western and Eastern notions of practice, such as meditation. The term *dialectical* results from the exchange between patient and therapist or clinician, as well as the need for the patient to go back and forth between rationality and emotionality. As one might expect, addressing self-harm is a priority, which is why it is an important intervention for use with women who have BPD. With this in mind, a key focus of DBT for the patient is on her becoming aware of emotions, learning how to be socially appropriate in relationships, being able to cope effectively, and learning how to regulate emotions.

## SFT

SFT is an approach that integrates CBT and other techniques from other psychotherapeutic approaches (Young et al., 2003). The main objective of this approach is to help women alter self-defeating behaviors by simultaneously changing how they think, feel, and behave in particular situations. This approach builds on the notion of schema identified in the work of Piaget. While SFT focuses on the individual, especially on traumatic childhood experiences, it also emphasizes how the individual functions in her daily life apart from therapy. Compared to DBT, SFT has only modest research support.

### TFT

TFT is a controversial intervention for BPD that focuses on addressing the underlying causes of BPD (Clarkin et al., 2007). The premise of this intervention is that, once the causes are identified, females with BPD can learn and build new behaviors via transference with the therapist or clinician. In this instance, transference means that in the therapeutic relationship a patient can transfer to the clinician the negative or unhealthy behaviors she has with others in her daily life. The belief is that in the therapeutic relationship the clinician can communicate with the patient to help her correct old behaviors and build new ones. While Clarkin et al. (2007) found this approach to be effective in a randomized clinical trial, Giesen-Bloo et al. (2006) found this not to be the case in another randomized clinical trial.

## Summary

Several themes in this chapter have salience for social workers. First, given the extent to which heredity contributes to BPD, social workers may want to critically think about the weight they give family dynamics, trauma experiences in childhood, and intimate partner violence in the lives of poor and low-income women. Second, social workers may want to consider how to collaborate with primary care physicians, who often see women with BPD for other medical reasons. If a social worker suspects BPD and validates the diagnosis via screening, the social worker might ask the consumer for written permission to speak and work with the physician. The collaborative approach identified in the chapter on depression might be very useful. Third, it is essential that social workers take into account the lethality associated with BPD and the strong tendency of women with BPD to complete suicide, particularly in terms of screening for BPD, BPS, and suicidal ideation among women who may have no access to mental health or substance abuse services. Last, social workers would benefit from attending a DBT training workshop, and similarly, departments or schools of social work should seriously consider offering a DBT course in clinical concentrations, especially given that DBT is often integrated into the treatment of SUD among women.

### Discussion Topics

1. Explain why BPD might be prevalent among poor women, and discuss the comorbidity of the disorder with PTSD, depression, and SUD.

2. Identify the diagnostic issues associated with BPD.

3. Explain the lethality associated with suicidal behavior and completion and the importance of communicative gestures relative to suicide attempts.

4. Debate the internal processes and environmental stressors associated with BPD, and how those aspects influence screening for and treatment of the disorder.

5. Consider how BPD might place poor women at risk of interpersonal violence.

---

## CASE STUDY 6.1

Tina's mother is confused about what is happening to Tina. Tina is a 25-year-old white female who worked at Walmart until she was let go. Her mother states that Tina is manipulative and often lies to friends and family. The mother believes that this is why Tina lost the Walmart job as well as previous jobs. Tina currently lives at home with her mother and a younger sibling because she has no source of income. Tina has threatened suicide on numerous occasions and in fact most recently overdosed after taking her mother's bottle of Motrin. While Tina's mother first noticed Tina's anger outbursts and mood swings when Tina was 18, she remembers that Tina was distractible, very active, and impulsive as a child. As an afterthought, Tina's mother indicated that Tina had been sexually abused once by an adolescent male neighbor when she was four.

### Case Questions

Which of Tina's behaviors suggests a possible diagnosis of BPD?

What in Tina's social history would also indicate that she might have BPD?

Why would it be important to screen for this disorder as early as possible in the lifespan of females?

To what extent should one be concerned with her communicative gestures?

Given her background and experiences, which particular evidence-based interventions presented in this chapter might be most effective in working with Tina?

# Illustrative Reading

## Acceptance and Change

*The Integration of Mindfulness-Based Cognitive Therapy Into Ongoing Dialectical Behavior Therapy in a Case of Borderline Personality Disorder With Depression*

Debra B. Huss

Ruth A. Baer
*University of Kentucky, Lexington*

Both dialectical behavior therapy (DBT) and mindfulness-based cognitive therapy (MBCT) include training in mindfulness skills and address the synthesis of acceptance and change. DBT is a comprehensive treatment for borderline personality disorder (BPD). MBCT was developed for prevention of relapse in individuals with a history of depressive episodes. Both have considerable empirical support for their efficacy. Many individuals with BPD also suffer from depressive episodes, which can interfere with motivation to participate in DBT. In such cases, it may be helpful to integrate strategies designed to prevent recurrence of depressive episodes. This case study describes integration of MBCT into ongoing DBT in the treatment of an individual with BPD and a history of depressive episodes. Findings suggest that MBCT can be successfully integrated into ongoing DBT in cases in which prevention of depressive episodes is an important goal. Findings also suggest that mindfulness skills may be very helpful in enhancing the efficacy of traditional cognitive-behavioral treatment approaches.

**Keywords**: mindfulness-based cognitive therapy; dialectical behavior therapy; mindfulness; acceptance and change

### Theoretical and Research Basis

Dialectical behavior therapy, (DBT; Linehan, 1993a, 1993b) and mindfulness-based cognitive therapy (MBCT; Segal, Williams, & Teasdale, 2002) both belong to the recently described expansion of the cognitive-behavioral tradition known as the third wave (Hayes, 2004; Hayes, Follette, & Linehan, 2004), after traditional behavior therapy and cognitive therapy. Third wave treatments generally include concepts such as mindfulness, acceptance, and dialectics and address the relationship between acceptance and change, often through training in mindfulness skills. Mindfulness can be described as the self-regulation of attention to nonjudgmentally focus on particular stimuli, including bodily sensations, perceptions (sights, sounds), cognitions, and emotions (Kabat-Zinn, 1990). Participants learn to observe these phenomena without evaluating their truth, importance, or value and without trying to

*(Continued)*

(Continued)

escape, avoid, or change them. Development of mindfulness skills is believed to lead to increased self-awareness and self-acceptance, reduced reactivity to thoughts and emotions, and improved ability to cope with problematic situations (Linehan, 1993a, 1993b).

DBT was developed for the treatment of borderline personality disorder (BPD) and emphasizes the synthesis of acceptance and change. It includes a wide range of behavioral and cognitive strategies designed to help individuals change their behaviors, emotions, and thoughts. To encourage acceptance of one's history and current experiences, including discomfort associated with change. DBT also incorporates training in mindfulness skills, including observation, description, and acceptance of current experiences (e.g., sensations, cognitions, and emotions) without evaluation or self-criticism and participation in current activities with undivided attention. DBT has strong empirical support for its efficacy (Robins & Chapman, 2004).

MBCT is an 8-week, manualized group program based largely on the mindfulness-based stress reduction program (MBSR) developed by Kabat-Zinn (1982, 1990). MBCT was developed for the prevention of depressive relapse and has been shown in randomized trials to be effective for individuals with a history of three or more major depressive episodes (Ma & Teasdale, 2004; Teasdale et al., 2000). MBCT includes mindfulness practices designed to cultivate nonjudgmental observation and acceptance of bodily sensations, cognitions, and emotions. Participants learn to engage in sustained observation of these phenomena, with an attitude of interest and curiosity, and to accept them as they are, without trying to change or escape them. MBCT also includes elements of cognitive therapy that are consistent with nonjudgmental acceptance of current experience. A decentered view of thoughts is emphasized, in which participants are encouraged to view their thoughts as transient mental events rather than as aspects of themselves or as necessarily accurate reflections of reality or truth.

Several mechanisms by which mindfulness may lead to symptom reduction and improved functioning have been suggested (Kabat-Zinn, 1982; Linehan, 1993a, 1993b; Segal et al., 2002). Sustained observation of aversive thoughts and feelings may function as exposure to these phenomena and lead to reduced emotional reactivity and fewer maladaptive escape and avoidance behaviors. Mindfulness also may encourage a particular perspective on internal events: that thoughts are just thoughts, are numerous and transient, may not be true or important, and do not necessitate specific behaviors. Mindfulness also may lead to improved self-observation, which may promote better recognition of internal states and ability to use adaptive coping skills. Thus, mindfulness skills may be applicable to a wide range of disorders.

Although DBT and MBCT share an emphasis on mindfulness, important differences can be noted. Linehan's (1993a) biosocial theory of BPD assumes that many individuals with BPD have grown up in severely dysfunctional environments in which they could not learn important skills. For this reason, DBT includes explicit instruction in a wide range of skills, including emotion regulation, interpersonal effectiveness, distress tolerance, problem solving, and behavioral analysis strategies. MBCT, in contrast, assumes that bringing mindfulness awareness to current experience will enable individuals to cope adaptively with difficulties by using skills already in their repertoires. Thus, MBCT places much less emphasis on teaching skills for behavior change. In addition, MBCT is an 8-week protocol with a clear agenda for each session and a focused goal: to teach mindfulness skills necessary to prevent relapse of depressive episodes. Standard outpatient DBT, in contrast, generally involves a 1-year commitment to treatment involving both group and individual sessions and encompasses a much broader array of goals tailored to the needs of the client. Finally, MBCT teaches mindfulness skills primarily through the practice of lengthy meditation exercises, in which participants spend up to 45 minutes sitting or lying quietly and directing their attention in specific ways. Linehan (1994) argues that many individuals with severe BPD are unable or unwilling to meditate this extensively. For this reason, DBT does not use extended meditation practices but rather provides a wide range of much shorter exercises for the practice of specific mindfulness skills, such as nonjudgmentally observing and describing.

Many individuals with BPD also suffer from depressive episodes *(Diagnostic and Statistical Manual of Mental Disorders,* American Psychiatric Association, 2000). Although depressive episodes can be treated effectively, the risk of relapse is high and increases with each episode. Prevention of relapse is a central challenge in the treatment of depression (Segal, Teasdale, & Williams, 2004). Depression is likely to interfere with motivation to participate in DBT, a rigorous and demanding treatment. Thus, for individuals with both BPD and a history of depressive episodes, it may be useful to include treatment strategies designed to prevent depressive relapse. MBCT has been shown to be effective for this purpose and may be beneficial for those clients willing and able to engage in the necessary meditation exercises.

The following case study describes the integration of MBCT into ongoing DBT in the treatment of an individual with BPD and a history of depressive episodes and other symptoms. When the client presented for treatment, her symptoms and skills deficits made her an excellent candidate for DBT. After she had learned a number of DBT skills and gained particular benefits from the mindfulness skills, it became clear that MBCT was consistent with her goals to become more aware of her emotions and to prevent additional depressive episodes. We hypothesized that MBCT could be integrated into the structure of ongoing DBT and would provide the client with tools helpful in maintaining her mental health over the long term. As described in the following sections, however, we also found that the mindfulness skills learned in MBCT showed more immediate benefits in facilitating the client's progress in DBT.

## Case Presentation

Ann was a Caucasian female in her mid-50s with one grown child living outside the home. She had been married for 10 years but had separated from her husband just before beginning the therapy described herein. She held a bachelor's degree in early childhood education but had been unemployed for 10 years because of poor mental health. She relied on financial support from her husband despite their marital difficulties. Ann spent her days sleeping, tending to her house, engaging in arts and crafts, and taking care of her pregnant daughter who was on bed rest. Although Ann was not living with her husband, she frequently visited him to cook and clean the house, despite feelings of sadness and anger when she spent time around him.

### Presenting Complaints

Ann presented for treatment with many of the symptoms of BPD (see assessment section below for more information). She was particularly troubled by symptoms of depression

*(Continued)*

(Continued)

and anxiety and reported severe insomnia. She also reported that she sometimes felt "numb" and wanted to become more in touch with her emotions. She stated that her social network was limited to individuals who also suffered from mental illness and that she provided more support to them than they provided to her. She wanted to improve her relationships by learning interpersonal skills that would enable her to give support to others while asserting her own needs and preferences. Ann had frequent interactions with her parents but desired less contact with them, as they often triggered memories of sexual abuse, particularly her father (see history section below). However, she was unable to communicate her wishes to them. Finally, Ann wanted to reduce her financial dependence on her husband by attaining employment, and she was interested in returning to school.

### History

Ann had a significant psychiatric history and a family history of mental illness. All of her immediate family members (parents and 7 siblings) had histories of mood disorders and all had attempted suicide. Ann's brothers and her father were alcoholics. Between the ages of 6 and 12, Ann had been sexually abused by her father, a brother, and her uncle. When the current therapy began, she had no ongoing relationships with any of her siblings.

Ann reported a history of frequent depressive episodes beginning in childhood. She had been participating intermittently in outpatient psychotherapy, primarily cognitive-behavioral therapy (CBT), since the age of 32. She reported two 1-week hospitalizations during the preceding 3 years for depression and suicidal ideation with a plan. She had participated briefly in our clinic's DBT program 1 year before the treatment described here, but shortly after starting, she missed four consecutive sessions because of circumstances including her husband's hospitalization for anxiety, her own hospitalization for depression, and her daughter's wedding. In accordance with standard DBT procedures, which had been carefully explained to her, these four consecutive absences resulted in her termination from the DBT program and she was referred to other sources of treatment. Several months later, Ann completed a voluntary, intensive, 10-week treatment at a psychiatric hospital, where she received some exposure to DBT skills along with treatment for post-traumatic stress disorder (PTSD), depression, anxiety, and insomnia. Throughout her psychiatric treatment history, Ann had been prescribed numerous psychotropic medications. When she began the current treatment, she was taking Trazadone, Buspar, and Lexapro.

## Assessment

### Intake Interview

Ann requested readmittance to the clinic's DBT program 1 year after her previous termination and following completion of inpatient treatment. She stated that she was now able to attend sessions regularly and motivated to participate actively in DBT. In accordance with the clinic's standard procedures, she attended an intake session focusing on her presenting complaints, her social and psychological history, the nature of DBT, and her goals for therapy. The BPD section of the Structured Clinical Interview for *DSM-IV,* (First, Spitzer, Williams, & Gibbon, 1997) was administered. Ann met 5 of the 9 diagnostic criteria for BPD, including an unstable sense of self, impulsive binge eating and reckless spending, chronic feelings of emptiness, affective instability, and dissociation in response to stress. Ann also was questioned about her other reported symptoms, and met criteria for chronic major depressive disorder (MDD), PTSD, and primary insomnia. Ann also completed the standard intake packet, which included the Beck Depression Inventory-II (BDI-II; Beck, 1996) and the Beck Anxiety Inventory (BAI; Beck & Steer, 1993). Her pretreatment scores on these measures were 13 and 24, respectively, indicating mild levels of depression and moderate levels of anxiety symptoms. Her BDI score was surprisingly low given that she had endorsed all the symptoms of MDD during the clinical interview and presented with flat affect and psychomotor retardation. However, it may be consistent with lack of awareness of her emotions and behavior sometimes observed early in treatment.

**Figure 1**  Minnesota Multiphasic Personality Inventory-2 Pretreatment and Posttreatment Results

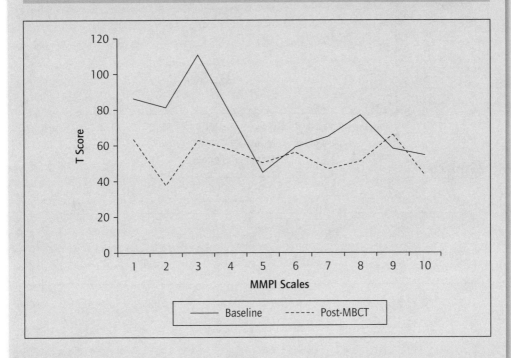

**Additional Assessment**

All clients at our clinic are asked to complete the Minnesota Multiphasic Personality Inventory-2 (MMPI-2; Hathaway & McKinley, 1989) and the Revised NEO Personality Inventory (NEO PI-R; Costa & McCrae, 1992) within 4 weeks of beginning therapy. On the

*(Continued)*

(Continued)

MMPI-2, Ann's validity scales were within normal limits, but she had significant elevations on 6 of the clinical scales (Scales 1, 2, 3, 4, 7, and 8; see Figure 1). Elevations on Scales 1, 2, and 3 were consistent with her reported symptoms of anxiety, depression, and sleep disturbance (Graham, 2000). The high score on Scale 3 also suggested lack of insight into how her bodily sensations, emotions, and environmental stresses are related. Elevation of Scale 8 suggested that she felt socially and emotionally isolated and had very little confidence in her abilities. On the NEO PI-R, Ann's neuroticism score fell in the very high range. Her openness to experience score fell in the high range, agreeableness in the average range, and extraversion and conscientiousness in the low range. Although Ann endorsed high levels of depression, anxiety, self-consciousness, and vulnerability, her scores suggested willingness to try new experiences and consider new ideas. Ann completed the BDI-II and BAI several times during her therapy. These scores can be seen in Figures 2 and 3 and are discussed in later sections.

**Figure 2**    Beck Depression Inventory-II Scores

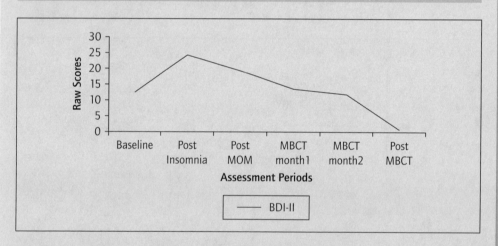

**Figure 3**    Beck Anxiety Inventory Scores

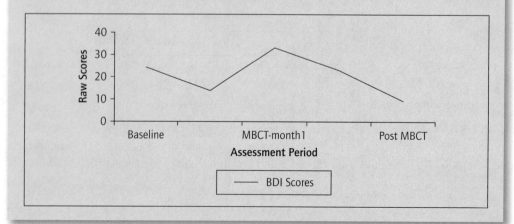

## Case Conceptualization

As Ann met diagnostic criteria for BPD, she was an excellent candidate for DBT. Ann's symptoms and history were clearly consistent with the biosocial theory of BPD, which states that BPD is a dysfunction of the emotion-regulation system brought on by the transaction over time of an emotionally vulnerable temperament and an invalidating environment (see Linehan, 1993a, for more detail). DBT views sexual abuse, which Ann had experienced for several years, as an extreme case of invalidation. Ann's history of invalidation was seen as a major factor in her pattern of ignoring or suppressing her emotional states and her tendency to be guarded in relationships, to worry about others perceptions of her, and to be overly accommodating to others' wishes without asserting her own needs and preferences. These tendencies appeared to be important factors in her depressed mood, as was sleep deprivation because of sleep apnea and insomnia.

Within DBT, case conceptualization is strongly guided by the hierarchy of targets, which prioritizes treatment goals (Koerner & Linehan, 1997). Several general principles are reflected in this hierarchy. Life-threatening and self-harming behaviors are the first targets of treatment, as the patient's death or serious injury will prevent progress in life improvement. Behavioral problems that interfere with participation in treatment, such as skipping sessions or failing to complete homework, are addressed next, as progress requires active participation in treatment. As Ann did not present with life-threatening or therapy-interfering behavior, she was able to progress immediately to the third step in the hierarchy, which involves learning skills for improving quality of life and managing emotional states. The hierarchy dictates that post-traumatic stress is not addressed until the patient has developed more stability in her life and mastered emotion-regulation and distress tolerance skills. These skills are seen as essential for managing the negative affect that inevitably will be elicited when childhood traumas are discussed. In Ann's case, this principle appeared especially important, as she had a significant trauma history and severe deficits in skills for managing negative affect. As case conceptualization is an ongoing process in DBT, evolving as targets are addressed and progress is made, additional material about our conceptualization of Ann's case is integrated into the following treatment section.

## Course of Treatment and Assessment of Progress

Treatment was conducted at an outpatient training clinic operated by the doctoral program in clinical psychology at the University of Kentucky. Therapy is provided by doctoral students who are supervised by licensed clinical psychologists. Ann was admitted to the DBT program and began attending weekly skills group and individual therapy sessions. The skills group is co-led by two doctoral students, whereas individual therapy is conducted by one doctoral student. For the first 6 months of Ann's participation in DBT, her individual therapist was also one of the skills group leaders. All DBT therapists meet weekly with the faculty supervisor to discuss clients' progress, facilitating continuity between individual and group components of the program.

Skills group meetings last 2.5 hours and include review of homework and didactic presentation and discussion of new skills. Four modules are covered: core mindfulness

*(Continued)*

(Continued)

interpersonal effectiveness, emotion regulation, and distress tolerance. The mindfulness module, which requires two or three sessions, is reviewed after each of the other modules. Completion of all four modules requires about 6 months, at which point the entire sequence is repeated. As most clients commit to participating in DBT for a minimum of 1 year, they will experience each module twice, with several additional reviews of the mindfulness module. The group is continuously ongoing, and new members are allowed to join whenever a new module is beginning. Ann joined just as the core mindfulness module was beginning.

The initial sessions of individual therapy focus on orientation to DBT, commitment, and goal setting. Ann expressed strong commitment to participation in DBT. The hierarchy of targets was reviewed. As Ann was not engaging in self-harming, life-threatening, or therapy-interfering behaviors, work began with problems interfering with her quality of life. In DBT, this category of targets is potentially very broad and can include problems related to health, finances, school or work, relationships, substance use, or other Axis I disorders. When appropriate, empirically supported and manualized treatment approaches for specific problems or disorders can be incorporated into this phase of treatment. For several reasons, Ann and her therapist agreed to address her insomnia as the first target of treatment. Sleep deprivation can have a substantial negative impact on mood, cognitions, and motivation and can interfere with concentration and energy levels. Thus, we hoped that improvement in Ann's sleep might have wide-ranging positive effects. In addition, CBT for insomnia has been shown to be effective (Jacobs, Pace-Schott, Stickgold, & Otto, 2004; Smith & Neubauer, 2003) and can often be accomplished in a few sessions, potentially providing an initial experience of success and mastery for the client.

An important element of DBT is development of a diary card, on which patients monitor target behaviors daily. The diary card is brought to each individual session and used for organizing the session and monitoring progress. As Ann's initial goal was to reduce insomnia, she and her therapist developed a sleep diary, on which she recorded the time she went to bed, latency to falling asleep, number of awakenings, hours slept, naps taken during the day, and type and dosage of sleeping medications used. She also rated the quality of her sleep and how refreshed she felt in the morning. Ann and her therapist also developed a more general diary card on which to monitor behaviors related to her other treatment goals. On this diary card, Ann recorded her meals, exercise, social activities, other enjoyable activities, and moods. Ann was very conscientious about completing both of these monitoring devices each day and often included additional detailed information she felt was important, such as negative thoughts or feelings or insights she had regarding her treatment goals.

## Treatment of Insomnia

CBT for insomnia generally includes educating the client about physiological, cognitive, and affective factors that may lead to insomnia, teaching the client to recognize maladaptive thoughts that may exacerbate sleep problems and developing and engaging in a sleep hygiene routine to reduce physiological arousal at bedtime and environmental reinforcers for wakefulness (e.g., food and caffeine consumption before bedtime, reading or watching TV in bed, etc.). We used an unpublished manual developed for an unrelated project (Beacham, Carlson, & Philips, 2001), which was based on similar approaches described in the literature and provided comprehensive treatment during three sessions (Jacobs et al., 2004).

To promote continuity between individual and group components of DBT, individual sessions generally include monitoring of progress in group. Although not part of the insomnia manual, the mindfulness skills that Ann was learning in group appeared very useful during this phase of treatment. These skills include nonjudgmentally observing and describing experiences and allowing them to be as they are and to come and go as they will. Ann reported using these skills at bedtime and noticing several factors related to her difficulties in falling asleep, including muscle tension, worries about stressors (e.g., marital difficulties, relationships with family members), and PTSD symptoms (e.g., flashbacks, bodily sensations related to abuse, and physiological arousal that made it difficult to relax) she experienced while lying in bed that were preventing her from falling asleep. Ann reported that her anxiety decreased if she observed and labeled these experiences without self-judgment or criticism and allowed them to come and go.

## Outcome of Insomnia Treatment

Prior to treatment, Ann's average latency to sleep onset was at least 2 hours. After three sessions, she was able to fall asleep within 15 to 20 minutes, on average. Ann's bedtime and wake time became more consistent, as did her structured bedtime routine. The benefits of this routine appeared to inspire her to increase the structure of her daytime routine as well, as she began planning her meals and activities in advance. During subsequent months, as treatment shifted to other goals, Ann continued to use a sleep diary and maintained her ability to fall asleep quickly at night, with only occasional, brief lapses.

Ann's improvements in insomnia appeared primarily related to her changed sleep hygiene behaviors and her application of mindfulness skills before falling asleep. Although the mindfulness skills reduced her anxiety at bedtime, they also increased her awareness of depressed mood and negative thinking, and her BDI-II score increased to 24. Unfortunately, it became apparent that Ann lacked skills for modifying maladaptive thoughts, in spite of her history of cognitive therapy. Ann and her therapist agreed that strengthening these skills would be beneficial in helping to reduce her depressive symptoms and began work on the Mind Over Mood workbook (MOM; Greenberger & Padesky, 1995), a structured manual based on the principles of cognitive therapy.

## Implementation of MOM

The MOM workbook focuses on recognizing automatic thoughts, identifying evidence for and against the thoughts, developing more balanced, rational thoughts, and recognizing core beliefs that lead to maladaptive thoughts. During the next 2 months, Ann worked diligently on these skills, completing thought records each week and bringing them to individual sessions for discussion. During this process, Ann identified several core beliefs

*(Continued)*

(Continued)

that she had developed early in life that contributed to her depressive thinking. She recognized that she had grown up believing that she had to take care of others to survive and be loved and therefore evaluated herself according to how others viewed her. In addition, she recognized that her core belief that she did not deserve happiness was at the center of her guilt feelings, her tendency to prioritize others over herself, and her inability to assertively and effectively communicate her wants and needs to her family and friends.

Although not part of the MOM workbook, the mindfulness skills learned in skills group again appeared very helpful in facilitating this work. Whenever Ann experienced a mood change during a session, she and the therapist practiced a brief mindfulness exercise together in which they observed their thoughts for several minutes. Ann was also encouraged to use mindfulness skills to increase awareness of her internal experiences between sessions. These skills appeared to help Ann to identify the thoughts related to her emotions and physical sensations.

### Outcomes of MOM Workbook

At the conclusion of working with MOM, Ann's BDI-II and BAI scores had declined to 12 and 14, respectively, indicating mild to minimal symptoms. Ann demonstrated substantially increased ability to recognize and modify maladaptive thoughts and had reduced her high rates of catastrophizing and of negative overgeneralizations about herself. At this point in treatment, Ann stated that her most important goals were to become more aware and less avoidant of her emotions and to learn skills for preventing the relapse of depression. MBCT has been shown effective for this purpose in a group format and seemed likely to increase her ability to experience and accept her emotions. Moreover, Ann had already shown benefit from and enjoyment of the mindfulness exercises taught in DBT. Ann was not referred to MBCT group treatment for several reasons. At the time, no MBCT groups were available in the area. Moreover, Ann was already committed to 1 year of the DBT program, which required her to attend weekly individual and group sessions. Attendance at another weekly group would have been unrealistic for Ann. As a result, the therapist considered adapting MBCT for individual therapy and incorporating it into the DBT program. Although clinical trials have established the efficacy of MCBT in group format, a recent case study with an individual with binge eating disorder suggests the feasibility of adaptation to individual therapy (Baer, Fischer, & Huss, 2005). For these reasons, Ann and her therapist agreed to work on the MBCT protocol as the next phase of treatment.

### Implementation of MBCT

MBCT is designed as an 8-week group intervention with 2-hour sessions. Initial adaptations for Ann's case included lengthening the duration of this phase of therapy from 8 to 10 sessions and expanding individual sessions from 50 to 90 minutes to allow sufficient time for reviewing the diary card, addressing any other treatment issues that might arise, and then working on the MBCT material. The MBCT portion of each session began with a 20- to 30-minute mindfulness meditation that the therapist led and in which both participated. At the conclusion of this exercise, Ann and the therapist discussed the meditation experience, addressing themes from the MBCT manual. Ann's experience of homework practice during the preceding week also was discussed, as was application of mindfulness skills to issues Ann was facing during the upcoming week. New material then was discussed, and homework for the following week was assigned.

Sessions 1 to 5 of MBCT included a wide variety of meditation exercises. During mindful eating (Session 1), Ann and the therapist slowly ate a few raisins, focusing attention on the sensations and movements associated with eating and on thoughts and emotions that arise while eating. In the body scan (Sessions 1 and 2), attention is focused sequentially on numerous parts of the body, and sensations are nonjudgmentally observed. When thoughts and emotions arise, these are noted briefly, and then attention is returned to the body. Mindful stretching (Session 3) and walking (Session 5) encourage awareness of internal experiences during slow, gentle movements. In sitting meditation (Sessions 3–5), awareness is focused sequentially on the sensations and movements of breathing, sensations in the body, sounds in the environment, thoughts, and emotions that may arise. Generalization of mindfulness to daily life was encouraged with the 3-minute breathing space (taught in Session 3), which involves practicing mindful awareness of internal experience for short periods during the day.

Cognitive therapy elements of MBCT include a discussion of how thoughts about situations influence our feelings about them and the crucial concept that thoughts are not facts (Session 2). In Session 4, symptoms of depression were reviewed, and automatic thoughts related to depression (e.g., "I'm no good"; "I'm a failure") were discussed. Ann was encouraged to notice these thoughts and allow them to come and go rather than becoming absorbed in them, believing them, or acting in accordance with them. The primary goals of these sessions were to increase nonjudgmental awareness of present moment experience and to recognize how often our minds are on automatic pilot and how this lack of awareness can lead to negative thinking and rumination, which in turn may lead to a relapse of depression.

The remaining sessions of MBCT focused on cultivating a different relationship to unpleasant experiences, accepting all internal experiences (pleasant or unpleasant), using the breathing space to bring mindful awareness to mood shifts, and developing a relapse prevention plan. Beginning in Session 6, the sitting meditation encouraged Ann intentionally to bring to mind a problem or difficulty she experienced and to observe the resulting sensations, emotions, and thoughts without trying to change or eliminate them. Given Ann's longstanding tendency to shut out all aversive thoughts and emotions, two additional sessions were added to the program at this point (bringing the total number of sessions for the MBCT protocol to 12) to allow Ann more opportunities to practice awareness and acceptance of unpleasant internal experiences. During this phase of treatment, the 3-minute breathing space was expanded to include practicing it during times of stress by focusing on unpleasant internal experiences with openness, willingness, and acceptance. This mindfulstance allowed Ann to make more adaptive choices about how to respond to stressful situations. In later sessions, Ann identified and increased her participation in activities that led to feelings of pleasure and mastery (e.g., babysitting and crafts) while decreasing participation in activities associated with negative thoughts and moods (e.g., interactions with her parents and husband). In the final two sessions, Ann developed

*(Continued)*

(Continued)

a relapse prevention plan that included identifying her depressive triggers, using a breathing space to observe them without maladaptive, impulsive attempts to avoid or escape them, and then choosing what to do next. Ann generated a list of DBT skills and cognitive change skills from which she could choose to help cope with her triggers.

Although the mindfulness approach to thoughts (nonjudgmentally observing them without changing them) appears to differ from the cognitive therapy approach to thoughts (changing distorted thoughts to more rational thoughts), integrating these two approaches was not difficult in Ann's case. Bringing nonjudgmental awareness to internal experience was described as the initial step in coping with mood changes. Once Ann became aware and accepting of her current experience, she could decide if additional steps were needed to cope with her current state. If Ann determined that change was necessary, one of her options was to use the cognitive restructuring skills learned from the MOM workbook to change her thoughts, thereby changing her behavior and mood. However, another option was to allow thoughts to come and go as they are while practicing other DBT skills (e.g., emotion regulation, distress tolerance) to address her current state. Ann readily understood these two options and found them useful in her step-by-step approach to coping with mood changes.

### Outcomes of MBCT

As MBCT progressed, Ann reported increased awareness of how her bodily sensations, thoughts, and emotions are related to each other and to environmental stressors. Increased self-awareness allowed Ann to recognize triggers that change her mood and to take necessary steps to prevent a negative mood from escalating. By the conclusion of 12 weeks of MBCT, Ann reported increased ability to notice changes in her current internal experience (moods, sensations, or thoughts) and to engage in a 3-minute breathing space to nonjudgmentally observe the experience. The therapist also observed that Ann was more readily aware of her thoughts, moods, and sensations and how they were related. Bringing mindful awareness to her experience enabled Ann to decide effectively how to cope with the change. At times, recognition and acceptance of the experience was sufficient. That is, on these occasions, Ann decided that an adaptive response was to allow the experience as it was, even if this meant accepting some inevitable unpleasantness. On other occasions, Ann was able to make adaptive decisions about which DBT skills to utilize to cope with the experience. This appeared to be a significant change. Prior to completing MBCT, Ann's choice of DBT skills to use in times of stress often appeared haphazard, as she generally described using the first skill that came to mind or the one most recently discussed in skills group, regardless of its applicability to the situation. However, after completing MBCT, Ann regularly described using a breathing space or practicing a short sitting meditation and then choosing a DBT skill well suited to the situation. For example, when Ann received a phone call from her father that resulted in an increase in anxiety, using a breathing space allowed Ann to identify the anxiety and accept it without becoming more alarmed. Although she noted that mindful observation alone significantly reduced her anxiety, she also identified the need to engage in relaxation and self-statements that she was safe.

By the conclusion of MBCT, Ann's BDI-II and BAI scores had declined from 12 to 1 and from 14 to 9, respectively, indicating no significant depressive or anxiety symptoms, and her MDD was in remission. In addition, Ann consistently reported experiencing a range of positive and negative emotions, rather than recognizing only intense, extreme emotion. It should be noted that Ann experienced an increase in anxiety symptoms (BAI = 33) early in her work on the MBCT protocol. This appeared related to an increase in awareness in bodily sensations and emotions and an increase in environmental stressors. As MBCT progressed, her symptoms steadily decreased. The MMPI-2 was readministered after completion of MBCT, and significant declines in previously elevated scales were noted. Although interpersonal interactions are not addressed by the MBCT protocol, Ann continued to attend the DBT skills group, which includes interpersonal effectiveness skills. During this period, Ann began engaging in more effective communication with her parents and friends and began taking steps to improve her social network. She was also engaging much more consistently in behaviors that promote a positive mood while reducing her vulnerability to emotional instability, such as eating, sleeping, and exercising regularly.

## Complicating Factors

Ann had previously been diagnosed with several medical conditions, including fibromyalgia, hypertension, asthma, hypothyroidism, and sleep apnea. When she began treatment, she reported that most of these conditions were reasonably well controlled but that sleep apnea was causing significant fatigue. Although her primary insomnia was substantially improved during treatment, Ann continued to have frequent nighttime awakenings because of sleep apnea. During the subsequent months of therapy, Ann worked closely with her physician to request that her insurance company pay for surgery for sleep apnea. On several occasions, she used the interpersonal effectiveness skills taught in DBT to talk with her physician and insurance company and also wrote several appropriate letters regarding the matter. At the present time, the surgery has been approved and scheduled. Ann uses distress tolerance skills to cope with fatigue and maintains good sleep hygiene behaviors.

### Managed Care Considerations

Managed care considerations are not an issue at our clinic. Like many doctoral training clinics, we use a sliding fee scale and require payment at each session. However, Comtois, Levensky, and Linehan (1999) note that since the publication of controlled trials showing DBT's efficacy (see Robins & Chapman, 2004, for a recent update), many behavioral health maintenance organizations, and some state departments of mental health, have become willing to fund DBT, in spite of the expense associated with its length and complexity.

### Follow-Up

Ann has completed about 8 months of her 1-year commitment to DBT. She remains in therapy and is working on additional treatment goals. Although she no longer meets criteria for MDD or primary insomnia, she continues to suffer from fatigue related to her

*(Continued)*

(Continued)

sleep apnea and perhaps her fibromyalgia. However, she has increased her physical activity, her social interactions, and her ability to concentrate despite her level of fatigue. In addition, although Ann continues to endorse symptoms of BPD, their frequency and severity have decreased. Perhaps her most significant presenting complaint that has not resolved is her PTSD. She reports flashbacks, nightmares, and anxiety resulting from trauma-related triggers at least once per month. However, Ann notes that the symptoms are less intense and less distressing as a result of her increased awareness, acceptance, and understanding of them and her increased repertoire of mindfulness, distress tolerance, and emotion-regulation skills. As noted earlier, DBT does not address PTSD until clients are consistently and successfully using the many skills taught in group to ensure that they will be able to manage the distress likely to arise when early traumas are discussed. Ann is currently working on increasing her social support network, increasing her participation in mastery-related and pleasant activities, and finding employment while continuing to practice her skills. When she is ready to address PTSD, she and her therapist will discuss a new commitment to this phase of therapy, which very likely will extend her participation in DBT beyond her initial 1-year commitment.

Strong conclusions about the efficacy of MBCT for preventing a relapse of depression in Ann's case cannot be drawn for quite a few months. However, Ann's improved ability to recognize mood changes and engage in healthy coping strategies suggests that she now has the skills necessary for preventing the escalation of negative moods into depressive relapse. Moreover, Ann's DBT and mindfulness skills also enable her to engage in adaptive behaviors that increase positive emotions while decreasing negative emotions. As randomized clinical trials cited earlier indicate that the likelihood of a depressive relapse within the year following MBCT is reduced by 50%, Ann's prognosis for relapse prevention is encouraging.

### Treatment Implications of the Case

This case study illustrates that MBCT can be integrated into ongoing DBT for BPD clients who have incorporated DBT skills into their repertoires and are willing to engage in meditation exercises. Although the intense negative affect common in many BPD clients may reduce their willingness to meditate, in Ann's case these exercises proved tolerable and useful. Their length was reduced from 45 minutes (typical in MBCT) to 20 to 30 minutes. In addition, Ann reported that she found the 3-minute breathing space at least as helpful as the lengthier meditations and regularly practiced this skill in her daily life.

This case also suggests the potential utility of mindfulness skills in increasing the effectiveness of CBT for a range of problems. Ann presented with a complex symptom picture. Despite her extensive history of mental health treatment, Ann was still disconnected from her thoughts, emotions, and bodily sensations. CBT generally includes monitoring of such experiences, and Ann realized that she needed to become more aware of them but lacked the skills to do so. Teaching mindfulness skills provided her with the tools she needed to observe and recognize her sensations, thoughts, and emotions, to understand how these are related to each other and to environmental stimuli, and to become more accepting of her moment-to-moment experiences, regardless of how pleasant or unpleasant it was.

This case also highlights the utility of integrating acceptance and change. During Ann's initial months of DBT, she was so averse to negative affect that she habitually searched for a "quick fix" to change how she was feeling. This often resulted in haphazard choice of DBT skills to use, which led to disappointment in their effectiveness, a sense of failure, and self-invalidation of her emotions. The longer mindfulness practices (20–30 minutes) that occurred during MBCT sessions facilitated the development of acceptance of emotions. Exposure to negative affect during these practices reduced her fear of these experiences as she realized that negative affect did not lead to catastrophic outcomes. During discussions of mindfulness practices, the therapist had opportunities to validate Ann's feelings and to emphasize that all emotions, thoughts, and sensations are a natural part of life and can help us develop insight if we attend to them carefully. Such validation appeared more meaningful to Ann when she had just spent 20 to 30 minutes closely observing her internal experiences.

The meditation practices also helped Ann to learn that change is not always required, even in unpleasant circumstances, and that acceptance may sometimes be more adaptive than immediate attempts to change things. Finally, the highly experiential nature of the mindfulness meditations taught in MBCT appeared helpful in facilitating acceptance. When Ann came to a session in a distressed mood and then completed a 20- to 30-minute meditation, she consistently reported that she now understood her distress, was less upset about it, and knew what (if anything) to do about it. The insights she gained from this practice appeared more powerful to her than the understandings gleaned from thought records or from discussions with the therapist about her emotional states.

MBCT and DBT differ substantially in the number of behavior-change skills taught. As noted earlier, DBT assumes that clients may have significant skills deficits and therefore includes reining in a broad array of skills. MBCT, in contrast, focuses primarily on mindfulness meditation practices designed to teach acceptance of experience as it is and assumes that "staying present with what is unpleasant in our experience . . . allows the process to unfold, lets the inherent 'wisdom' of the mind deal with the difficulty, and allows more effective solutions to suggest themselves" (Segal et al., 2002, p. 190). Thus, MBCT does not teach interpersonal interaction, emotion regulation, or problem-solving skills. The course of therapy with Ann suggests the potential utility of both approaches. When she presented for the therapy described here, Ann had significant skills deficits and was an excellent candidate for DBT skills training. However, after she had spent several months learning these skills, the value of the MBCT approach became very clear. That is, bringing mindful awareness to difficult situations allowed Ann to choose wisely from skills within her repertoire.

Several limitations of this case study should be noted. One limitation of adapting the MBCT manual for individual therapy is the loss of group support, which is likely an important factor in the success of MBCT (Segal et al., 2002). Although the therapist practiced

*(Continued)*

(Continued)

all the meditation exercises both during the sessions and during the week and discussed her experiences of the practice at every session, Ann did not have the opportunity to receive the support and feedback from other clients regarding MBCT practices that group format would have provided. Although she was participating in group mindfulness practice and receiving group support from the DBT skills group, it is not clear whether the DBT group was an adequate substitute for the group support in MBCT, especially given the much longer duration of meditation practices in MBCT. More research is needed to investigate the importance of the group experience in the outcome of MBCT.

Because Ann was simultaneously learning mindfulness skills in DBT skills group and from MBCT in individual therapy, another limitation of this case study is that the influence of these two programs on Ann's outcomes cannot be separately evaluated. However, as noted earlier, it appeared that the lengthier meditation practices of MBCT had beneficial effects that had not been observed during Ann's initial months in DBT. Research investigating the effects of different types of mindfulness exercises might clarify this question. Although conclusions cannot be drawn regarding which aspects of the two treatments had the greatest impact on the clinical outcomes, the integration of these two treatments, with their differing emphases on acceptance and change-based strategies, appeared very useful in this case.

## Recommendations to Clinicians and Students

This case study suggests that, in appropriate cases, MBCT can be integrated into ongoing DBT and that mindfulness skills can contribute substantially to the efficacy of cognitive-behavioral approaches. Development of mindfulness appears to enable clients to become more aware of their internal experiences, less distressed by them, and more accepting of them. This state of nonjudgmental awareness appears to facilitate making adaptive choices about skills and strategies to use in coping with problematic situations. More rigorous research is needed to clarify the effects of incorporating both acceptance and change-based strategies in the treatment of presenting problems and the prevention of relapses.

Clinicians and students interested in these treatment approaches may wish to pursue professional training that is available through a variety of workshops nationwide. Information about DBT workshops is available at www.behavioraltech.com. MBCT training is occasionally offered at the Omega Institute (www.eomega.org). In addition, MBCT stipulates that therapists have their own regular mindfulness practice. Thus, interested professionals may wish to learn about beginning a mindfulness meditation practice. Suggestions for pursuing this option can be found in Segal et al. (2002).

## References

American Psychiatric Association. (2000). *Diagnostic and statistical manual of mental disorders* (4th ed. text revision). Washington, DC: Author.

Baer, R. A., Fischer. S., & Huss, D. B. (2005). Mindfulness-based cognitive therapy applied to binge eating disorder: A case study. *Cognitive and Behavioral Practice, 12*(3), 351–358.

Beacham, A. O., Carlson. C., & Philips. B. A. (2001). *A good night's sleep: Nonpharmacological treatment for insomnia.* Unpublished manual. Lexington, KY.

Beck, A. T. (1996). *Beck Depression Inventory-II manual.* San Antonio, TX: The Psychological Corporation.

Beck. A. T., & Steer, R. A. (1993). *Beck Anxiety Inventory manual.* San Antonio, TX: The Psychological Corporation.

Comtois, K. A., Levensky. E. R., & Linehan. M. M. (1999). Behavior therapy. In M. Hersen & A. S. Bellack (Eds.), *Handbook of comparative interventions for adult disorders* (2nd ed., pp. 555–583). New York: John Wiley.

Costa, P. T., & McCrae, R. R. (1992). *Revised NEO Personality Inventory (NEO PI-R) and NEO Five-Factor Inventory (NEO-FFI): Professional manual.* Odessa, FL: Psychological Assessment Resources.

First. M. B., Spitzer. R. L., Williams. J. B. W., & Gibbon, M. (1997). *Structured Clinical Interview for DSM-IV disorders (SCID).* Washington, DC: American Psychiatric Press.

Graham, J. R. (2000). MMPI-2: Assessing personality and psychopathology (3rd ed.). New York: Oxford University Press.

Greenberger, D., & Padesky, C. A. (1995). *Mind over mood: Change how you feel by changing the way you think.* New York: Guilford.

Hathaway, S. R., & McKinley, J. C. (1989). *MMPI-2 (Minnesota Multiphasic Personality Inventory-2) manual for administration and scoring.* Minneapolis: University of Minnesota Press.

Hayes, S. C. (2004). Acceptance and commitment therapy, relational frame theory, and the third wave of behavioral and cognitive therapies. *Behavior Therapy, 35,* 639–665.

Hayes, S. C., Follette, V. M., & Linehan, M. M. (Eds.). (2004). *Mindfulness and acceptance: Expanding the cognitive-behavioral tradition.* New York: Guilford.

Jacobs, G. D., Pace-Schott, E. R., Stickgold, R., & Otto, M. W. (2004). Cognitive behavior therapy and pharmacotherapy for insomnia: A randomized controlled trial and direct comparison. *Archives of Internal Medicine, 164,* 1888–1897.

Kabat-Zinn, J. (1982). An outpatient program in behavioral medicine for chronic pain patients based on the practice of mindfulness meditation: Theoretical considerations and preliminary results. *General Hospital Psychiatry, 4,* 33–47.

Kabat-Zinn, J. (1990). *Full catastrophe living: Using the wisdom of your body and mind to face stress, pain, and illness.* New York: Delacorte.

Koerner, K., & Linehan, M. M. (1997). Case formulation in dialectical behavior therapy for borderline personality disorder. In T. D. Eells (Ed.), *Handbook of psychotherapy case formulation* (pp. 340–367). New York: Guilford.

Linehan, M. M. (1993a). *Cognitive-behavioral treatment of borderline personality disorder.* New York: Guilford.

Linehan, M. M. (1993b). *Skills training manual for treating borderline personality disorder.* New York: Guilford.

Linehan, M. M. (1994). Acceptance and change: The central dialectic in psychotherapy. In S. C. Hayes, N. S. Jacobson, V. M. Follette & M. J. Dougher (Eds.), *Acceptance and change: Content and context in psychotherapy* (pp. 73–86). Reno, NV: Context Press.

Ma, S. H., & Teasdale, J. D. (2004). Mindfulness-based cognitive therapy for depression: Replication and exploration of differential relapse prevention effects. *Journal of Consulting and Clinical Psychology, 72,* 31–40.

Robins, C. J., & Chapman, A. L. (2004). Dialectical behavior therapy: Current status, recent developments, and future directions. *Journal of Personality Disorders, 18,* 73–89.

Segal, Z. V., Teasdale, J. D., & Williams, J. M. G. (2004). Mindfulness-based cognitive therapy: Theoretical rationale and empirical status. In S. C. Hayes, V. M. Follette, & M. M. Linehan (Eds.), *Mindfulness and acceptance: Expanding the cognitive-behavioral tradition* (pp. 45–65). New York: Guilford.

*(Continued)*

(Continued)

Segal, Z. V., Williams, J. M. G., & Teasdale, J. D. (2002). *Mindfulness-based cognitive therapy for depression: A new approach to preventing relapse.* New York: Guilford.

Smith, M. T., & Neubauer, D. N. (2003). Cognitive behavior therapy for chronic insomnia. *Clinical Cornerstone, 5,* 28–40.

Teasdale, J. D., Williams, J. M., Soulsby, J. M., Segal, Z. V., Ridgeway, V. A., & Lau. M. A. (2000). Prevention of relapse/recurrence in major depression by mindfulness-based cognitive therapy. *Journal of Consulting and Clinical Psychology, 68,* 615–623.

## About the Authors

**Debra B. Huss**, MA, is a 5th-year clinical psychology graduate student at the University of Kentucky. She is interested in clinical outcome research, health psychology, pediatric psychology, and mindfulness and acceptance-based interventions.

**Ruth A. Baer**, PhD, is a faculty member in the Department of Psychology at the University of Kentucky. She is interested in mindfulness and acceptance-based interventions and the assessment and conceptualization of mindfulness.

# 7

# Toward Effective Practice With Low-Income Women

In this book, we have examined the mental disorders most prevalent among low-income women. In this process, we learned that considerable evidence is emerging that suggests that particular biochemical processes and genetic factors contribute in unique and significant ways to the disorders, though violence is an external stressor that exacerbates those predispositions. We also learned that the use of age-appropriate, ethnically sensitive, valid, and reliable screening measures can increase the likelihood that low-income women will be screened as early as possible in the lifespan. Last, we found that CBT and its variations are the most effective interventions to use in addressing the mental health disorders most prevalent among low-income women. Unfortunately, there is a significant gap between the demand for psychosocial interventions and mental health services available to low-income women. We are encouraged that the National Institutes of Health has identified the effects of poverty on women's mental health as a national priority, thus facilitating study of clinical interventions that might be effective in addressing mental health disorders in low-income women (Substance Abuse and Mental Health Services Administration, 2009).

## Directions for Social Work Practice With Low-Income Women

Within the context of the cumulative and cyclical interdependencies model of poverty, it is imperative that social workers develop programs and services that enhance the self-sufficiency of women who live in or near poverty. In order to do this, social workers must understand that the intersection of poverty and violence affects the mental health of low-income women in unique and negative ways. As such, there is a need for the programs and services developed to serve low-income women to focus first and foremost on the traumatic experiences in their lives. Given the lack of resources and staff in many areas of the United States, there is also a need for programs and services that utilize stepped and collaborative care in the most efficient ways to address the mental health problems of low-income women. Relative to the well-documented association between childhood sexual abuse and intimate partner violence (IPV), there is a need for gender-specific violence prevention programs in schools that address trauma experiences of low-income females as early as possible. In the following sections, we provide examples of how social workers can be proactive rather than reactive in addressing the mental health of low-income women.

# Integrative and Survivor-Centered Programs and Services

Given the intersection of poverty and IPV, programs and services developed to address the mental health needs of low-income women should be integrative, trauma-focused, and survivor-centered. For example, encouraging low-income women in IPV situations to use problem-solving coping as a means of managing the stress in their lives may actually cause them more distress due to the lack of available resources to address either IPV or poverty (Goodman, Smyth, Borges, & Singer, 2009). Instead, low-income women in violent situations utilize "survival focused coping" (p. 318), which means that they survive in the moment and meet basic needs. In this regard, a low-income woman who is in an abusive situation may concentrate on keeping herself and her children safe from moment to moment rather than on the fact that she is actually in an abusive relationship (Goodman et al., 2009). It is difficult for many laypersons and service providers to comprehend this coping strategy, and in turn, to understand why low-income women stay in abusive situations.

In addition, many low-income women with some combination of disorders identified in this text have experienced trauma in both childhood and adulthood. As a result, several groups of researchers have emphasized the importance of trauma in the lives of low-income women and that trauma-informed programs and services are warranted to address the mental health concerns of low-income women (Cocozza et al., 2005; Elliott, Bjelajac, Fallot, Markoff, & Reed, 2005; Markoff, Reed, Fallot, Elliott, & Bjelajac, 2005). Elliott et al. (2005) identified the following ten principles of trauma-focused services:

- Trauma is a core event that affects women's sense of self, coping skills, and views of the world.
- Services must create an atmosphere that is respectful of survivors' need for safety.
- Services must engage consumers in the use of services.
- Services must employ an empowerment perspective toward helping women who have often been disenfranchised.
- Services must be woman centered.
- Women consumers must be able to give informed consent to the services they receive.

- Services must be oriented towards relationship and collaboration.
- Services should emphasize women's strengths, focusing on adaptation and resilience.
- Service providers must acknowledge the uniqueness of each female consumer.
- Consumers should be involved in the design, implementation, and evaluation of services.

Cocozza et al. (2005) also noted the need for advocacy, parenting, and integrated counseling services. Specifically, Davies, Lyon, and Monti-Catania (1998) suggested the use of "woman-defined advocacy" that relies on the perspective of the client regarding the need for and goal of advocacy.

Markoff et al. (2005) proposed that trauma-focused programs must be comprehensive, integrated, trauma-informed, and involve consumer/survivor/ recovering (CSR) women in service delivery. As such, they stress how important it is to understand that trauma is often at the core of women's mental health problems, especially low-income women who have experienced IPV. It is important as well to provide women with a safe environment, and to this end, it is best to avoid asking women about symptoms and disclosure, but rather to focus on women's experiences, identifying ways to work collaboratively with CSR women using their strengths as survivors. Outreach that assures women that they will have trusting relationships with service providers is needed in light of the possibility that many women have had negative experiences with service providers where there is no trauma focus. Last, service providers should be cautious in screening beyond the need for safety and a history of trauma, primarily due to the shame and stigma that women may feel if asked directly about past violent experiences.

In terms of service provision, crisis intervention and peer-led services can be especially helpful in addressing the mental health problems of low-income, survivor women. In the case of a service provider who has already established a relationship with a CSR woman, the two of them can develop a crisis plan that includes identifying under what circumstances the plan is to be implemented; the type of safe environment that will be needed, such as detoxification; specific facilities to be used; transportation needed; conditions for returning home; child accommodations; expectations of the service provider; and expectations of CSR woman. With involvement of the CSR woman in planning, the crisis plan is similar to an advanced directive (Massachusetts Department of Health, 1996).

By comparison, peer-led services can insure that women are empowered to take control over their lives (see Brown & Worth, 2002; Prescott, 2001). With assistance, women can develop services that meet their needs. The advantages of those services include:

- Participants are both helpers and those who are helped.
- No one person has the answers.
- Participants can safely accept responsibility.

- Services are inexpensive in terms of cost.
- Numerous problems and needs can be addressed.

Twelve-step programs can be helpful as well, with the caveat that they must include the trauma focus and the notion of powerlessness must be addressed relative to the notion of empowerment (see Davis-Kasl, 1992).

In order to enhance the mental health care for low-income survivor women, social workers will need to move toward trauma-informed programs and services, and this will require modifications at the mezzo and macro levels of practice. At the agency (mezzo) level, leadership is warranted to move away from traditional services with no trauma focus and toward trauma-focused mental health services for women. In addition, service providers/staff require cross-training to address the intersection of poverty, traumatic experiences, and mental health disorders. In turn, agency policies and procedures should reflect the provision of trauma-informed services, and this *must* include women survivors in the planning for and implementing of services. At the policy (macro) level, funding, licensing, and regulations must reflect the importance of trauma focused education and training for professionals. See Figure 7.1.

**Figure 7.1**   Trauma-Focused Services for Low-Income Women

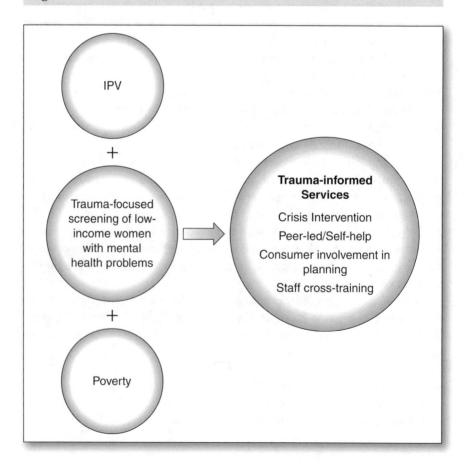

## Stepped and Collaborative Care

The two main features of stepped care are that (a) treatment for an individual should be the least restrictive from among the evidence-based treatments that are likely to result in mental health gains for the individual and that (b) the care can change to a more restrictive step of care based on the need of the consumer (Bower & Gilbody, 2005). Despite the finding that CBT and its variations are the most evidence-based interventions for use in treating post-traumatic stress disorder (PTSD), depression, generalized anxiety disorder (GAD), substance use disorder (SUD), and borderline personality disorder (BPD), it is likely that less intensive interventions used individually or in some combination might result in mediating the problem or problems prior to using CBT. Those include problem solving, interpersonal therapy, group treatments, and self-help interventions.

The key consideration in using a stepped care model of service delivery is identifying the number of steps that can be provided to consumers (Bower & Gilbody, 2005). This is contingent to a large extent on the interventions available in particular areas and on defining the uppermost stepped care as that used in traditional services (e.g., some form of CBT in most instances). In rural areas, for example, there may be a minimum of services available, and the only service provider who is trained to use CBT is an itinerant professional who serves several communities. In this situation, the care must be stepped down whenever possible to a professional in the service delivery model who can work on problem-solving skills.

The primary intent of stepped care is to increase efficiency in service delivery and reduce more intensive interventions that tend to be more costly within the context of behavioral health management. A second intent of stepped care is to make care available to more individuals. With these intentions in mind, decisions about service provision should be based on data collected during the screening and assessment process or within treatment. Although rapid screening and/or assessment measures are recommended for use in measuring outcomes because they are inexpensive and can be easily standardized, the judgment of the clinician and consumer regarding the step of care needed should be considered as well.

It is critical that the step of care not be so low that it results in treatment failure (Bower & Gilbody, 2005). In the first or lowest step of care, for example, the use of books on the topic of child abuse and neglect as a means of addressing depression in a woman whose children have been removed due to neglect will likely be ineffective in both the short term and the long term. This is due primarily to the lengthy period of time it will take her to earn the right to have her children returned to the home. By comparison, the use of books on the topic of divorce as a means of addressing situational depression in a newly divorced woman might be useful. In either case, the perspectives of both the clinician and the consumer, as well as a measure of depression, will help determine which step of care is needed.

Stepped care is predicated on three assumptions. The first assumption is that overall consumer progress made in using stepped care is equivalent to consumer progress made in using traditional, more intensive therapies immediately. The second and third assumptions are that using minimal interventions will allow resources to be used more efficiently and that the interventions used are acceptable to both professionals and consumers. Despite the need for more research that validates the overall stepped care process, it is once again important to note that many poor women who experience PTSD, depression, GAD, SUD, BPD, or some combination of these disorders currently have no access to any mental health services.

In sum, the model of stepped care developed in a particular community or region will depend on the available resources, and especially on the education and training of staff in various social service agencies. For example, if there are no psychiatrists available to prescribe medications, then care is stepped to primary care physicians or general practitioners. We believe that social workers can be involved in providing mental health care for low-income women that is preventive, though this will require collaboration and creativity. The example of a stepped care model illustrated in Figure 7.2

**Figure 7.2**    Proposed Basic Stepped Care Approach to Mental Health Intervention with Low-Income Women

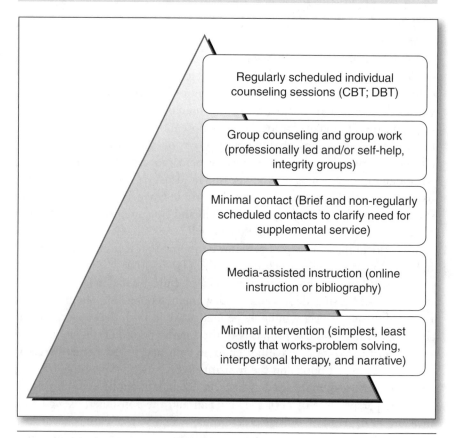

*Source:* Model adapted from Black and Hultsman (1989).

can be adapted to the provision of stepped care for treating the mental health needs of low-income women (Black & Hultsman, 1989, p. 29).

## Gender-Specific Violence Prevention Programs

Gender-specific programs and services for females are needed early in the developmental process to address mental health problems among low-income women, primarily because society socializes girls differently than boys. As a result, girls often lack a sense of worth, especially girls who have been victimized in some way. In turn, the lack of self-worth and power that develops among girls who have been victimized may result in their being aggressive. Some may seek power through their own aggressive behavior, though the acquisition of power in this way is temporary and results in continued lack of self-worth (Artz, 1998).

By comparison, most statistics on childhood sexual abuse suggest that many females keep sexual victimization secret and internalize the stress associated with the victimization. In the context of secrecy and nondisclosure, girls often develop mental health problems, including depression, anxiety, or both. Because females tend to internalize feelings and ruminate as a means of coping with stress, those who have been or are being physically or sexually abused in the home are often not referred for services in the school setting, primarily because they present with fewer acting-out behaviors that come to the attention of educational personnel.

Whether the outcome of victimization is externalization or internalization of feelings, violence prevention programs designed specifically for girls seem warranted in the preadolescent years. In particular, these types of programs seem needed for girls who reside in low-income neighborhoods, where violence tends to occur more frequently than in high income neighborhoods. In this regard, Girls Incorporated of Metro Denver identified the need for programs that (a) take the feelings and thoughts of girls seriously; (b) foster diversity; (c) provide opportunities for active involvement with peers acquiring new information, practicing new skills, and advocating for change; and (d) allow girls to establish relationships with adults who understand their needs and strengths, challenge them to take risks, and maintain high standards for their achievement. (go to www .girlsincdenver.org).

Social workers in schools and communities can be instrumental in implementing trauma-focused and violence prevention programs with females in schools, especially as early as the program is appropriate. The easiest way for social workers to implement these types of programs and to measure the extent to which programs are effective is to use a wait-list experimental design, such as that illustrated in Figure 7.3. In doing so, social workers and educational personnel can answer the following two questions: (1)What is the difference in outcomes between students in the experimental group and

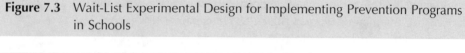

**Figure 7.3**  Wait-List Experimental Design for Implementing Prevention Programs in Schools

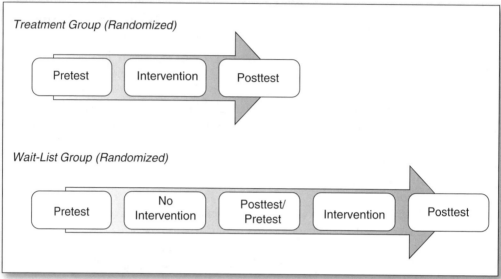

students in the wait-list (control) group? (2)What is the difference in outcomes between students in the experimental group and students in the wait-list group after they receive the intervention?

# Summary

We have provided students with the evidence regarding the mental health disorders most prevalent among low-income women, though much of the evidence regarding effective practice in addressing those disorders in women has resulted from studies in clinical studies. We have also highlighted the intersections of poverty, IPV, and women's mental health. Given these factors, we envision that social workers can be involved in enhancing the mental health of low-income women in unique and creative ways that go beyond the clinical setting. When one considers that social workers practice with low-income women in numerous settings, including community human service agencies, schools, domestic violence shelters, rape crisis centers, hospitals, clinics, and child welfare and community mental health facilities, we believe that they can (a) develop and implement trauma-focused services (see Anderson, 2010), (b) create stepped care models of practice that most effectively (and efficiently) address the mental health needs of low-income women in particular locations, and (c) implement gender-specific violence prevention programs in schools as early as seems warranted.

Moreover, social workers are trained to design, deliver, and evaluate social work practice strategies with individuals, families, groups, and communities. Thus, they have the opportunity to intervene directly with individual clients and also to develop and implement programs and policy initiatives that can prevent, minimize, or in other ways ameliorate mental health problems within their communities. We strongly encourage social workers and other professionals in helping disciplines to make appropriate use of the data we have presented and explained within this volume and also to create policies and programs that will allow them to intervene as early as possible to prevent and address mental health disorders among low-income women.

# References

Abramovitz, M. (1996). *Regulating the lives of women.* Boston: South End Press.

Abramson, L., Alloy, L., Hankin, B., Haeffel, G., MacCoon, D., & Gibb, B. (2002). Cognitive vulnerability-stress models of depression in a self-regulatory and psychobiological context. In I. Gotlieb & C. Hammen (Eds.), *Handbook of depression* (pp. 268–294). New York: Guilford Press.

Agrawal, A., & Lynskey, M. (2006). The genetic epidemiology of cannabis use, abuse, and dependence. *Addiction, 101*(6), 801–812. doi:10.1111/j.1360–0443 .2006.01399.x

Alastair, F. (2005). Generalized anxiety disorder in elderly patients: Epidemiology, diagnosis and treatment options. *Drugs & Aging, 22*(2), 101–114.

Alexander, L., LaRosa, J., & Bader, H. (2001). *New dimensions in women's health* (2nd ed.). Sudbury, MA: Jones and Bartlett.

Alinsky, S. (1945). *Reveille for radicals.* Chicago: University of Chicago Press.

*American heritage dictionary* (3rd ed.). (1990). Boston: Houghton Mifflin.

American Psychiatric Association. (1994). *Diagnostic and statistical manual of mental disorders* (4th ed., Text revision). Washington, D.C.: Author.

Amott, T., & Matthaei, J. (1996). *Race, gender, and work: A multicultural economic history of women in the United States* (3rd ed.). Boston: South End Press.

Anderson, K. (2010). *Enhancing resilience in survivors of family violence.* New York: Springer.

Anderson, S., & Gryslak, B. (2002). Social work advocacy in the post-TANF research studies. *Social Work, 47*(3), 301–314.

Anguelova, M., Benkelfat, C., & Turecki, G. (2003). A systematic review of association studies investigating genes coding for serotonin receptors and the serotonin transporter: Suicidal behavior. *Molecular Psychiatry, 8*, 646–653. doi:10.1038/ sj.mp.4001336

Ansseau, M., Fischler, B., Dierick, M., Albert, A., Leyman, S., & Mignon, A. (2008). Socioeconomic correlates of generalized anxiety disorder and major depression in primary care: The GADIS II study. *Depression and Anxiety, 25*(6), 50613. doi:10.1002/da.20306

Antony, M., Orsillo, S., & Roemer, L. (Eds.). (2001). *Practitioner's guide to empirically based measures of anxiety.* New York: Kluwer Academic/Plenum Publishers.

Arria, A., Derauf, C., LaGasse, L., Grant, P., Shah, R., Smith, L., et al. (2006). Methamphetamine and other substance use during pregnancy: Preliminary estimates from the Infant Development, Environment, and Lifestyle (IDEAL) Study. *Maternal and Child Health Journal, 10*(3), 293–302. doi:10.1007/ s10995–005–0052–0

Artz, S. (1998). Where have all the schoolgirls gone? Violent girls in the schoolyard. *Child and Youth Care Forum, 27*(2), 77–107.

Asen, R. (2002). *Visions of poverty: Welfare policy and political imagination.* East Lansing: Michigan State University Press.

Azid, N. (1999). Cultural sensitization and clinical guidelines for mental health professionals working with Afghan immigrant/refugee women in the United States. *Dissertation Abstracts International,* 60 (3-B). (UMI No. 95018–237)

Baer, J., Kivlahan, D., Blume, A., McKnight, P., & Marlatt, G. (2001). Brief intervention for heavy-drinking college students: Four-year follow-up and natural history. *American Journal of Public Health, 91*(8), 1310–1316.

Bandelow, B., Krause, J., Wedekind, D., Broocks, A., Hajak, G., & Ruther, E. (2005). Early traumatic life events, parental attitudes, family history, and birth risk factors in patients with borderline personality disorder and healthy controls. *Psychiatric Research, 134,* 169–174. doi:10.1016/j.psychres.2003.07.008

Barr, C., Newman, T., Schwandt, M., Shannon, C., Dvoskin, R., & Lindell, S. (2004). Sexual dichotomy of an interaction between early adversity and the serotonin trans- porter gene promoter variant in rhesus macaques. *Proceedings of the National Academy of Science, 101,* 12354–12363. doi:10.1073/pnas.0403763101

Barry, L., Allore, H., Guo, Z., Bruce, M., & Gill, T. (2008). Higher burden of depres- sion among older women: The effect of onset, persistence, and mortality over time. *Archives of General Psychiatry, 65*(2), 172–178. doi:10.1001/archgen psychiatry.2007.17

Barusch, A., Taylor, M., Abu-Bader, S., & Derr, M. (1999). *Understanding families with multiple barriers to self-sufficiency.* Salt Lake City, UT: Social Research Institute.

Bassuk, E. L., Buckner, J. C., Perloff, J. N., and Bassuk, S. S. (1998). Prevalence of mental health and substance use disorders among homeless and low-income housed mothers. *American Journal of Psychiatry, 155,* 1561–1564.

Bazanis, E., Rogers, R., Dowson, J., Taylor, P., Meux, C., Staley, C., et al. (2002). Neurocognitive deficits in decision-making and planning of patients with DSM-III-R borderline personality disorder. *Psychological Medicine, 32,* 1395–1405. doi:10.1017/S0033291702006657

Beck, A. (1967). *Depression.* Philadelphia: University of Pennsylvania Press.

Beck, A., Epstein, N., Brown, G., & Steer, R. (1988). An inventory for measuring clinical anxiety: Pyschometric properties. *Journal of Consulting and Clinical Psychology, 56,* 893–897. doi:10.1037/0022–006X.56.6.893

Beck, A. (1996). *Beck Depression Inventory.* New York: Harcourt.

Beck, A., Steer, R., & Brown, G. (1996). *Beck Depression Inventory (BDI-II).* Boston: Pearson Education.

Beck, A., Weissman, A., Lester, D., & Trexler, L. (1974). The measurement of pessimism: The hopelessness scale. *Journal of Consulting and Clinical Psychology, 42,* 861–865. doi:10.1037/h0037562

Bekker, M., & van Mens-Verhulst, J. (2007). Anxiety disorders: Sex differences in prevalence, degree, and background, but gender-neutral treatment. *Gender Medicine, 4*(Suppl. 2), S178–193.

Belle, D., & Doucet, J. (2003). Poverty, inequality, and discrimination as sources of depression among U.S. women. *Psychology of Women Quarterly, 27*(2), 101–113.

Ben-Noun, L. (1998). Generalized anxiety disorder in dysfunctional families. *Journal of Behavior Therapy & Experimental Psychiatry, 29*(2), 115–122.

Benishek, L., Bieschke, K., Stoffelmayr, B., Mavis, B., & Humphreys, K. (1992). Gender differences in depression and anxiety among alcoholics. *Addictive Behavior, 4,* 235–245.

Bernstein, G., Layne, A., Egan, E., & Tennison, D. (2005). School-based interventions for anxious children. *Journal of the American Academy of Child and Adolescent Psychiatry, 44*(11), 1118–1127. doi:10.1097/01.chi.0000177323 .40005.a1

Bernstein, J., Bernstein, E., Tassiopoulos, K., Heeren, T., Levenson, S., & Hingson, R. (2005). Brief motivational intervention at a clinic visit reduces cocaine and heroin use. *Drug and Alcohol Dependence, 77*(1), 49–59.

Berrick, J. (1997). *Faces of poverty: Portraits of women and children on welfare.* New York: Oxford University Press.

Bhui, K., & Dinos, S. (2008). Health beliefs and culture: Essential considerations for outcome measurement. *Disease Management & Health Outcomes, 16*(6), 411–419.

Birnbaum, H. G., Leong, S. A., & Greenberg P. E. (2003). The economics of women and depression: An employer perspective. *Journal of Affective Disorders, 74*(1), 15–22. doi:10.1016/S0165–03279(02)00427–5

Bisson, J., & Andrew, J. (2007). Psychological treatment of post-traumatic stress disorder (PTSD). *Cochrane Database of Systematic Reviews, 3,* Article No. CD003388. doi:10.1002/146551858.CD003388.pub3

Bisson, J., Ehlers, A., & Matthews, R. (2007). Review: Trauma-focused psychological treatments to improve post-traumatic stress disorder symptoms. *British Journal of Psychiatry, 190,* 97–104. doi:10.1192/bjp.bp.106.021402

Black, D., & Hultsman, J. (1989). The Purdue Stepped Approach Model: Groups as a symbiosis of career development and mental health counseling. *The Counseling Psychologist, 16,* 647–667. doi:10.1177/0011000088164007.

Blair, R., Colledge, E., Murray, L., & Mitchell, D. (2001). A selective impairment in the processing of sad and fearful expressions in children with psychopathic tendencies. *Journal of Abnormal Psychology, 29,* 491–498.

Blake, D., Weathers, F., Nagy, L., Kaloupek, D., Klauminzer, G., Charney, D., et al. (1990). A clinician rating scale for assessing current and lifetime PTSD: The CAPS-1. *The Behavior Therapist, 13,* 187–188.

Blank, R. (2003). Selecting among anti-poverty policies: Can an economist be both critical and caring? *Review of Social Economy, 61*(4), 447–471.

Bledsoe, S., & Grote, N. (2006). Treating depression during pregnancy and the postpartum: A preliminary meta-analysis. *Research on Social Work Practice, 2,* 641–645. doi:10.1177/1049731505282202

Bleiberg, K., & Markowitz, A. (2005). A pilot study of interpersonal psychotherapy for posttraumatic stress disorder. *American Journal of Psychiatry, 158,* 181–183. doi:10.1176/appi.ajp.162.1.181

Blumenthal, J., Babyak, M., Moore, K., Craighead, W., Herman, S., Khatri, P., et al. (1999). Effects of exercise training on older patients with depression. *Archives of Internal Medicine, 159,* 2349–2356. doi:10.1001/archinte.159.19.2349

Bond, F. W., & Bunce, D. (2003). The role of acceptance and job control in mental health, job satisfaction, and work performance. *Journal of Applied Psychology, 88*, 1057–1067. doi:10.1037/0021–9010.88.6.1057

Borkovec, T. D., Alcaine, O., & Behar, E. (2004). Avoidance theory of worry and generalized anxiety disorder. In R. G. Heimberg, C. L. Turk, & D. S. Mennin (Eds.), *Generalized anxiety disorder: Advances in research and practice* (pp. 77–108). New York: Guilford Press.

Bornovalova, M., Gratz, K., Delany-Brumsey, A., Paulson, A., & Lejuez, C. (2006). Temperamental and environmental risk factors for borderline personality disorder among inner-city substance users in residential treatment. *Journal of Personality Disorders, 20*(3), 218–231. doi:10.1521/pedi.2006.20.3.218

Bower, P., & Gilbody, S. (2005). Stepped care in psychological therapies: Access, effectiveness, and efficiency. [Narrative literature review.] *British Journal of Psychiatry, 186*, 11–17. doi:10.1192/bjp.186.1.11

Bradley, R., Greene, J., Russ, E., Dutra, L., & Westen, D. (2005). A multidimensional meta-analysis of psychotherapy for PTSD. *American Journal of Psychiatry, 162*, 214–227. doi:10.1176/appi.ajp.162.2.214

Bradshaw, T. (2007). Theories of poverty and anti-poverty programs in community development. *Community Development, 38*(1), 7–25.

Brady, T. M., & Ashley, O. S. (Eds.). (2005). *Women in substance abuse treatment: Results from the Alcohol and Drug Services Study (ADSS)*. (DHHS Publication No. SMA 04–3968, Analytic Series A-26). Rockville, MD: Substance Abuse and Mental Health Services Administration, Office of Applied Studies.

Bremner, M., Narayan, M., Staib, L., Southwick, S., McGlashan, T., & Charney, D. (1999). Neural correlates of memories of childhood sexual abuse in women with and without posttraumatic disorder. *American Journal of Psychiatry, 156*, 1787–1795.

Breslau, N., & Davis, G. (1992). Posttraumatic stress disorder in an urban population of young adults: Risk factors for chronicity. *American Journal of Psychiatry, 149*, 671–675.

Breslau, N., Chilcoat, H., Peterson, E., & Schultz, L. (2000). Gender differences in major depression: The role of anxiety. In E. Frank (Ed.), *Gender and its effects on psychopathology* (pp. 131–150), Washington, DC: American Psychopathological Association.

Breslau, N., Davis, G., Andreski, P. Peterson, E., & Schultz, L. (1997). Sex differences in posttraumatic stress disorder. *Archives of General Psychiatry, 54*, 1044–1048.

Brewin, C., & Holmes, E. (2003). Psychological theories of posttraumatic stress disorder. *Clinical Psychology Review, 23*(3), 339–376.

Bride, B. (2001). Single-gender treatment of substance abuse: Effect on treatment retention and completion. *Social Work Research, 25*, 223–232.

Briere, J., Scott, C., & Weathers, F. (2005). Peritraumatic and persistent dissociation in the presumed etiology of PTSD. *American Journal of Psychiatry, 162*, 2295–2301. doi:10.1176/appi.ajp.162.12.2295

Brooks, S., Krulewicz, S., & Kutcher, S. (2003). The Kutcher Adolescent Depression Scale: Assessment of its evaluative properties over the course of an 8-week pediatric pharmacotherapy trial. *Journal of Child Psychopharmacology, 13*, 337–349.

Brown, B. (2000). Outcome in female patients with both substance use and posttraumatic stress disorders. *Alcohol Treatment Quarterly, 18*, 127–135.

Brown, V., & Worth, D. (2002). *Recruiting, training, and maintaining consumer staff: Strategies used and lessons learned.* Culver City, CA: Prototypes Systems Change Center.

Brown, V., Melchior, L., & Huba, G. (1995). Level of burden among women diagnosed with severe mental illness and substance abuse. *Journal of Psychoactive Drugs, 31,* 31–40.

Browne, A., & Bassuk, S. (1997). Intimate violence in the lives of homeless and poor housed women : Prevalence and patterns in an ethnically diverse sample. *American Journal of Orthopsychiatry, 67*(2), 261–278. doi:10.1037/h0080230

Bryant, R. (2006). Acute stress disorder. *Psychiatry, 5*(7), 238–239.

Burden, D., & Gottlieb, N. (Eds.). (1987). *The woman client: Providing human services in a changing world.* New York: Tavistock.

Butler, A., & Beck, J. (2001). Cognitive therapy outcomes: A review of meta-analyses. *Tidsskrift for Norsk Psykologforening, 38*(8), 698–706.

Butler, A., Chapman, J., Forman, E., & Beck, A. (2006). The empirical status of cognitive-behavioral therapy: A review of meta-analyses. *Clinical Psychology Review, 26*(1), 17–31. doi:10.1016/j.cpr.2005.07.003

Cancian, M. (2001). The rhetoric and reality of work based welfare reform. *Social Work 46*(4), 309–314.

Cancian, M., Haveman, R., Meyer, D., & Wolfe (2002). Before and after TANF: The economic well-being of women leaving welfare. *Social Service Review, 76*(4), 603–641. doi:10.1086/342997.

Carroll, K., Ball, S., Nich, C., Martino, S., Frankforter, T., & Farentinos, C. (2006). Motivational interviewing to improve treatment engagement and outcomes in individuals seeking treatment for substance abuse: A multisite effectiveness study. *Drug and Alcohol Dependence, 81*(3), 301–312.

Caspi, A., Sugden, K., Moffitt, T., Taylor, A., Craig, I., Harrington, H, et al. (2003). Influence of life stress on depression: Moderation by a polymorphism in the 5-HTT gene. *Science, 301,* 386–389. doi:10.1126/science.1083968

Castle, D., Kulkarni, J., & Abel, K. (Eds.). (2006). *Mood and anxiety disorders in women.* New York: Cambridge University Press.

Caudle, D., Senior, A., Wetherell, J., Rhoades, H., Beck, J., Kunik, M., et al. (2007). Cognitive errors, symptom severity, and response to cognitive behavior therapy in older adults with generalized anxiety disorder. *American Journal of Geriatric Psychiatry, 15*(8), 680–689. doi:10.1097/JGP.0b013e31803c550d

Cawthorne, A. (October 8, 2008). *The straight facts on women in poverty.* Washington, DC: Center for American Progress.

Centers for Disease Control. (2008). *HIV/AIDS among women.* Atlanta, GA: Department of Health and Human Services.

Chaturvedi, A., Chiu, C., & Viswanathan, M. (2009). Literacy, negotiable fate, and thinking style among low income women in India. *Journal of Cross-Cultural Psychology, 40*(5), 880–893.

Chubb, J., & Moe, T. (1996). Politics, markets, and equality in schools. In M. R. Darby (Ed.), *Reducing poverty in America: Views and approaches* (pp. 121–133). Thousand Oaks, CA: Sage.

Clark, C., Ryan, L., Kawachi, I., Canner, M., Berkman, L., & Wright, R. (2008). Witnessing community violence in residential neighborhoods: A mental health hazard for urban women. *Journal of Urban Health, 85*(1), 22–38.

Clarkin, J., Levy, K., Lenzenweger, M., & Kenberg, O. (2007). Evaluating three treatments of borderline personality disorder: A multi-wave study. *American Journal of Psychiatry, 164,* 922–928. doi:10.1176/appi.ajp.164.6.922

Cocca, C. (2002). From "welfare queen" to "exploited teen": Welfare dependency, statutory rape. *NSWE Journal, 14*(2), 56–79.

Cocozza, J., Jackson, E., Hennigan, K., Morissey, J., Reed, B., Fallot, R., et al. (2005). Outcomes for women with co-occurring disorders and trauma: Program level effects. *Journal of Substance Abuse Treatment, 28,* 109–119. doi:10.1016/j.jsat2004.08.010

Coehlo, H., Cooper, P., & Murray, L. (2007). A family study of co-morbidity between generalized social phobia and generalized anxiety disorder in a non-clinical sample. *Journal of Affective Disorders, 100* (1-3), 103–113.

Coffman, S., Martell, C., Dimidjian, S., Gallop, R., & Hollon, S. (2007). Extreme non-response in cognitive therapy: Can behavioral activation succeed where cognitive therapy fails? *Journal of Consulting and Clinical Psychology, 75,* 531–541.

Cohen, J., Deblinger, E., & Mannarino, A. (2004). Trauma-focused cognitive behavioral therapy for sexually abused children. *Psychiatric Times, 21*(10), 743–765.

Cohen, L., Altshuler, L., Harlow, B., Nonacs, R., Newport, D., Viguera, A., et al. (2006). Relapse of major depression during pregnancy in women who maintain or discontinue antidepressant treatment. *JAMA: The Journal of the American Medical Association, 295*(5), 499–507. doi:10.1001/jama.295.1.65

Coiro, M. (2001). Depressive symptoms among women receiving welfare. *Women & Health, 32*(1–2), 1–23.

Condelli, W., Koch, M., & Fletcher, B. (2000). Treatment refusal/attrition among adults randomly assigned to programs at a drug treatment campus. *Substance Abuse Treatment, 18,* 395–407.

Connelly, D. (2000). *Homeless mothers: Face to face with women and poverty.* Minneapolis: University of Minnesota Press.

Conway K., Compton, W., Stinson, S., & Grant, B. (2006). Lifetime comorbidity of DSM-IV mood and anxiety disorders and specific drug use disorders: Results from the National Epidemiologic Survey on Alcohol and Related Conditions. *Journal of Clinical Psychiatry, 67*(2), 247–257.

Cook, J., Mock, L., Jonikas, J., Burke-Miller, J., Carter, T., Taylor, A., et al. (2009). Prevalence of psychiatric and substance use disorders among single mothers nearing lifetime welfare eligibility limits. *Archives of General Psychiatry, 66*(3), 249–258. doi:10.1001/archgenpsychiatry.2008.539

Corcoran, M., Danziger, S., & Tolman, R. (2003). Long term employment of African American and White welfare recipients and the role of persistent health and mental health problems. *Women & Health, 39*(4), 1–23.

Cordozo, C., & Sussman, L. (2001). *Mental health needs of women in transition from welfare to work.* Boston: Center for Women in Politics and Public Policy, John W. McCormack Institute of Public Affairs, University of Massachusetts Boston.

Cougle, J., Keough, M., Riccardi, C., & Sachs-Ericcson, N. (2009). Anxiety disorders and suicidality in the National Comorbidity Survey-Replication. *Journal of Psychiatric Research, 43*(9), 825–829.

Cougle, J., Reardon, D., & Coleman, P. (2005). Generalized anxiety following unintended pregnancies resolved through childbirth and abortion: A cohort study of the 1995 National Survey of Family Growth. *Journal of Anxiety Disorders, 19,* 137–142.

Cox, J., Holden, J., & Sagovsky, R. (1987). Detection of postnatal depression: Development of the 10-item Edinburgh Postnatal Depression Scale. *British Journal of Psychiatry, 150,* 782–786. doi:10.1192/bjp.150.6.782

Cuijpers, P., van Straten, A., & Warmerdam, L. (2007). Behavioral activation treatments of depression: A meta-analysis. *Clinical Psychology Review, 27,* 318–326.

Cyranowski, J., & Frank, E. (2006). Targeting populations of women for prevention and treatment of depression. In C. Mazure and G. Keita (Eds.), *Understanding depression in women: Applying empirical research to practice and policy* (pp. 71–112). Washington, DC: American Psychological Association.

Dansky, B., & Kilpatrick, D. (1997). Effects of sexual harassment. In W. O'Donohue (Ed.), *Sexual harassment: Theory, research, and treatment* (pp. 152–174). Boston: Allyn & Bacon.

Danziger, S. K., Kalil, A., & Anderson, N. J. (2001). Human capital, health, and mental health of welfare recipients: Co-occurrence and correlates. *Journal of Social Issues, 54*(4), 637–656.

Davidson, P. R., & Parker, K. C. H. (2001). Eye movement desensitization and reprocessing (EMDR): A meta-analysis. *Journal of Consulting and Clinical Psychology, 69,* 305–316. doi:10.1037/0022–006X.69.2.305

Davies, J., Lyon, E., & Monti-Catania, D. (1998). *Safety planning with battered women: Complex lives/difficult choices.* Thousand Oaks, CA: Sage.

Davis-Kasl, C. (1992). *Many roads one journey: Moving beyond the twelve steps.* New York: HarperPerennial.

Davis, L. (Ed.). (1994). *Building on women's strengths: A social work agenda for the twenty-first century.* New York: Haworth Press.

Davis, S. (1994). Drug treatment decisions of chemically-dependent women. *International Journal of Addiction, 29,* 1287–1304.

Deblinger, E., Lippman, J., & Steer, R. (1996). Sexually abused children suffering posttraumatic stress symptoms: Initial treatment outcome findings. *Child Maltreatment, 1,* 310–321. doi:10.1177/1077559596001004003

Dennis, C. (2005). Psychosocial and psychological interventions for prevention of postnatal depression: Systematic review. *BMJ (British Medical Journal), 15*(2), 331. doi:10.1136/bmj.331.7507.15

Dennis, C., Ross, L., & Grigoriadis, S. (2009). Psychosocial and psychological interventions for treating antenatal depression. *Cochrane Database of Systematic Reviews, 3,* Article No. CD006309. doi:10.1002/14651858.CD006309

Desai, R., Harpaz-Rotem, I., Najavits, L., & Rosenheck, R. (2008). Impact of the Seeking Safety Program on clinical outcomes among homeless female veterans with psychiatric disorders. *Psychiatric Services, 59,* 996–1003. doi:10.1176/appi.ps.59.9.996

Dick, D., Pagan, J., Viken, R., Purcell, S., Kaprio, J., Pulkkinen, L., et al. (2007). Changing environmental influences on substance use across development. *Twin Research in Human Genetics, 10*(2), 315–326.

Dobie, D., Kivlahan, D., Maynard, C., Bush, K., Davis, T., & Bradley, K. (2004). Posttraumatic stress disorder in female veterans: Association with self-reported health problems and functional impairment. *Archives of Internal Medicine, 164,* 394–400. doi:10.1001/archinte.164.4.394

Dreher, J., Schmidt. P., Kohn, P., Furman, D., Rubinow, D., & Berman, K. (2007). Menstrual cycle phase modulates reward-related neural function in women. *Proceedings of the National Academy of Sciences, 104*(7), 2465–2470.

Dubro, A., Wetzler, S., & Kahn, M. (1988). A comparison of three self-report questionnaires for the diagnosis of DSM-III personality disorders. *Journal of Personality Disorders, 2,* 256–266.

Dutton, S. (2002). Marital relationship functioning in a clinical sample of generalized anxiety disorder clients. *Dissertation Abstracts International, 62* (9-B). (UMI No. 95006–084)

Eberhard-Gran, M., Eskild, A., Tambs, K., Opjordsmoen, S., & Samuelsen, S. (2001). Review of validation studies of the Edinburgh Postnatal Depression Scale. *Acta Psychiatrica Scandinavica 104*(4), 243–249. doi:10.1034/j.1600–0447.2001.00187.x

Edmond, T., Rubin, A., & Wambach, K. (1999). The effectiveness of EMDR with adult female survivors of childhood sexual abuse. *Social Work Research, 23,* 103–116.

Edmond, T., Sloan, L., & McCarty, D. (2004). Sexual abuse survivors' perceptions of the effectiveness of EMDR and eclectic therapy: A mixed-methods study. *Research on Social Work Practice, 14,* 259–272. doi:10.1177/1049731504265830

Ehrenreich, B. (1996). *Nickel and dimed: On (not) getting by in America.* New York: Henry Holt.

Elliot, D., Mok, D., & Briere, J. (2004). Adult sexual assault: Prevalence, symptomatology, and sex differences in the general population. *Journal of Traumatic Stress, 17,* 203–211.

Elliott, D., Bjelajac, P., Fallot, R., Markoff, L., & Reed, B. (2005). Trauma informed or trauma-denied: Principles, competencies, and implementation of trauma-informed services for women. *Journal of Community Psychology, 33*(4), 461–475.

Elton, C. (2009, July 20). The melancholy of motherhood: Would it help or hurt to screen all mothers for postpartum depression? *Time, 174*(2), 55–56.

Ersche, K., Clark, L., London, M., Robbins, T., & Sahakian, B. (2006). Profile of executive and memory function associated with amphetamine and opiate dependence. *Neuropsychopharmacology, 31*(5), 1036–1047. doi:10.1038/sj.npp.1300889

Eubanks-Carter, C., Burckell, L., & Goldfried, M. (2005). Enhancing therapeutic effectiveness with lesbian, gay, and bisexual clients. *Clinical Psychology: Science and Practice, 12*(1), 1–18.

Evans-Campbell, T., Lindhorst, T., Huang, B., & Walters, K. (2006). Interpersonal violence in the lives of urban American Indian and Alaska Native women: Implications for health, mental health, and help-seeking. *American Journal of Public Health, 96,* 1416–1422. doi:10.2105/AJPH.2004.054213

Ewing, J. (1984). Detecting alcoholism: The CAGE Questionnaire. *Journal of the American Medical Association, 252,* 1905–1907.

Fava, G., Ruini, C., Rafanelli, C., Finos, L., Salmaso, L., Mangelli, L., et al. (2005). Well-being therapy of generalized anxiety disorder. *Psychotherapy and Psychosomatics, 74*(1), 26–30.

Fiorentine, R., & Hillhouse, M. (1999). Drug treatment effectiveness and client-counselor empathy. *Journal of Drug Issues, 29,* 59–74.

Fischer, J., & Corcoran, K. (1994). *Measures for clinical practice: A sourcebook* (Vol. 2). New York: Free Press.

Foa, E. B., Rothbaum, B. O., Riggs, D. S., & Murdock, T. B. (1991). Treatment of posttraumatic stress disorder in rape victims: A comparison between cognitive-behavioral procedures and counseling. *Journal of Consulting and Clinical Psychology, 59*(5), 715–723. doi:10.1037/0022–006X.59.5.715

Foa, E., & Jaycox, L. (1999). Cognitive-behavioral theory and treatment of post-traumatic stress disorder. In D. S. Spiegel (Ed.), *Efficacy and cost effectiveness of psychotherapy*. Washington, DC: American Psychological Association.

Foa, E., Cashman, L., Jaycox, L., & Perry, K. (1997). The validation of a self-report measure of post-traumatic stress disorder : The Posttraumatic Diagnostic Scale. *Psychological Assessment, 9*(4), 445–451. doi:10.1037/1040–3590.9.4.445

Foa, E., Dancu, C., Hembree, E., Jaycox, L., Meadows, E., & Street, G. (1999). A comparison of exposure therapy, stress inoculation training, and their combination for reducing posttraumatic stress disorder in female assault victims. *Journal of Consulting and Clinical Psychology, 67*, 194–200.

Foa, E., Riggs, D., Dancu, C., & Rothbaum, B. (2005). Reliability and validity of a brief instrument for assessing post-traumatic stress disorder. *Journal of Traumatic Stress, 6*(4), 459–473.

Freeman, E., Sammel, M., Lin, H., & Nelson, D. (2006). Associations of hormones and menopausal status with depressed mood in women with no history of depression. *Archives of General Psychiatry, 63*(4), 375–382. doi:10.1001/archpsyc.63.4.375

Friedman, S. (Ed.). (1997). *Cultural issues in the treatment of anxiety*. New York: Guilford Press.

Friedman, S. (2001). Cultural issues in the assessment of anxiety disorders. In M. Antony, S. Orsillo, & L. Roemer (Eds.), *Practitioner's guide to empirically based measures of anxiety* (pp. 37–41). New York: Kluwer Academic/Plenum Pubishers.

Gallagher, S., Allen, J., Hitt, S., Schnyer, R., & Manber, R. (2001). Six-month depression relapse rates among women treated with acupuncture. *Complementary Therapies in Medicine, 9*, 216–218. doi:10.1054/ctim.2001.0470

Gambrill, E. (1999). Evident-based practice: An alternative to authority-based practice. *Families in Society, 80*, 341–350.

Gambrill, E. (2001). Social work: An authority-based profession. *Research on Social Work Practice, 11*(2), 166–175. doi:10.1177/104973150101100203

Gatz, M., & Fiske, A. (2003). Aging women and depression. *Professional Psychology: Research and Practice, 34*, 3–9.

Gatz, M., Brown, V., Hennigan, K., Rechberger, E., O'Keefe, M., Rose, T., et al. (2007). Effectiveness of an integrated trauma-informed approach to treating women with co-occurring disorders and histories of trauma. *Journal of Community Psychology, 35*, 863–878. doi:10.1002/jcop.20186

Gellis, Z., & Kenaley, B. (2008). Problem-solving therapy for depression in adults: A systematic review. *Research on Social Work Practice, 18*(2), 117–131.

Giesen-Bloo, J., Van Dyck, R., Spinhoven, P., Van Tilburg, W., Dirksen, C., Van Asselt, T., et al. (2006). Outpatient psychotherapy for borderline personality disorder: Randomized trial of schema-focused therapy vs. transference-focused psychotherapy. *Archives of General Psychiatry, 63*, 649–658. doi:10.1001/archpsyc.64.5.610

Gilbertson, M., Shenton, M., Ciszewski, A., Kasai, K., Lasko, N., Orr, S., et al. (2002). Smaller hippocampal volume predicts pathologic vulnerability to psychological trauma. *Nature and Neuroscience, 5*, 1242–1247.

Gilbody, S., Bower, P., Fletcher, J., Richards, D., & Sutton, A. (2006). Collaborative care for depression: A cumulative meta-analysis and review of longer-term outcomes. *Archives of Internal Medicine, 166*, 2314–2321. doi:10.1001/archinte.166.21.2314

Gilgun, J. (2005). The four cornerstones of evidence-based practice in social work. *Research on Social Work Practice*, 15(1), 52–61. doi:10.1177/10497315042 69581.

Golding, J. (1999). Intimate partner violence as a risk factor for mental disorders: A meta-analysis. *Journal of Family Violence*, 14, 99–132.

Goldsmith, W., & Blakely, E. (1992). *Separate societies: Poverty and inequality in American cities*. Philadelphia: Temple University Press.

Goodman, L., Smyth, K., Borges, A., & Singer, R. (2009). When crises collide: How intimate partner violence and poverty intersect to shape women's mental health and coping? *Trauma, Violence, & Abuse*, 10(4), 306–329. doi:10.1177/15248 38009339754

Goodwin, R., Fergusson, D., & Horwood, L. (2004). Early anxious/withdrawn behaviors predict later internalizing disorders. *Journal of Child Psychology and Psychiatry*, 45(4), 874–883.

Grant, B., Chou, P., Goldstein, R., Huang, B., Stinson, F., Saha, T., et al. (2008). Prevalence, correlates, disability, and comorbidity of DSM-IV Borderline Personality Disorder: Results from the Wave 2 National Epidemiologic Survey on Alcohol and Related Conditions. *Journal of Clinical Psychiatry*, 69(4), 533–545. doi:10.4088/JCP.v69n0511

Grant, B., Hasin, D., Stinson, F., Dawson, D., Ruan, J., Goldstein, R., et al. (2005). Prevalence, correlates, comorbidity, and comparative disability of DSM-IV generalized anxiety disorder in the USA: Results from the National Epidemiologic Survey on Alcohol and Related Conditions. *Psychological Medicine*, 35, 1747–1759.

Green, C., Polen, M., Dickinson, D., Lynch, F., & Bennett, M. (2002). Gender differences in predictors of initiation, retention, and completion in an HMO-based substance abuse treatment program. *Journal of Substance Abuse Treatment*, 23, 285–295.

Green, C., Polen, M., Lynch, F., Dickinson, D., & Bennett, M. (2004). Gender differences in outcomes in an HMO-based substance abuse treatment program. *Journal of Addictive Disorders*, 23, 47–70.

Greenberg, P., Kessler, R., Birnbaum, H., Leong, S., Lowe, S., Berglund, P., et al. (2003). The economic burden of depression in the United States: How did it change between 1990 and 2000? *Journal of Clinical Psychiatry*, 64, 1465–1475.

Greenfield, S., Brooks, A., Gordon, S., Green, C., Kropp, F., McHugh, K., et al. (2007). Substance abuse treatment entry, retention, and outcome in women: A review of the literature. *Drug and Alcohol Dependence*, 86, 1–21. doi:10.1016/j. drugalcdep.2006.05.012

Greenfield, S., Hufford, M., Vagge, L., Muenz, L., Costello, M., & Weiss, R. (2000). The relationship of self-efficacy expectancies to relapse among alcohol dependent men and women: A prospective study. *Journal of Studies of Alcoholism*, 61, 345–351.

Greenfield, S., Kolodziej, M., Sugarman, D., Muenz, L., Vagge, L., He, D., et al. (2002). History of abuse and drinking outcomes following inpatient alcohol treatment: A prospective study. *Drug and Alcohol Dependence*, 67, 227–234.

Greenfield, S., Sugarman, D., Muenz, L., Patterson, M., He, D., & Weiss, R. (2003). The relationship between educational attainment and relapse among alcohol-dependent men and women: A prospective study. *Alcohol: Clinical and Experimental Research*, 27, 1278–1285.

Greenfield, S., Weiss, R., Muenz, L., Vagge, L., Kelly, J., Bello, L., et al. (1998). The effect of depression on return to drinking: A prospective study. *Archives of General Psychiatry, 55*, 259–265. doi:10.1001/archpsyc.55.3.259

Guarnaccia, P., & Rogler, L. (1999). Research on culture bound syndromes. *American Journal of Psychiatry, 156*, 1322–1327.

Gunderson, J., & Ridolfi, M. (2001). Borderline personality disorder: Suicidality and self-mutilation. *Annals of the New York Academy of Sciences, 932*, 61–77.

Gunderson, J., Kolb, J., & Austin, V. (1981). The diagnostic interview for borderline patients. *American Journal of Psychiatry, 138*, 896–903.

Gutek, B., & Done, R. (2001). Sexual harassment. In R. K. Unger (Ed.), *Handbook of the psychology of women and gender* (pp. 367–387). New York: John Wiley.

Gutierrez, L., & Lewis, E. (Eds.). (1999). *Empowering women of color.* New York: Columbia University Press.

Gwartney, J., & McCaleb, T. (1985). Have anti-poverty programs increased poverty? *Cato Journal, 5*(5), 1–16.

Gwynn, H. G., McQuistion, H., McVeigh, K., Garg, R., Frieden, T., & Thorpe, L. (2008). Prevalence, diagnosis, and treatment of depression and generalized anxiety disorder in a diverse urban community, *Psychiatric Services, 59*, 641–647. doi:10.1176/appi.ps.59.6.641

Hakistan, A., & McLean, P. (1989). Brief Screen for Depression. *Psychological Assessment, 1*, 139–141.

Hale, W., Engels, R., & Meeus, W. (2006). Adolescent's perceptions of parenting behaviors and its relationship to adolescent generalized anxiety disorder. *Journal of Adolescence, 29*(3), 407–417.

Haller, D., & Miles, D. (2004). Psychopathology is associated with completion of residential treatment in drug dependent women. *Journal of Addictive Disorders, 23*(1), 17–28.

Halligan, S., Michael, T., Clark, D., & Ehlers, A. (2003). Post-traumatic stress disorder following assault: Role of cognitive processing, trauma memory, and appraisals. *Journal of Consulting and Clinical Psychology, 71*(3), 419–431.

Hamilton, M. (1960). A rating scale for depression. *Journal of Neurology, Neurosurgery and Psychiatry, 23*, 56–62.

Han, B., Gfroerer, J., Colliver, J., & Penne, M. (2009). Substance use disorder among older adults in the United States in 2020. *Addiction, 104*, 88–96. doi:10.1111/j.1360-0443.2008.02411.x

Hanmer, J., & Statham, D. (1989). *Women and social work: Towards a woman-centered practice.* Chicago: Lyceum Books.

Hazen, R., Vasey, M., & Schmidt, N. (2009). Attentional retraining: A randomized clinical trial for pathological worry. *Journal of Psychiatric Research, 43*(6), 627–633.

Heim, C., Newport, D., Heit, S., Graham, Y., Wilcox, M., Bonsall, R., Miller, A., & Nemeroff, C. (2000). Pituitary-adrenal and autonomic responses to stress in adult women with sexual and physical abuse in childhood. *JAMA: The Journal of the American Medical Association, 284*, 592–597.

Henskens, R., Mulder, C., & Garretsen, H. (2005). Gender differences in problems and needs among chronic, high risk crack abusers: Results of a randomized controlled trial. *Journal of Substance Abuse, 10*(2-3), 128-140.

Herman, J. (1992). *Trauma and recovery.* New York: Basic Books.

Heron, J., O'Connor, T., Evans, J., Golding, J., & Glover, V. (2004). The course of anxiety and depression through pregnancy and the postpartum in a community sample. *Journal of Affective Disorders, 80*(1), 65–73.

Herrman, N., Mittman, N., Silver I., Shulman, K., Busto, U., Shear, N., et al. (1996). Validation study of the geriatric depression scale short form. *International Journal of Geriatric Psychiatry, 11*, 457–460.

Hettema, J., Neale, M., & Kendler, K. (2001). A review of meta-analyses of the genetic epidemiology of anxiety disorders. *American Journal of Psychiatry, 158*, 1568–1578.

Hien, D., Cohen, L., Litt, L., Miele, G., & Capstick, C. (2004). Promising empirically supported treatments for women with co-morbid PTSD and substance use disorders. *American Journal of Psychiatry, 161*, 1426–1432. doi:10.1176/appi.ajp.161.8.1426

Hinshaw, S. (2003). Impulsivity, emotion regulation, and developmental psychopathology: Specificity versus generality of linkages. *Annals of the New York Academy of Science, 1008*, 149–159. doi:10.1196/annals.1301.016

Hodnett, D. (2007). Psychosocial and psychological interventions for treating postpartum depression. *Cochrane Database of Systematic Reviews, 4*, Article No. CD006116. doi:10.1002/14651858.CD006116.pub2

Holbrook, T., Hoyt, D., Stein, M., & Sieber, W. (2002). Gender differences in long-term post-traumatic stress disorder outcomes after major trauma: Women are at higher risk of adverse outcomes than men. *The Journal of Trauma: Injury, Infection, and Critical Care, 53*(5), 882–888.

Holdcraft, L. C., & Comtois, K. A. (2002). Description of and preliminary data from a women's dual diagnosis community mental health program. *Canadian Journal of Community Mental Health, 21*, 91–109.

Hollon, S. (2000, October). *Psychotherapy for women with depression.* Paper presented at the American Psychological Association Summit 2000 on Women and Depression, Queensland, MD.

Holm, A., & Severinsson, E. (2008). The emotional pain and distress of borderline personality disorder: A review of the literature. *International Journal of Mental Health Nursing, 17*(1), 27–35.

Holroyd, M., & Clayton, A. (2002). Measuring depression in the elderly: Which scale is best? *Medscape General Medicine, 2*(4), 1–8.

Holwerda, T., Schoevers, R., Dekker, R., Jack, D., Dorly, J., Jonker, C., et al. (2007). The relationship between generalized anxiety disorder, depression, and mortality in old age. *International Journal of Geriatric Psychiatry, 22*(3), 241–249.

Hser, Y., Evans, E., & Huang, Y. (2005). Treatment outcomes among women methamphetamine abusers in California. *Journal of Substance Abuse Treatment, 28*(1), 77–85. doi:10.106/j.jsat.2004.10.009

Hughes, P., Coletti, S., Neri, R., Urmann, C., Stahl, S., Sicilian, D., et al. (1995). Retaining cocaine-abusing women in a therapeutic community: The effect of a child live-in program. *American Journal of Public Health, 85*, 1149–1152. doi:10.2105/AJPH.85.8_Pt_1.1149

Hunot, V., Churchill, R., Teixeira, V., & Silva de Lima, M. (2009). Psychological therapies for generalized anxiety disorder. *Cochrane Database of Systematic Reviews, 3*, 1–88.

Hyler, S. (1994). *PDQ-4 and PDQ-4+: Instructions for use.* Unpublished manuscript, Columbia University.

Hyler, S., Lyons, M., Rieder, R., Young, L., Williams, J., & Spitzer, R. (1990). The factor structure of self-report DSM-III Axis II symptoms and their relationship to clinicians' ratings. *American Journal of Psychiatry, 147*, 751–757.

Hyman, S. (2006). Foreword: The importance of studying women and depression. In C. Mazure and G. Keita (Eds.), *Understanding depression in women: Applying empirical research to practice and policy* (pp. 3–7). Washington, DC: American Psychological Association.

Hypericum Depression Trial Study Group. (2002). Effect of Hypericum perforatum (St. John's wort) in major depression disorder: A randomized controlled trial. *JAMA: The Journal of the American Medical Association, 287*, 1807–1814.

Irle, E., Lange, C., & Sachsse, U. (2005). Reduced size and abnormal asymmetry of parietal cortex in women with borderline personality disorder. *Biological Psychiatry, 57*(2), 173–182. doi:10.1016/j.biopsych.2004.10.004

Jaberghaderi, N., Greenwald, R., Rubin, A., Dolatabadim S., & Zand, S. O. (2004). A comparison of CBT and EMDR for sexually abused Iranian girls. *Clinical Psychology and Psychotherapy, 11*, 358–368.

Jacobson, J., & Jacobson, A. (Eds.). (2001). *Psychiatric Secrets* (2nd ed.). Philadelphia: Hawley & Belfus.

Jayakody, R., Danziger, S., & Pollack, H. (2000). Welfare reform, substance abuse, and mental health. *Journal of Health Politics, Policy and Law, 25*(4), 623–651. doi:10.1215/03616878-25-4-623

Jencks, C. (1996). Can we replace welfare with work? In M. R. Darby (Ed.), *Reducing poverty in America* (pp. 69–81). Thousand Oaks, CA: Sage.

Jiang, Y. (2004). *Demographic factors, life stress and depression among minority women.* Paper presented at the annual meeting of the American Sociological Association at the Hilton San Francisco & Renaissance Parc 55 Hotel in San Francisco, CA on August 8, 2004. Retrieved from http://www.allacademic.com/meta/p109569_index.html

Johnson, J., & Bornstein, R. (1992). Utility of the Personality Diagnostic Questionnaire-Revised in a nonclinical sample. *Journal of Personality Disorders, 6*, 450–457.

Johnson, P., Hurley, R., Benkelfat, C., Herpertz, S., & Taber, K. (2003). Understanding emotion regulation in borderline personality disorder: Contributions of neuroimaging. *Journal of Neuropsychiatry and Clinical Neuroscience, 15*, 397–402.

Jordan, C., & Franklin, C. (2003). *Clinical assessment for social workers: Quantitative and qualitative methods* (2nd ed.). Chicago: Lyceum Books.

Kail, B., & Elberth, M. (2002). Moving the Latina substance abuser toward treatment: The role of gender and culture. *Journal of Ethnicity and Substance Abuse, 1*, 3–16.

Kaiser, M., & Hays, B. (2005). Health-risk behaviors in a sample of first-time pregnant adolescents. *Public Health Nursing, 22*(6), 483–493. doi:10.1111/j.0737-1209.2005.220611.x

Kaskutas, L., Zhang, L., French, M., & Witbrodt, J. (2005). Women's programs versus mixed-gender day treatment: Results from a randomized study. *Addiction, 100*, 60–69. doi:10.1111/j.1360-0443.2005.00914.x

Kehle, S. (2008). The effectiveness of cognitive behavioral therapy for generalized anxiety disorder in a frontline service setting. *Cognitive Behavior Therapy, 37*(3), 192–198.

Keita, G. (2007). Psychosocial and cultural contributions to depression in women: Considerations for women midlife and beyond. *Journal of Managed Care Pharmacy, 13*(9 S-a), s12–s13.

Kelly, P., Blacksin, B., & Mason, E. (2001). Factors affecting substance abuse treatment completion for women. *Issues in Mental Health Nursing, 22*(287–304). doi:10 .1080/01612840152053110

Kendall, P., Hudson, J., Gosch, E., Flannery-Schroeder, E., & Suveg, C. (2008). Cognitive-behavioral therapy for anxiety disordered youth: A randomized clinical trial evaluating child and family modalities. *Journal of Consulting and Clinical Psychology, 76*(2), 282–297.

Kendler, K., & Prescott, C. (1999). A population based twin study of lifetime major depression in men and women. *Archives of General Psychiatry, 56*, 39–44.

Kendler, K., Gardner, C., Gatz, M., & Pedersen, N. (2007). The sources of co-morbidity between major depression and generalized anxiety disorder in a Swedish national twin sample. *Psychological Medicine, 37*, 453–462.

Kendler, K., Gardner, C., Neale, M., & Prescott, C. (2001). Genetic risk factors for major depression in men and women: Similar or different heritabilities and same or partly distinct genes? *Psychological Medicine, 31*, 605–616.

Kendler, K., Thornton, L., & Prescott, C. (2001). Gender differences in the rates of exposure to stressful life events and sensitivity to their depressogenic effects. *American Journal of Psychiatry, 158*, 587–593.

Kessler, R., Barker, P., Colpe, L., Epstein, J., Gfroerer, J., Hiripi, E., et al. (2003). Screening for serious mental illness in the general population. *Archives of General Psychiatry, 60*(2), 184–189.

Kessler, R., Berglund, P., Demler, O., Jin, R., Koretz, D., Merikangas, K., & Rush, A. (2003). The epidemiology of major depressive disorder: results from the National Comorbidity Survey Replication (NCS-R). *JAMA: The Journal of the American Medical Association, 289*(3), 3095–3105.

Kessler, R., McGonagle, K., Swartz, M., Blazer, D., & Nelson, C. (1993). Sex and depression in the National Comorbidity Survey 1: Lifetime prevalence, chronicity, and recurrence. *Journal of Affective Disorders, 29*, 85–96.

Kilpatrick, D., Edmunds, C., & Seymour, A. (1992). *Rape in America: A report to the nation.* Charleston, SC: Crime Victims Research and Treatment Center.

Kilpatrick, D., Resnick, H., & Saunders, B. (1998). Rape, other violence against women, and post-traumatic stress disorder. In B. Dohrenwend, (Ed.), *Adversity, stress, and psychopathology* (pp. 161–176). New York: Oxford University Press.

Kimerling, R., Ouimette, P., & Wolfe, J. (Eds.). (2002). *Gender and PTSD.* New York: Guilford Press.

King-Casas, B., Sharp, C., Lomax-Bream, L., Lohrenz, T., Fonagy, P., & Montague, P. (2008). The rupture and repair of cooperation in borderline personality disorder. *Science, 321*, 806–809. doi:10.1126/science.1156902

King, A., & Canada, S. (2004). Client-related predictors of early treatment drop-out in a substance abuse clinic exclusively employing individual therapy. *Journal of Substance Abuse Treatment, 26*, 189–195.

Klein, J., Jacobs, R., & Reinbeck, M. (2007). Cognitive-behavioral therapy for adolescent depression: A meta-analytic investigation of changes in effect-size estimates. *Journal of the American Academy of Child and Adolescent Psychiatry, 46*(11), 1403–1413.

Koons, C., Robins, C., Tweed, J., Lynch, T., Gonzales, A., Morse, J., et al. (2001). Efficacy of dialectical behavior therapy in women veterans with borderline personality disorder. *Behavior Therapy, 32*, 371–390. doi:10.1016/S0005-894(01)80009-5

Kornør, H., Winje, D., Ekeberg, O., Weisæth, L., Kirkehei, I., Johansen, K., et al. (2008). Early trauma-focused cognitive-behavioural therapy to prevent chronic post-traumatic stress disorder and related symptoms: A systematic review and meta-analysis. *BMC Psychiatry, 8*(81), http://www.biomedcentral.com/1471–244X/8/81

Kornstein, S. (2002). Chronic depression in women. *Journal of Clinical Psychiatry, 63,* 602–609.

Kornstein, S., Schatzberg, A., Thase, M., Yonkers, K., McCullough, K., Keitner, G., et al. (2002). Gender differences in chronic major and double depression. *Journal of Affective Disorders, 60,* 1–11.

Koss, M., Bailey, J., Yuan, N., Herrera, V., & Lichter, E. (2003). Depression and PTSD in survivors of male violence: Research and training initiatives to facilitate recovery. *Psychology of Women Quarterly, 27,* 130–142.

Kovacs, M. (2003). *Children's depression inventory: Technical manual.* Toronto: Multi-Health Systems.

Kovacs, M., Obrosky, D., & Sherrill, J. (2003). Developmental changes in the phenomenology of depression in girls compared to boys from childhood onward. *Journal of Affective Disorders, 74,* 33–48.

Kroenke, K., Spitzer, J., Williams, J., Monahan, P., & Lowe, B. (2007). Anxiety disorders in primary care: Prevalence, impairment, co-morbidity, and detection. *Annals of Internal Medicine, 146,* 317–325.

Kronenberger, W., & Meyer, R. (2001). *The child clinician's handbook.* Needham Heights, MA: Allyn & Bacon.

Kubany, E., Hill, E., & Owens, J. (2003). Cognitive behavioral therapy for battered women with PTSD: Preliminary findings. *Journal of Traumatic Stress, 16*(1), 81–91.

Kubany, E., Hill, E., Owens, J., Iannce-Spencer, C., McCaig, M., Tremayne, K., & Williams, P. (2004). Cognitive behavioral therapy for battered women with PTSD. *Journal of Consulting and Clinical Psychology, 72*(1), 3–18. doi:10.1037/0022–006X.72.1.3

Kubiak, S. (2005). Trauma and cumulative adversity in women of a disadvantaged social location. *American Journal of Orthopsychiatry, 75*(4), 451–465.

Lara, M., Navarro, C., & Rubi, N. (2003). Two levels of intervention in low income women with depressive symptoms: Compliance and programme assessment. *International Journal of Social Psychiatry, 49*(1), 43–57.

Le, H., Munoz, R., Ippen, C., & Stoddard, J. (2003). Treatment is not enough: We must prevent major depression in women. *Prevention & Treatment, 6*(2), 1–43. doi:10.1037/1522-3736.6.0010a

Lens, V. (2002). TANF: What went wrong and what to do next. *Social Work, 47*(3), 279–290.

Lenzenweger, M., Clarkin, J., Fertuck, E., & Kernberg, O. (2004). Executive neurocognitive functioning and neurobehavioral systems indicators in borderline personality disorder: A preliminary study. *Journal of Personality Disorders, 18,* 421–438. doi:10.1521/pedi.18.5.421.51323

Lesher, E., & Berryhill, J. (1994). A validation study of the Geriatric Depression Scale-Short Form. *Journal of Clinical Psychology, 50,* 256–260.

Lewis, O. (1998). The culture of poverty. *Society, 35*(2), 7–9.

Lex, B. (1991). Some gender differences in alcohol and poly-substance abusers. *Health Psychology, 10,* 121–132. doi:10.1037/0278–6133.10.2.121

Lieb, R., Becker, E., & Altamura, C. (2005). The epidemiology of generalized anxiety disorder in Europe. *European Neuropsychopharmacology, 15*(4), 445–452.

Linehan, M. M. (1993). *Cognitive-behavioral treatment of borderline personality disorder*. New York: Guilford Press.

Linehan, M. M. (1995). *Understanding borderline personality disorder: The dialectical approach program manual*. New York: Guilford Press.

Linehan, M. M., Comtois, K., Murray, A., Brown, M., Gallop, R., Heard, H., et al. (2006). Two-year randomized controlled trial and follow-up of dialectical behavior therapy vs therapy by experts for suicidal behaviors and borderline personality disorder. *Archives of General Psychiatry, 63*(7), 757–766. doi:10.1001/archpsyc.63.7.757

Livesley, W., Jang, K., & Vernon, P. (1998). Phenotypic and genetic structure of traits delineating personality disorder. *Archives of General Psychiatry, 55,* 941–948.

Lonstein, J. (2007). Regulation of anxiety during the postpartum period. *Frontiers in Microbiology, 28*(2–3), 115–141.

Loseke, D. (1992).*The battered woman and shelters: The social construction of wife abuse*. Albany: State University of New York Press.

Lown, E. A., Schmidt, L., & Wiley, J. (2006). Interpersonal violence among women seeking welfare: Unraveling lives. *American Journal of Public Health, 96*(8), 1409–1415. doi:10.2105/AJPH.2004.057786

Lucas, S., & Weatherington, C. (2005). Sex- and gender-related differences in the neurobiology of drug abuse. *Clinical Neuroscience Research, 5*(2–4), 75–87.

Luo, W., Liu, H., & Mei, S. (2007). Clinical study on "Jin's three-needling" in treatment of generalized anxiety disorder. *Chinese Journal of Integrated Traditional and Western Medicine, 27*(3), 201–203.

Lynch, T., Rosenthal, M., Kosson, D., Cheavens, J., Lejuez, C., & Blair, R. (2006). Heightened sensitivity to facial expressions of emotion in borderline personality disorder. *Emotion, 6,* 647–655. doi:10.1037/1528–3542.6.4.647

Lyons-Ruth, K., Holmes, B., Sasvari-Szekely, M., Ronai, Z., Nemoda, Z., & Pauls, D. (2007). Serotonin transporter polymorphism and borderline/antisocial traits among low-income young adults. *Psychiatric Genetics, 17*(6), 339–343. doi:10.1097/YPG.013e328ac237e

Maciejewski, P., Prigerson, H., & Mazure, C. (2001). Sex differences in event-related risk for major depression. *Psychology of Medicine, 31,* 593–604. doi:10.1017/S0033291701003877

Manber, R., Allen, J., & Morris, M. (2002). Alternative treatments for depression: Empirical support and relevance to women. *Journal of Clinical Psychiatry, 63,* 628–640.

Markoff, L., Reed, B., Fallot, R., Elliott, D., & Bjelajac, P. (2005). Implementing trauma-informed alcohol and other drug and mental health services for women: Lessons learned in a multi-site demonstration project. *American Journal of Orthopsychiatry, 75*(4), 525–539. doi:10.1037/0002–9432.75.4.525

Martin, E., Taft, C., & Resick, P. (2006). A review of marital rape. *Aggression and Violent Behavior, 12*(3), 329–347.

Masi, G., Millepiedi, S., Mucci, M., Poli, P., Bertini, N., & Milantoni, L. (2004). Generalized anxiety disorder in referred children and adolescents. *Journal of the American Academy of Child and Adolescent Psychiatry, 43*(6), 752–760.

Maskovsky, J. (2001). Afterword: Beyond the privatist consensus. In J. Goode & J. Maskovsky (Eds.), *The new poverty studies*. New York: New York University Press.

Massachusetts Department of Health. (1996). *Report of the Massachusetts task force on the restraint and seclusion of persons who have been physically or sexually abused.* Boston: Author.

Mazure, C., Bruce, M., Maciejewski, P., & Jacobs, S. (2000). Adverse life events and cognitive-personality characteristics in the prediction of major depression and antidepressant response. *American Journal of Psychiatry, 157,* 896–903.

Mazure, C., & Keita, G. (2006). *Understanding depression among women: Applying empirical research to practice and policy.* Washington, DC: American Psychological Association

McCollough, J. (2000). *Treatment of chronic depression: Cognitive Behavioral Analyses system of psychotherapy (CBASP).* New York: Guilford Press.

McCollough, J. (2006). *Treating chronic depression with disciplined personal involvement: CBASP.* New York: Springer-Verlag.

McDermott, B., Quanbeck, C., & Frye, M. (2007). Co-morbid substance use disorder in women with bipolar disorder associated with criminal arrest. *Bipolar Disorders, 9*(5), 536–540. doi:10.1111/j.1399–5618.2007.00346.x

Mcnelis-Domingos, A. (2004). *Cognitive behavioral skills training for persons with co-occurring posttraumatic stress disorder and substance abuse.* Thesis submitted for the degree of Master of Social Work, Southern Connecticut State University, New Haven.

Meara, E. (2006). Welfare reform, employment, and drug and alcohol use among low-income women. *Harvard Review of Psychiatry, 14*(4), 223–232. doi:10.1080/10673220600883150

Mertens, J., & Weisner, C. (2000). Predictors of substance abuse treatment retention among women and men in an HMO. *Alcoholism: Clinical and Experimental Research, 24,* 1525–1533.

Meyer, C. (1992). Social work assessment: Is there an empirical base? *Research on Social Work Practice, 2*(3), 297–305.

Meyer, T., Miller, R., Metzger, R., & Borkovec, T. (1990). Development and validation of the Penn State Worry Questionnaire. *Behavioral Research & Therapy, 28,* 487–495.

Mezzich, J., Kleinman, A., Fabrega, H., & Parron, D. (1996). *Culture and psychiatric diagnosis: A DSM-IV perspective.* Washington, DC: American Psychiatric Press.

Miller, M., Mastuera, M., Chao, M., & Sadowski, K. (2004). *Pathways out of poverty: Early lessons of the Family Independence Initiative.* Oakland, CA: Family Independence Initiative.

Miller, W., & Rollnick, S. (2002). *Motivational interviewing: Preparing people for change* (2nd ed.). New York: Guilford Press.

Mineka, S., & Zinbarg, R. (2006). A contemporary learning theory perspective on the etiology of anxiety disorders: It's not what you thought it was. *American Psychologist, 61*(1), 10–26.

Minnen, A., & Kampman, M. (2001). The interaction between anxiety and sexual functioning: A controlled study of sexual functioning in women with anxiety disorders. *Sexual and Relationship Therapy, 15*(1), 47–57.

Miranda, J. (2006). Improving services and outreach for women with depression. In C. Mazure and G. Keita (Eds.), *Understanding depression in women: Applying empirical research to practice and policy* (pp.113–135). Washington, DC: American Psychological Association.

Miranda, J., Bernal, G., Lau, A., Kohn, L., Huang. W., & LaFromhouse, T. (2005). State of the science on psychosocial interventions for ethnic minorities. *Annual Review of Clinical Psychology, 1,* 113–142. doi:10.1146/annurev.clinpsy.1 .102803.143822

Moffitt, T., Caspi, A., Harrington, H., Milne, B., Melchior, M., Goldberg, D., et al. (2007). Generalized anxiety disorder and depression: Childhood risk factors in a birth cohort followed to age 32. *Psychological Medicine, 37,* 441–452. doi:10.1017/S0033291706009640

Mohlman, J. (1999). What kind of attention is necessary for fear reduction? An empirical test of the emotional processing model. *Dissertation Abstracts International, 59* (7-B), 3704. (UMI No. 95002–342)

Mojtabai, R. (2005). Use of specialty substance abuse and mental health services in adults with substance use disorders. *Drug and Alcohol Dependence, 78,* 345–354.

Mollica, R., & Caspi-Yavin, Y. (1994). Measuring torture and torture-related symptoms. *Psychological Assessment: Journal of Consulting and Clinical Psychology, 3,* 581–587.

Montgomery, S., & Asberg, M. (1979). A new depression scale designed to be sensitive to change. *British Journal of Psychiatry, 134,* 382–389. doi:10.1192/bjp .134.4.382

Montoya, I., Bell, D., Atkinson, J., Nagy, C., & Whitsell, N. (2002). Mental health, drug abuse, and the transition from welfare to work. *The Journal of Behavioral Health Services & Research, 29* (2), 144–156.

Moore, K. A., & Vandivere, S. (2000). *Stressful family lives: Child and parent well-being.* Washington, DC: The Urban Institute.

Morgenstern, J., Blanchard, K., McCrady, B., McVeigh, K., Morgan, T., & Pandina, R. (2006). Effectiveness of intensive case management for substance-dependent women receiving Temporary Assistance for Needy Families. *American Journal of Public Health, 96*(11), 2016–2023. doi:10.2105/AJPH.2005.076380

Morgenstern, J., Neighbors, C., Kuerbis, A., Riordan, A., Blanchard, K., McVeigh, K., et al. (2009). Improving 24-month abstinence and employment outcomes for substance-dependent women receiving Temporary Assistance for Needy Families with intensive case management. *American Journal of Public Health, 99*(2), 328–333. doi:10.2105/AJPH.2007.133553

Munk-Jorgensen, P., Allgulander, C., Dahl, A., Foldager, L., Holm, M., Rasmussen, I., et al. (2006). Prevalence of generalized anxiety disorder in general practice in Denmark, Finland, Norway, and Sweden. *Psychiatric Services, 57,* 1738–1744. doi:10.1176/appi.ps.57.12.1738

Munoz, R., Le, H., Ippen, C., Diaz, M., Urizar, G., Soto, J., et al. (2007). Prevention of postpartum depression in low-income women: Development of the Mamas y Bebe/Mothers and Babies Course. *Cognitive and Behavioral Practice, 14*(1), 70–83. doi:10.1016/j.cbpra.2006.04.021

Murray J., Ehlers A., & Mayou R. A. (2002). Dissociation and posttraumatic stress disorder: Two prospective studies of motor vehicle accident survivors. *British Journal of Psychiatry, 180,* 363–368. doi:10.1192/bjp.180.4.363

Mynors-Wallis, L. (2005). *Problem solving treatment for anxiety and depression: A practical guide.* Oxford, UK: Oxford University Press.

Nabkasorn, C., Miyai, N., Sootmongkol, A., Junprasert, S., Yamamoto, H., Arita, M., et al. (2006). Effects of physical exercise on depression: Neuroendocrine stress hormones and physiological fitness in adolescent females with depressive symptoms. *The European Journal of Public Health, 16*(2), 179–184.

Najavits, L., (2002). *Seeking safety: A treatment manual for PTSD and substance abuse.* New York: Guilford Press.

Najavits, L., Gallop, R., & Weiss, R. (2006). Seeking Safety therapy for adolescent girls with PTSD and substance abuse: A randomized controlled trial. *Journal of Behavioral Health Services & Research, 33,* 453–463. doi:10.1007/s11414–006–9034–2

Najavits, L., Rosier, M., Nolan, A., & Freeman, M. (2007). A new gender-based model for women's recovery from substance abuse: Results of a pilot outcome study. *American Journal of Drug and Alcohol Abuse, 33,* 5–11.

Najavits, L., Weiss, R., Shaw, S., & Muenz, L. (1998). "Seeking Safety": Outcome of a new cognitive behavioral psychotherapy for women with post traumatic stress disorder and substance dependence. *Journal of Traumatic Stress, 11,* 437–456.

National Institute of Mental Health. (2004). *Setting priorities for basic brain & behavioral science at NIMH: Final report of the National Advisory Mental Health Council's Workgroup on Basic Sciences.* Washington, DC: United States Department of Health and Human Services.

Nelson-Zlupko, L., Dore, M., Kauffman, E., & Kaltenbach, K. (1996). Women in recovery: Their perceptions of treatment effectiveness. *Journal of Substance Abuse Treatment, 13,* 51–59.

Nemeroff, C., Bremner, D., Foa, E., Mayberg, H., North, C., & Stein, M. (2006). Posttraumatic stress disorder: A state-of-the-science review. *Journal of Psychiatric Research, 40,* 1–21. doi:10.1176/appi.ajp.159.1.3

Ness, R. (1978). The old hag phenomenon as sleep paralysis: A bio-cultural interpretation. *Culture, Medicine, and Psychiatry, 2*(1), 15–39. doi:10.1007/BF00052448

New, A., Triebwasser, J., & Charney, D. (2008). The case for shifting borderline personality disorder to Axis I. *Biological Psychiatry, 64,* 653–659. doi:10.1016/j.biopsych.2008.04.020

Newman, E., Weathers, F., Nader, K., Kaloupek, D., Pynoos, R., Blake, D., et al. (2004). *Clinician-administered PTSD scale for children and adolescents (CAPS-CA) interviewer's guide.* Los Angeles: Western Psychological Services.

Nixon, R., Resick, P., & Griffen, M. (2004). Panic following trauma: The etiology of acute posttraumatic arousal. *Journal of Anxiety Disorders, 18,* 193–210.

Nolen-Hoeksema, S. & Jackson, B. (2001). Mediators of the gender difference in rumination. *Psychology of Women Quarterly, 25*(1), 37–47. DOI: 10.1111/1471-6402.00005.

Nolen-Hoeksema, S. (2004). The response styles theory. In C. Papageorgiou & A. Wells (Eds.), *Depressive rumination: Nature, theory, and treatment* (pp. 107–124). New York: Wiley.

Nolen-Hoeksema, S. (2006). The etiology of gender differences in depression. In C. Mazure and G. Keita (Eds.), *Understanding depression in women: Applying empirical research to practice and policy* (pp.113–135). Washington, DC: American Psychological Association.

Novick, J., Stewart, J., Wisniewski, S., Cook, I., Manev, R., Nierenberg, A., et al. (2006). Clinical and demographic features of atypical depression in outpatients with major depressive disorder: Preliminary findings from STARD. *Journal of Clinical Psychiatry, 67*(6), 996–997.

O'Hara, M., & Swain, A. (1996). Rates and risk of postpartum depression: A meta-analysis. *International Review of Psychiatry, 8,* 37–54. doi:10.3109/09540269609037816

Oldham, J. (2005). Guideline watch: Practice guideline for the treatment of patients with borderline personality disorder. *Focus, 3*, 396–400.

Ouimette, P., Cronkite, R., Henson, B., Prins, A., Gima, K., & Moos, R. (2004). Posttraumatic stress disorder and health status among female and male medical patients. *Journal of Traumatic Stress, 17*, 1–9.

Ozer, E., Best, S., Lipsey, T., & Weiss, D. (2003). Predictors of posttraumatic stress disorder and symptoms in adults: A meta-analysis. *Psychological Bulletin, 129*(1), 52–73. doi:10.1037/0033–2909.129.1.52

Paris, J. (1997). Childhood trauma as an etiological factor in the personality disorders. *Journal of Personality Disorder, 11*, 34–49.

Paris, J. (2003). Personality disorders over time. Washington, DC: American Psychiatric Press.

Paris, J. (2005). Syntheses: Borderline personality disorder. *Canadian Medical Association Journal, 172*(2), 1579–1587. doi:10.1503/cmaj.045281

Paris, J., & Zweig-Frank, H. (2001). A 27-year follow-up of patients with borderline personality disorder. *Comprehensive Psychiatry, 42*, 482–487. doi:10.1053/comp2001.26271

Parker, G., Parker, I., Brotchie, H., & Stuart, S. (2006). Interpersonal psychotherapy for depression? The need to define its ecological niche. *Journal of Affective Disorders, 95*(1-3), 1–11.

Patel, V., Araya, R., Chatterjee, S., Chisholm, D., Cohen, A., DeSilva, et al. (2007). Treatment and prevention of mental disorders in low-income and middle-income countries. *The Lancet, 370*(9591), 991–1005.

Patrick, J., Links, P., Van Reekum, R., & Mitton, M. (1995). Using the PDQ-R BPD scale as a brief screening measure in the differential diagnosis of personality disorder. *Journal of Personality Disorders, 9*, 266–274.

Peele, R., & Kadekar, S. (2007). Dimensional models of personality disorders: Refining the research agenda for DSM-V [Book review]. *Psychiatric Services, 58*, 1016–1017. doi:10.1176/appi.ps.58.7.1016

Pelissier, B., & Jones, N. (2005). A review of gender differences among substance abusers. *Crime and Delinquency, 51*(3), 343–372. doi:10.1177/0011128704270218

Pennix, B. (2006). Women's aging and depression. In C. Keyes & S. Goodman (Eds.), *Women and depression: A handbook for the social, behavioral, and biomedical sciences.* New York: Cambridge University Press.

Peterson, J., & Lieberman, A. (Eds.). (2001). *Building on women's strengths: A social work agenda for the 21st century* (2nd ed.). Binghamton, NY: Haworth Press.

Pharm, B., Simoni-Wastila, L., & Yang, H. (2006). Psychoactive drug abuse in older adults. *The American Journal of Geriatric Pharmacotherapy, 4*(4), 380–394.

Phillips, N., Hammen, C., Brennan, P., Najman, J., & Bor, W. (2005). Early adversity and the prospective prediction of depressive and anxiety disorders in adolescents. *Journal of Abnormal Psychology, 33*(1), 13–24.

Phillipsen, A., Limberger, M., Lieb, K., Feige, B., Kleindienst, N., Ebner-Priemer, U., et al. (2008). Attention-deficit hyperactivity disorder as a potentially aggravating factor in borderline personality disorder. *British Journal of Psychiatry, 192*, 118–123.

Pirard, S., Estee, S., & Kang, S. (2005). Prevalence of physical and sexual abuse among substance abuse patients and impact on treatment outcomes. *Drug and Alcohol Dependence, 78*(1), 57–64. doi:10.1016/j.drugalcdep.2004.09.005

Pollack, H., & Reuter, P. (2006). Welfare receipt and substance abuse treatment among low-income mothers: The impact of welfare reform. *American Journal of Public Health, 96*(11), 2024–2031. doi:10.2105/AJPH.2004.061762

Posner, M., Rothbart, M., Vizueta, N., Levy, K., Evans, D., Thomas, K., et al. (2002). Attentional mechanisms of borderline personality disorder. *PNAS: Proceedings of the National Academy of Sciences of the United States of America, 99*, 16366–16370. doi:10.1073/pnas.252644699

Prescott, L. (2001). *Consumer/survivor/recovering women: A guide for partnerships in collaboration.* Delmar, NY: Policy Research Associates.

Pruitt, L. (2007). Missing the mark: Welfare reform and rural poverty. *Journal of Race, Gender, and Justice, 10*(3), 443–477.

Pynoos, R. S., Frederick, C., Nader, K., Arroyo, W., Steinberg, A., Eth, S., et al. (1987). Life threat and posttraumatic stress in school-age children. *Archives of General Psychiatry, 44*, 1057–1063.

Quigley, W. (2003). *Ending poverty as we know it.* Philadelphia: Temple University Press.

Quinn, P. (2005). Treating adolescent girls and women with ADHD: Gender-specific issues. *Journal of Clinical Psychology, 61*(5), 579–587. doi:10.1002/jclp.20121

Radloff, L. (1977). The CES-D scale: A self-report depression scale for research in the general population. *Applied Psychological Measurement, 1*, 385–401. doi:10.1177/014662167700100306

Raphael, J. (2000). *Saving Bernice: Battered women, welfare, and poverty.* Lebanon, NH: University of New England Press.

Resick, P., Neshith, T., Weaver, M., Astin, M., & Fuer, C. (2002). A comparison of cognitive-processing therapy with prolonged exposure and a waiting condition for the treatment of chronic posttraumatic stress disorder in female rape victims. *Journal of Consulting and Clinical Psychology, 70*, 867–879. doi:10.1037/0022–006X.70.4.867

Revicki, D., Brandenburg, N., Matza, L., Hornbrook, M., & Feeny, D. (2008). Health-related quality of life and utilities in primary-care patients with generalized anxiety disorder. *Quality of Life Research: An International Journal of Quality of Life Aspects of Treatment, Care & Rehabilitation, 17*(10), 1285–1294. doi:10.1007/s11136–008-9406–6

Reynolds, C., Frank, E., Perel, J., Imber, S., Cornes, C., Miller, M., et al. (1999). Nortriptyline and interpersonal psychotherapy as maintenance therapies for recurrent major depression: a randomized controlled trial in patients older than 59 years. *JAMA: The Journal of the American Medical Association, 281*(1), 39–45. doi:10.1001/jama.281.1.39

Reynolds, W. (2005). *Reynolds adolescent depression scale* (2nd ed., Short Form.). Lutz, FL: PAR.

Reynolds, W., & Graves, A. (1989). Reliability of children's reports of depressive symptomatology. *Journal of Abnormal Child Psychology, 17*(6), 647–655.

Riolo, S., Nguyen, A., Greden, J., & King, C. (2005). Prevalence of depression by race/ethnicity: Findings from the National Health and Nutrition Examination Survey III. *American Journal of Public Health, 95*, 998–1000. doi:10.2105/AJPH.2004.047225

Riskind, J., & Williams, N. (2005). The looming cognitive style and generalized anxiety disorder: Distinctive danger schemas and cognitive phenomenology. *Cognitive Therapy and Research, 29*(1), 7–27. doi:10.1007/s10608–005–1645-z

Roberts, A. (Ed.). (1998). *Battered women and their families: Intervention strategies and treatment programs*. New York: Springer.

Roberts, A., & Nishimoto, R. (1996). Predicting treatment retention of women dependent on cocaine. *American Journal of Alcohol and Drug Abuse, 22*, 313–333.

Roemer, L., Orsillo, S., & Salters-Pedneault, K. (2008). Efficacy of an acceptance-based therapy for generalized anxiety disorder: Evaluation in a randomized controlled trial. *Journal of Consulting and Clinical Psychology, 76*(6), 1083–1089. doi:10.1037/a0012720

Rose, R., Dick, D., Viken, R., & Kaprio, J. (2001). Gene-environment interaction in patterns of adolescent drinking: Regional residency moderates longitudinal influences on alcohol use. *Alcoholism: Clinical and Experimental Research, 25*, 637–643. doi:10.1111/j.1530–0277.2001.tb02261.x

Rose, R., Dick, D., Viken, R., Pulkkinen, L., & Kaprio, J. (2001). Drinking or abstaining at age 14: A genetic epidemiological study. *Alcoholism: Clinical and Experimental Research, 25*, 1594–1604. doi:10.1111/j.1530–0277.2001.tb02166.x

Rose, R., Viken, R., Dick, D., Bates, J., Pulkkinen, L., & Kaprio, J. (2003). It does take a village: Non-familial environments and children's behavior. *Psychological Science, 14*, 273–277. doi:10.1111/1529–1006.03434

Rosen, A., & Proctor, E. (2002). Standards for evidence-based social work practice: The role of replicable and appropriate interventions, outcomes, and practice guidelines. In A. R. Roberts & G. J. Greene (Eds.), *Social workers' desk reference* (pp. 743–747). New York: Oxford University Press.

Rosen, D., Tolman, R., & Warner, L. (2004). Low-income women's use of substance abuse and mental health services. *Journal of Health Care for the Poor in the United States, 15*, 206–219.

Ross, L., & McLean, L. (2006). Anxiety disorders during pregnancy and the postpartum period: A systematic review. *Journal of Clinical Psychology, 67*(8), 1285–1298.

Rothbaum, B., Astin, M., & Marsteller, F. (2005). Prolonged exposure versus eye movement desensitization and reprocessing (EMDR) for PTSD rape victims. *Journal of Traumatic Stress, 18*(6), 607–616. doi:10.1002/jts.20069

Ruscio, A., Chiu, W., Roy-Byrne, P., Stang, P., Stein, D., Wittchen, H., et al. (2007). Broadening the definition of generalized anxiety disorder: Effects on prevalence and association with other disorders in the National Co-morbidity Survey Replication. *Journal of Anxiety Disorders, 21*(5), 662–676.

Russel, M., Martier, S., Sokol, R., Mudar, P., Bottoms, S., Jacobson, S., & Jacobson, J. (1994). Screening for pregnancy risk-drinking. *Alcoholism Clinical and Experimental Research, 18*(5), 1156–1161.

Ryff, C. (1989). Happiness is everything, or is it? Explorations on the meaning of psychological well-being. *Journal of Personality and Social Psychology, 57*, 1069–1081. doi:10.1037/0022–3514.57.6.1069

Sansone, R., Reddington, A., Sky, K., & Wiederman, M. (2007). Borderline personality symptomatology and history of domestic violence among women in an internal medicine setting. *Violence and Victims, 22*(1), 120–126. doi:10.1891/vv-v22i1a008

Sansone, R., Wiederman, M., & Sansone, L. (1998). The Self-Harm Inventory (SHI): Development of a scale for identifying self-destructive behaviors and borderline personality disorder. *Journal of Clinical Psychology, 54*(7), 973–983.

Satre, D., Mertens, J., Arean, P., & Weisner, C. (2003). Contrasting outcomes of older versus middle-aged and younger adult chemical dependency patients in a managed care program. *Journal of Studies on Alcohol, 64*, 520–530.

Saunders, B., Kilpatrick, D., Hanson, R., Resnick, H., & Walker, M. (1999). Prevalence, case characteristics, and long-term psychological correlates of child rape among women: A national survey. *Child Maltreatment, 4*, 187–200. doi:10.1177/1077559599004003001

Schiefelbein, V., & Susman, E. (2006). Cortisol levels and longitudinal cortisol change as predictors of anxiety in adolescents. *The Journal of Early Adolescence, 26*(4), 397–413.

Schmidt, L., Dohan, D., Wiley, J., & Zabkiewicz, D. (2002). Addiction and welfare dependency: Interpreting the connection. *Social Problems, 49*, 221–241. doi:10.1525/sp.2002.49.2.221

Schmidt, L., Zabkiewicz, D., Jacobs, L., & Wiley, J. (2007). Substance abuse and employment among welfare mothers: From welfare to work and back again? *Substance Abuse and Misuse, 42*(7), 1069–1087.

Schmidt, P., Nieman, L., Danaceau, M., Adams, L., & Rubinow, D. (1998). Differential behavioral effects of gonadal steroids in women with and in those without premenstrual syndrome. *New England Journal of Medicine, 338*(4), 209–216. doi:10.1056/NEJM199801223380401

Schwartz, G., Davidson, R., & Goleman, D. (1978). Patterning of cognitive and somatic processes in the self-regulation of anxiety: Effects of meditation versus exercise. *Psychosomatic Medicine, 40*(4), 323–328.

Scogin, F., Welsh, D., Hanson, A., Stump, J., & Coates, A. (2005). Evidence-based psychotherapies for depression in older adults, *Clinical Psychology: Science and Practice, 12*(3), 222–237.

Seefeldt, K., & Orzol, S. (2005). Watching the clock tick: Factors associated with TANF accumulation. *Social Work Research, 29*(4), 215–229.

Seekles, W., van Straten, A., Beekman, A., van Marwijk, H., & Cuijpers, P. (2009). Stepped care for depression and anxiety: From primary care to specialized mental health care: A randomized controlled trial testing the effectiveness of a stepped care program among primary care patients with mood or anxiety disorders. *BMC Health Services Research, 9*, 90. doi:10.1186/1472-6963-9-90

Segal, Z., Williams, J., & Teasdale, J. (2002). *Mindfulness-based cognitive therapy for depression: A new approach in preventing relapse.* New York: Guilford Press.

Seidler, G., & Wagner, F. (2006). Comparing the efficacy of EMDR and trauma-focused cognitive-behavioral therapy in the treatment of PTSD: a meta-analytic study. *Psychological Medicine, 36*(11), 1515–1522. doi:10.1017/S0033291706007963

Sen, A. (1999). *Development as freedom.* New York: Anchor.

Shaffer D., Scott, M., Wilcox, H., Hicks, R., Lucas, C., Garfinkel, R., & Greenwald, S. (2004). The Columbia Suicide Screen: validity and reliability of a screen for youth suicide and depression. *Journal of the American Academy of Child & Adolescent Psychiatry, 43*(1), 71–79. doi:10.1097/0000458 3-200401000-00016

Shansky, R., Glavis-Bloom, C., Lerman, D., McRae, P., Benson, C., Miller, K., et al. (2004). Estrogen mediates sex differences in stress-induced prefrontal cortex dysfunction. *Molecular Psychiatry, 9*, 531–538. doi:10.1038/sj.mp.4001435

Shapiro, (2002). MDR and the role of the clinician in psychotherapy evaluation: Towards a more comprehensive integration of science and practice. *Journal of Clinical Psychology, 58*(12), 1453–1463. doi:10.1002/jclp.10104

Shear, K., Jin, R., Ruscio, A., Walters, E., & Kessler, R. (2006). Prevalence and correlates of estimated DSM-IV child and adult separation anxiety disorders in the

National Comorbidity Survey Replication. *American Journal of Psychiatry, 163*(6), 1074–1083. doi:10.1176/appi.ajp.163.6.1074.

Shear, M., Feske, U., & Greeno, C. (2000). Gender differences in anxiety disorders: Clinical implications. In E. Frank (Ed.), *Gender and its effect on psychopathology* (pp. 151–168). Washington, DC: American Psychopathological Association.

Shors, T., & Leuner, B. (2003). Estrogen-mediated effects on depression and memory formation in females. *Journal of Affective Disorders, 74,* 85–96.

Shors, T., Miesegaes, G., Beylin, A., Zhao, M., Rydel, T., & Gould, E. (2001). Neurogenesis in the adult is involved in the formation of trace memories. *Nature, 410,* 372–376. doi:10.1038/35066584

Silberg, J., Pickles, A., Rutter, M., Hewitt, J., Simonoff, E., Maes, H., et al. (1999). The influence of genetic factors and life stress on depression among adolescent girls. *Archives of General Psychiatry, 56,* 225–232. doi:10.1001/archpsyc.56.3.225

Simmons, L., Braun, B., Charnigo, R., Havens, J., & Wright, D. (2008). Depression and poverty among rural women: A relationship of social causation or social selection. *Journal of Rural Health, 24*(3), 292–298. doi:10.1111/j.1748–0361.2008.00171.x

Simpson, D., Joe, G., Broome, K., Hiller, M., Knight, K., & Rowan-Szal, G. (1997). Program diversity and treatment retention rates in the Drug Abuse Treatment Outcome Study (DATOS). *Psychological and Addictive Behavior, 11*(4), 279–293.

Sinha, R., & Rush, A. (2006). Treatment and prevention of depression in women. In C. Mazure and G. Keita (Eds.), *Understanding depression in women: Applying empirical research to practice and policy* (pp.45–70). Washington, DC: American Psychological Association.

Skodal, A., & Bender, D. (2003). Why are women diagnosed borderline more than men? *Psychiatric Quarterly, 74,* 349–360. doi:10.1023/A.1026087410516

Smith, A. (2005). *Conquest: Sexual violence and American Indian genocide.* Boston: South End Press.

Smith, B. (2005). Battering, forgiveness, and redemption: Alternative models for addressing domestic violence in communities of color. In N. Sokoloff & C. Pratt (Eds.), *Domestic violence at the margins: Readings in race, class, gender, and culture* (pp. 321–339). Piscataway, NJ: Rutgers University Press.

Smith, D., & Seymour, R. (2001). Women in treatment: Addiction, abuse, and pregnancy and treating elderly patients. *Clinician's guide to substance abuse* (pp. 255–264). New York: McGraw-Hill.

Sokol, R. J., Martier, S. S., & Ager, J. W. The T-ACE questions: Practical prenatal detection of risk-drinking. (25 refs.) *American Journal of Obstetrics and Gynecology, 160*(4): 863–870, 1989.

Soloff, P., Fabio, A., Kelly, T., Malone, K., & Mann, J. (2005). High-lethality status in patients with borderline personality disorder. *Journal of Personality Disorders, 19*(4), 386–399. doi:10.1521/pedi.2005.19.4.386

Sonne, S., Back, S., Zuniga, C., Randall, C., & Brady, K. (2003). Gender differences in individuals with co-morbid alcohol dependence and post-traumatic stress disorder. *American Journal of Addiction, 12,* 412–413.

Spielberger, C., Gorsuch, R., Lushene, R., Vagg, P., & Jacobs, G. (1983). *Manual for the State-Trait Anxiety Inventory* (Form Y). Palo Alto, CA: Mind Garden.

Spijker, J., de Graaf, R., Bijl, R., Beekman, A., Ormel, J., & Nolen, W. (2002). Duration of major depressive episodes in the general population: Results from the Netherlands Mental Health Survey and Incidence Study (NEMESIS). *British Journal of Psychiatry, 181,* 208–213. doi:10.1192/bjp.181.3.208

Spinelli, M., & Endicott, J. (2003). Controlled clinical trial of interpersonal psychother-apy versus parenting education program for depressed pregnant women. *American Journal of Psychiatry, 160*(3), 555–562. doi:10.1176/appi.ajp.160.3.555

Spitzer, R., & Williams, J. (1985). *Structured clinical interview for DSM-III (SCID).* New York: Biometrics Research Division.

Spitzer, R., Kroenke, K., & Williams, J. (1999). Validation and utility of a self-report version of PRIME-MD: The PHQ Primary Care Study. *JAMA: The Journal of the American Medical Association 282*(18), 1737–1744. doi:10.1001/jama.282.18.1737

Spitzer, R., Kroenke, K., Williams, J., & Lowe, B. (2006). A brief measure for assessing generalized anxiety disorder. *Archives of Internal Medicine, 166*, 1092–1097. doi:10.1001/archinte.166.10.1092

Springer, K., Sheridan, J., Kuo, D., & Carnes, M. (2007). Long-term physical and mental health consequences of childhood physical abuse: Results from a large population-based sample of men and women. *Child Abuse & Neglect, 31*(5), 517–530. doi:10.1016/j.chiabu.2007.01.003

Stahler, G., Shipley, T., Kirby, K., Godboldte, C., Kerwin, M., Shandler, I., et al. (2005). Development and initial demonstration of a community-based interven-tion for homeless, cocaine-using, African American women. *Journal of Substance Abuse Treatment, 28*(2), 171–179. doi:10.1016/j.jsat.2004.12.003

Stanley, B., Molcho, A., Stanley, M., Winchel, R., Gameroff, M., & Parsons, B. (2000). Association of aggressive behavior with altered serotonergic function in patients who are not suicidal. *American Journal of Psychiatry, 157*, 609–614. doi.10.1176/appi.ajp.157.4.609

Stanley, M., Wilson, N., Novy, D., Rhoades, H., Wagener, P., Greisinger, A., et al. (2009). Cognitive behavior therapy for generalized anxiety disorder among older adults in primary care: A randomized clinical trial. *JAMA: Journal of the American Medical Association, 301*(14), 1460–1467. doi:10.1001/jama.2009.458

Stein, M., Jang, K., Taylor, S., Vernon, P., & Livesley, J. (2002). Genetic and environ-mental influences on trauma exposure and posttraumatic stress disorder symp-toms: A twin study. *American Journal of Psychiatry, 159*, 1675–1681. doi:10.1176/appi.ajp.159.10.1675

Sterling, R., Gottheil, E., Weinstein, S., & Serota, R. (2001). The effect of therapist/patient race- and sex-matching in individual treatment. *Addiction, 96*(7), 1015–1022. doi:10.1046/j.1360-0443.2001.967101511.x

Stout, K., & McPhail, B. (1998). *Confronting sexism and violence against women: A challenge for social work.* New York: Longman.

Straussner, S., & Brown, S. (Eds.). (2002). *The handbook of addiction treatment for women: Theory and practice.* San Francisco: Jossey-Bass.

Strickland, T. (2001). Substance abuse. In R. Braithwaite & S. Taylor (Eds.), *Health issues in the Black community* (pp.384–402). San Francisco: Jossey-Bass.

Substance Abuse and Mental Health Service Administration. (2007). *National Registry of Evidence-based Programs and Practices (NREPP).* Washington, DC: Government Printing Office.

Substance Abuse and Mental Health Services Administration. (2009). *Action steps for improving women's mental health.* Washington, DC: Department of Health and Human Services.

Substance Abuse and Mental Health Services Administration. (2009). *Results from the 2008 National Survey on Drug Use and Health: National findings.* Washington, DC: Government Printing Office.

Sullivan, G., Craske, M., Sherbourne, C., Edlund, M., Rose, R., Golinelli, D., et al. (2007). Design of the Coordinated Anxiety Learning and Management (CALM) study: Innovations in collaborative care for anxiety disorders. *General Hospital Psychiatry, 29*(3), 379–387. doi:10.1016/j.genhosppsych.2007.04.005

Sutter-Dallay, A., Giaconne-Marcesche, E., Glatigny-Dallay, E., & Verdoux, H. (2004). Women with anxiety disorders during pregnancy are at increased risk of intense postnatal depressive symptoms: A prospective survey of the MATQUID cohort. *European Psychiatry, 19*(8), 459–463.

Szuster, R., Rich, L., Chung, A., & Bisconer, S. (1996). Treatment retention in women's residential chemical dependency treatment: The effect of admission with children. *Substance Use and Misuse, 31*, 1001–1013.

Takeuchi, D., Chung, R., Lin, K., Shen, H., Kurasaki, K., Chun, C., et al. (1998). Lifetime and twelve-month prevalence rates of major depressive episodes and dysthymia among Chinese Americans in Los Angeles. *American Journal of Psychiatry, 155*, 1407–1414.

Thibault J., & Steiner R. (2004). Efficient identification of adults with depression and dementia. *American Family Physician, 70*(6), 1101–1110.

Tjaden, P., & Thoennes, N. (2000). *Full report of the prevalence, incidence, and consequences of violence against women.* Washington, DC: United States Department of Justice, Office of Justice Programs, National Institute of Justice.

Tolman, R., & Raphael, J. (2000). A review of research on welfare and domestic violence. *Journal of Social Issues, 56*, 655–682. doi:10.1111/0022–4537.00190

Tolman, R., Danziger, S., & Rosen, D. (2001). *Domestic violence and economic well-being of current and former welfare recipients.* Ann Arbor, MI: Program on Poverty and Social Policy.

Torgersen, S. (2000). Genetics of patients with borderline personality disorder. *Psychiatry for Clinicians of North America, 23*, 1–9. doi:10.1016/S0193–953X (05)70139–8

Trull, T., Sher, K., Minks-Brown, C., Durbin, J., & Burr, R. (2000). Borderline personality disorder and substance use disorders: A review and integration. *Clinical Psychology Review, 20*(2), 235–253. doi:10.1016/S0272–7358(99)00028–8

Tsuang, M., Bar, J., Stone, S., & Faraone, S. (2004). Gene-environment interactions in mental disorders. *World Psychiatry, 3*(2), 73–83.

Tucker, J., D'Amico, J., Wenzel, S., Golinelli, D., Elliott, M., & Williamson, S. (2005). A prospective study of risk and protective factors for substance use among impoverished women living in temporary shelter settings in Los Angeles County. *Drug and Alcohol Dependence, 80*(1), 35–43. doi:10.1016/j.drugalcdep .2005.03.008

Turner, L., Danziger, S., & Seefeldt, K. (2006). Failing the transition from welfare to work: Women chronically disconnected from employment and cash welfare. *Social Science Quarterly, 87*(2), 227–249. doi:10.1111/j.1540–6237.2006.00378.x

Twenge, J., & Nolen-Hoeksema, S. (2002). Age, gender, race, SES, and birth cohort differences on the Children's Depression Inventory: A meta-analysis. *Journal of Abnormal Psychology, 111*, 578–588. doi:10.1037/0021–843X.111.4.578

Tyrer, P., & Baldwin, D. (2009). Generalized anxiety disorder. *The Lancet, 368*(9553), 2156–2166.

Ullman, S., & Brecklin, L. (2003). Sexual assault history and health-related outcomes in a national sample of women. *Psychology of Women Quarterly, 27*, 46–57. doi:10.1111/1471–6402.t01–2-00006

United States Census Bureau. (2000). *Census 2000*. Washington, DC: U. S. Government Printing Office.

University of Michigan Depression Center. (2007). *Facts about depression in children and adolescents*. Retrieved Feburary 15, 2010 from www.med.umich.edu/depression/caph.htm

Valentine, C. (1968). *Culture and poverty*. Chicago: University of Chicago Press.

Van Den Bergh, N. (1995). *Feminist practice in the 21st century*. Washington, DC: NASW Press.

Van Den Bergh, N., & Cooper, L. (Eds.). (1986). *Feminist visions for social work*. Silver Spring, MD: NASW Press.

Van Wormer, K. (2001). *Counseling female offenders and victims: A strengths-restorative approach*. New York: Springer.

Van Wormer, K., & Bartollas, C. (2000). *Women and the criminal justice system*. Boston: Allyn & Bacon.

Vandergriff-Avery, A. (2002). Rural families speak: A qualitative investigation of stress protective and crisis recovery strategies utilized by rural low-income women and their families. *Dissertation Abstracts International, 62*(12), 4350-A–4351-A.

Vega, W., Kolody, B., Aguilar-Goxiola, S., Alderete, E., Catalano, R., & Caraveo-Anduaga, J. (1998). Lifetime prevalence of DSM-III-R psychiatric disorders among urban and rural Mexican Americans in California. *Archives of General Psychiatry, 55*, 771–778. doi:10.1001/archpsyc.55.9.771

Vega, W., Kolody, B., Anguilar-Gaxiola, S., & Catalano, R. (1999). Gaps in service utilization by Mexican Americans with mental health problems. *American Journal of Psychiatry, 156*, 928–934.

Verheul, R., Van Den Bosch, L. M., Koeter, M. W., de Ridder, M. A., Stijnen, T., & Van Den Brink, W. (2003). Dialectical behaviour therapy for women with border-line personality disorder: A 12-month randomized clinical trial in The Netherlands. *British Journal of Psychiatry, 182*, 135–140. doi:10.1192/bjb.182.2.135

Vesga-Lopez, O., Schneier, F., Wang, S., Heimberg, R., Liu, S., Hasin, D., et al. (2007). Gender differences in generalized anxiety disorder: Results from the National Epidemiologic Survey on Alcohol and Related Conditions (NESARC). *Journal of Clinical Psychiatry, 69*(10), 1606–1616.

Vitiello, B. (2009). Treatment of adolescent depression: What we have come to know. *Depression and Anxiety, 26*, 393–395. doi:10.1002/da.20572

Vogel, L., & Marshall, L. (2001). PTSD symptoms and partner abuse: Low income women at risk. *Journal of Traumatic Stress, 14*(3), 569–584. doi:10.1023/A1011116824613

Wagner, A., & Linehan, M. (1999). Facial expression recognition ability among women with borderline personality disorder: Implications for emotion regulation? *Journal of Personality Disorders, 13*, 329–344.

Walker, E., Katon, W., Russo, J., Ceichanowski, P., Newman, E., & Wagner, A. (2003). Healthcare costs associated with posttraumatic stress disorder symptoms in women. *Archives of General Psychiatry, 60*, 369–374. doi:10.1001/archpsyc.60.4.369

Watson, C., Juba, M., Manifold, V., Kucala, T., & Anderson, P. (1991). The PTSD interview: Rationale, descriptions, reliability, and concurrent validity of the DSM-III-based technique. *Journal of Clinical Psychology, 47*(2), 179–188.

Weathers, F., Litz, B., Herman, D., Huska, J., & Keane, T. (1993, October). *The PTSD checklist (PCL): Reliability, validity, and diagnostic utility*. Paper presented at the annual convention of the International Society for Traumatic Stress Studies, San Antonio, TX.

Webb, S. (2001). Some considerations on the validity of evidence-based practice in social work. *British Journal of Social Work, 31,* 57–79.

Weber, B., & Jensen, L. (2004). *Poverty and place: A critical review of rural poverty literature.* (Working Papers No. 18913). Corvallis, OR: Oregon State University, Rural Poverty Research Center.

Weber, M. (2001). *The Protestant ethic and the spirit of capitalism.* New York: Routledge.

Weisner, C. (1993). Toward an alcohol treatment entry model: A comparison of problem drinkers in the general population and in treatment. *Alcoholism: Clinical and Experimental Research, 17,* 746–752.

Weiss, D. (1994). The Impact of Event Scale–Revised. In J. Wilson & T. Keane (Eds.), *Assessing psychological trauma and PTSD* (pp. 168–169). New York City: Guilford Press.

Weiss, L. (September 10, 2009). *Unmarried women hit hard by poverty: Census shows most poor adults are women, particularly women on their own.* Washington, DC: Center for American Progress.

Weissman, J., & Levine, S. (2007). Anxiety disorders and older women. *Journal of Women & Aging, 19*(1–2), 70–101. doi:10.1300/J074v19n01_06

Wells, A. (2005). The metacognitive model of GAD: Assessment of meta-worry and relationship with DSM-IV generalized anxiety disorder. *Cognitive Therapy and Research, 29*(1), 107–121. doi:10.1007/s10608–005–1652–0

Wenzel, A., Haugen, E., Jackson, L., & Brendle, J. (2005). Anxiety symptoms and disorders at eight weeks postpartum. *Journal of Anxiety Disorders, 19*(3), 295–311. doi:10.1016/j.janxdis.2004.04.001

Wenzel, S., Tucker, J., Hambarsoomian, K., & Elliott, M. (2006). Toward a more comprehensive understanding of violence against impoverished women. *Journal of Interpersonal Violence, 21*(6), 820–839. doi:10.1177/0886260506288662.

Western, D. (1997). Divergences between clinical and research methods for assessing personality disorders: Implications for research and the evolution of Axis II. *American Journal of Psychiatry, 154,* 895–903.

White, C., Gunderson, J., Zanarini, M., & Hudson, J. (2003). Family studies of borderline personality disorder: A review. *Harvard Review of Psychiatry, 11,* 8–19. doi:10.1080.10673220303937

Widiger, T., & Rogers, J. (1989). Prevalence and comorbidity of personality disorders. *Psychiatric Annals, 19,* 132–136.

Widiger, T., Simonsen, E., Sirovatka, P., & Regier, D. (2007). *Dimensional models of personality disorders: Refining the research agenda.* Arlington, VA: American Psychiatric Publishing.

Wisner, K., Parry, B., & Piontek, C. (2002). Clinical practice: Postpartum depression. *New England Journal of Medicine, 347,* 194–199. doi:10.1056/NEJMcp011542

Witkin, S., & Harrison, W. (2001). Whose evidence and for what purpose? *Social Work, 46*(4), 293–296.

Wittchen, H. (2002). Generalized anxiety disorder: Prevalence, burden, and cost to society. *Depression and Anxiety, 14*(4), 162–171.

Wittchen, H., & Boyer, P. (1998). Screening for anxiety: Sensitivity and specificity of the Anxiety Screening Questionnaire (ASQ-15). *British Journal of Psychiatry, 173*(Suppl. 34), 10–17.

Work Group on Borderline Personality Disorder. (2001). Practice guideline for the treatment of patients with borderline personality disorder. *American Journal of Psychiatry, 158*, 1–2.

Yesavage, J., Brink, T., Rose, T., Lum, O., Huang, V., Adey, M., et al. (1983). Development and validation of a geriatric depression screening scale: A preliminary report. *Journal of Psychiatric Research, 17*, 37–49.

Yoshihama, M., Hammock, A. C., & Horrocks, J. (2006). Intimate partner violence, welfare receipt, and health status of low income African American women: A lifecourse analysis. *American Journal of Community Psychology, 37*(1–2), 95–109.

Young, J., Klosko, J., & Weishaar, M. (2003). *Schema therapy: A practitioner's guide.* New York: Guilford Press.

Young, S., Rhee, S., Stallings, M., Corley, R., & Hewitt, J. (2006). Genetic and environmental vulnerabilities underlying adolescent substance use and problem use: General or specific? *Behavior Genetics, 36*(4), 603–615. doi:10.1007/s10519-006-9066-7

Zanarini, M. (2000). Childhood experiences associated with the development of borderline personality disorder. *Psychiatric Clinicians of North America, 23*, 89–101. doi:10.1016/S0193-953X(05)70145.3

Zanarini, M., Frankenburg, F., Hennen, J., & Silk, K. (2003). The longitudinal course of borderline psychopathology: 6-year prospective follow-up of the phenomenology of borderline personality disorder. *American Journal of Psychiatry, 160*, 274–283. doi:10.1176/appi.ajp.160.2.274

Zanarini, M., Frankenburg, F., Hennen, J., Reich, B., & Silk, K. (2005). The McLean Study of Adult Development (MSAD): Overview and implications of the first six years of prospective follow-up. *Journal of Personality Disorders, 19*, 505–523. doi:10.1521/pedi.2005.19.5.505

Zanarini, M., Frankenburg, F., Hennen, J., Reich, B., & Silk, K. (2006). Prediction of the 10-year course of borderline personality disorder. *American Journal of Psychiatry, 163*, 827–832. doi:10.1176/appi.ajp.163.5.827

Ziegert, D., & Kistner, J. (2002). Response styles theory: Downward extension to children. *Journal of Clinical Child and Adolescent Psychology, 31*, 325–334.

Zigmond, A., & Snaith, R. (1983). The Hospital Anxiety and Depression Scale. *Acta Psychiatrica Scandinavica, 67*, 361–370.

Zimmerman, M., & Mattia, J. (1999). Axis I diagnostic comorbidity and borderline personality disorder. *Comprehensive Psychiatry, 4*, 245–252.

Zinbarg, R., Lee, J., & Yoon, K. (2007). Dyadic predictors of outcome in a cognitive-behavioral program for patients with generalized anxiety disorder in committed relationships: A "spoonful of sugar" and a dose of non-hostile criticism may help. *Behavior Research and Therapy, 45*(4), 699–713. doi:10.1016/j.brat.2006.06.005

Zlotnick, C., Najavits, L., & Rohsenow, D. (2003). A cognitive-behavioral treatment for incarcerated women with substance use disorder and posttraumatic stress disorder: Findings from a pilot study. *Journal of Substance Abuse Treatment, 25*, 99–105.

Zlotnick, C., Rothschild, L., & Zimmerman, M. (2002). The role of gender in the clinical presentation of patients with borderline personality disorder. *Journal of Personality Disorders, 16*, 277–282. doi:10.1521/pedi.16.3.277.22540

Zlotnik, C., Miller, I., Pearlstein, T., Howard, M., & Sweeney, P. (2006). A preventive intervention for pregnant women on public assistance at risk for postpartum depression. *American Journal of Psychiatry, 163*, 1443–1445. doi:10.1176/appi.ajp.163.8.1443

Zubenko, G., Hughes, H., Maher, B., Stiffler, J., Zubenko, W., & Marazita, M. (2002). Genetic linkage of region containing the CREB1 gene depressive disorders in women from families with recurrent, early onset major depression. *American Journal of Medical Genetics, 114*, 980–987. doi:10.1002/ajmg.b.10933

Zubenko, G., Hughes, H., Stiffler, J., Zubenko, W., & Kaplan, B. (2002). Genome survey for susceptibility loci for recurrent, early-onset major depression: Results at 10cM resolution. *American Journal of Medical Genetics, 114*, 413–422. doi:10.1002/ajmg.10381

Zucherbrot, R., Cheung, A., Jensen, P., Stein, R., Laraque, D., & the GLAD-PC steering group. (2007). Guidelines for Adolescent Depression in Primary Care (GLAD-PC): I. Identification, assessment, and initial management. *Pediatrics, 120*, e1299-e1312. doi:10.1542/peds.2007–1144

Zung, W. (1965). A self-rating depression scale. *Archives of General Psychiatry, 12*, 63–70.

# Index

# About the Authors

**Martha Markward** earned both her MSW and PhD from the University of Illinois-Urbana. She is currently an associate professor in the University of Missouri's School of Social Work in Columbia where she teaches policy, with focuses on women, poverty, and mental health; children's mental health; and evaluation of clinical practice. Although Dr. Markward's research and scholarly publications focus on women, children, and youth, much of her research on women is related to violence against women. She co-edited a book entitled *Reassessing Social Work Practice with Children* and has contributed chapters in six books. Dr. Markward is particularly interested in gender-specific violence prevention research with females who are in the prepubescent stage of development, especially in the ability of young females to cope with violence. Dr. Markward has practiced social work in hospital, public welfare, and school settings, primarily with low-income women and children who have physical and/or mental disabilities. In this regard, she also conducted a study on the sense of empowerment among parents of school-age children in Bulgaria.

**Bonnie Yegidis** currently serves as the director of the School of Social Work at the University of South Florida in Tampa and formerly served as dean of the School of Social Work at the University of Georgia. Dr. Yegidis is also an accomplished author, having cowritten several textbooks and contributed to chapters in eight books, as well as having produced numerous conference papers, book reviews, and articles published in peer-reviewed journals. Her areas of expertise include social work practice with families, practice with women, and international education for social work. Her book, *Research Methods for Social Workers,* is in its 6th edition and is widely used in schools of social work nationally, and she developed a measure to assess abuse among women. She has worked with women abused in intimate partner relationships, conducted research with women in the Ukraine, and is a certified family mediator in the state of Florida.

# SAGE Research Methods Online

## The essential tool for researchers

**Sign up now at www.sagepub.com/srmo for more information.**

### An expert research tool

- An **expertly designed taxonomy** with more than 1,400 unique terms for social and behavioral science research methods
- **Visual and hierarchical search tools** to help you discover material and link to related methods

- Easy-to-use navigation tools
- Content organized by complexity
- Tools for citing, printing, and downloading content with ease
- Regularly updated content and features

### A wealth of essential content

- The most comprehensive picture of quantitative, qualitative, and mixed methods available today
- More than **100,000 pages of SAGE book and reference material** on research methods as well as editorially selected material from SAGE journals
- More than **600 books** available in their entirety online

Launching 2011!

 **⑤SAGE** research methods online